Freedom to Move

Movement therapy for spinal pain and injuries

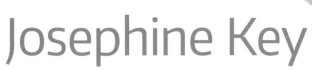

Josephine Key

Freedom to Move

Movement therapy for spinal pain and injuries

Forewords by
Ginger Garner
Elizabeth Larkam
Thomas W Myers

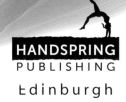

HANDSPRING
PUBLISHING

Edinburgh

HANDSPRING PUBLISHING LIMITED
The Old Manse, Fountainhall,
Pencaitland, East Lothian
EH34 5EY, Scotland
Tel: +44 1875 341 859
Website: www.handspringpublishing.com

First published 2018 in the United Kingdom by Handspring Publishing

ISBN 978-1-909141-92-6
ISBN (Kindle eBook) 978-1-909141-93-3

British Library Cataloguing in Publication Data
A catalogue record for this book is available from the British Library

Library of Congress Cataloguing in Publication Data
A catalog record for this book is available from the Library of Congress

Notice
Neither the Publisher nor the Authors assume any responsibility for any loss or injury and/or damage to persons or property arising out of or relating to any use of the material contained in this book. It is the responsibility of the treating practitioner, relying on independent expertise and knowledge of the patient, to determine the best treatment and method of application for the patient.

Commissioning Editor Sarena Wolfaard
Project Manager Morven Dean
Copy editor Ceinwen Sinclair
Designer Bruce Hogarth
Indexer Aptara, India
Typesetter DSM Soft, India
Printer Melita, Malta

The
Publisher's
policy is to use
paper manufactured
from sustainable forests

CONTENTS

FOREWORD *by Ginger Garner*

Our modern, busy lives can often lead us into a perpetual "fight, flight, or freeze" state – an appropriate response to short term stress, but inappropriate if it ends up being our long-term, habitual response to life. The way we respond to stress affects us in a myriad of ways, including the way we rest and digest food, the way we interact with ourselves and others, and ultimately, how we move.

Stress can be positive (eustress) as well as negative (distress), and it would seem that those who view stress as character building and strength cultivating often feel more content, and according to evidence, live longer and with less disease. How, then, do we get to that point of using stress to build strength?

Close your eyes, and think of the last time you felt totally at ease. *Freedom to Move*, by Josephine Key, is an invitation into that gracious space. An invitation to move with creative ease, with mindful fluidity, and with safety and efficacy. It is born from the author's experience, research, and freedom to experiment with her craft, physical therapy and human movement.

The human body is born to move. It is an incredible design. An ever-hopeful organism in persistent allostasis with unlimited potential. Our body is more than a complex machine, it is an enigma, and one to be embraced.

This text extends an invitation to move in a way that is congruent with the latest science, all the while acknowledging that there is no clear winner in the research when it comes to movement approaches. A pragmatic approach to explore the intricate, ever-layered potential that human movement harnesses, the individualized, biopsychosocial approach this book embraces has emerged as the best fit way to offer multiple entry points for healing and well-being. This text gives you the tools to tackle the "bio" portion of the model, and when it comes to chronic and persistent pain, the biopsychosocial model and its personalized, multidisciplinary team approach is the gold standard.

As a veteran physical therapist in sports medicine and women's health, I spend most of my time working on stress response and neuromuscular patterning with my patients, and the distinction between muscle strength and endurance from motor control is a key part of what can make this text so helpful for many. The icing on the cake is the inclusion of the complex role of fascia and our emerging understanding of the science of its function. Our robust "ception" system, from proprioception to neuroception to interoception (there are many more), is a "bio"-directional system that is intimately influenced by the gut microbiome and our cranial nerves and their subsequent vagal-driven pressure system. When we begin to appreciate polyvagal theory, for example, we begin to understand the deceptively "simple on the surface only" power of movement and its potential to transform the human experience. Key's text is once again a call to understand and experience the deeper layers of influence and potential in human movement.

Stephen Hawking said that we do not experience the world so much as we experience our own nervous system. We are not simply a vessel for information in and information out – we are capable of change in a profound way. We are "plastic," meaning that the human mind and body is elastic in a way that allows us to be in control of our own transformation. Since movement is a sensory experience, we can use it to change and alter the way we move and assume posture, which is the essential message of the text. Neuroplasticity is the key to transformation – which is good news for everyone who picks up this book. You have the potential to change your body's perception of and experience with pain!

We can change the pain experience, one movement and one thought at a time. It is why mindfulness is the key to effective physical training and recovery. Debunking back and spinal pain myths. Key presents the evidence in a way that clears the air of conflicting information – further vetting the biopsychosocial approach as a reliable and valid method for addressing the pain experience, while also paving the way for recognizing and teaching some key elements that movement must include.

For example, the child's song, "the hip bone's connected to the back bone, the back bone's connected to the rib bone, the rib bone's connected to the breathing 'bone'" holds a perennial truth. No, there is no "breathing bone," but the point is this – everything is connected. Breathing is connected to every intimate process in the body. And those connecting points between the shoulder, the spine, and the pelvis, are connected to breathing and one another. The concepts of autonomic function, impacting stress response, and regional interdependence, are but a few of the important issues in this text. Seemingly unrelated impairments in one area of the body can be influenced by or influence your primary pain or stress experience, which is important since the spine is connected to everything.

Affecting health through the three major diaphragms of the body (laryngeal, respiratory, and pelvic) through mindful movement and pressurization (intra-abdominal pressure, intra-thoracic, intra-pelvic, and subglottal pressures) is another key component of the exercises introduced in this text. Weaving in yogic breathing, for example using *ujjayi* as a glottal control technique, is an effective way not only to improve spinal

health and pressurization, but also to introduce meditation and mindfulness, which is requisite to changing movement behavior and impacting overall health.

The easiest way to understand the concept of pressurization is to imagine trying to pick up a young child who does not want to be picked up. She or he will do what I call "butter shoulders," or what I have heard others call going "boneless." When they were small, my own three children did it a thousand times if they did it once. Put simply, the child deflates and goes limp, which makes it hard to pick her up. While the analogy is not exact, you can see how if you are not "helping" your spine with proper breath and you go "limp" in your office chair or on your sofa, endlessly slumping and rounding the spine without introducing other movement periodically, you can end up with postural derangements, stuck and nonresponsive tissue that perceives threat, and a body that is increasingly difficult to control or move with ease.

Our habits of movement and/or a lack of movement, give us a clear picture into our state of being, of our mind–body allostasis. If we can move with creative ease, fluidity, and control, we are more likely to process stress well. And the reverse is also true. Affecting pain, especially spinal pain, is layered and complex, but this text will offer an innovative entry point for many. Tackling back pain is not about becoming a gym rat, doing crunches, sucking in your belly button, rigidly holding your abs, or targeting singular muscles for strength. It is about making a connection between a loss of fundamental movement patterns of the spine, thorax, and rib cage and subsequent loss of subtle and overt neuromuscular patterning, driven or exacerbated by poor respiration and nonoptimal stress response. *Freedom to Move* will help you understand basic, fundamental movement patterns in order to appreciate the complexity of movement – and how we must layer this knowledge with fascial science and autonomic impact or stress response. All of this makes the prescription of movement and exercise regionally interdependent – both psychobiologically and neurophysiologically.

This intersectionality offers a caveat. One of the most poignant aspects of the text is an appropriate warning shot to all mindful movement instructors, as the author suggests that movement pattern assessment reveals why some yoga and Pilates "mindfulness" movement programs can fail in their endeavors, as they take faulty neuromuscular patterns into gross movement, which reinforces the use of superficial muscles in the absence of deeper stability. Clients often rely on "tried and true" dominant strategies such as Key's "inferior tethers" which can lead to central sensitization when peripheral input is sustained. This is akin to the spinal paraspinals constantly firing and "running from the tiger," or staying in "fight/flight" mode all the time. The case studies included in this text also drive the point home well, and sound similar to cases I have experienced in clinical practice treating spinal pain.

The book is divided into two sections. The first provides a foundation for a deeper understanding and knowledge of the healthy and impaired spine. The second gets to work giving a method for assessment and intervention to rebuild essential spinal movement and patterns. I believe this book will be valuable and helpful to many people who have spinal pain, and for those who want to prevent it. The 60 movement exercises that are introduced in this text can be functionally applied to many mindful movement disciplines, providing a fundamental basis for conscious, effortless movement with sustainable control and ease. *Freedom to Move*'s mindful movement exercise program offers an entry point to rebuild foundational patterns of control for enhanced movement and to optimize self-regulation, making it an essential book for anyone helping those with, or seeking freedom from, spinal pain and injury. I look forward to seeing the benefits that many will reap in picking up this book.

Ginger Garner, DPT, ATC/L, PYT
Founder, Professional Yoga Therapy Institute
Author, *Medical Therapeutic Yoga*
Emerald Isle, NC, USA
July 2018

Josephine Key has created an essential resource for our times. Manual therapists, movement therapists, and movement educators from all disciplines will find unique, relevant guidance in *Freedom to Move: Movement therapy for spinal pain and injuries*. The explanations of fundamental patterns that lead to exercise design are valuable for every practitioner.

Each reader will appreciate that Josephine Key has thoroughly documented her life's work. She developed and perfected this evidence-based approach to a comprehensive, whole-body movement education program during decades of treating patients and moving through her own experiences with pain.

Today, Americans spend an average of 13 hours a day sitting.[1] The World Health Organization ranks physical inactivity – sitting too much – as the fourth biggest preventable killer globally, causing an estimated 3.2 million deaths annually.[2] Dr James Levine, professor of endocrinology at the Mayo Clinic, Phoenix, Arizona, writes, "Sitting is more dangerous than smoking, kills more people than HIV and is more treacherous than parachuting."[3]

People of all ages spend increasing amounts of time absorbing information from screens of all sizes – handheld devices, desktop devices, and large screen media devices. Focusing one's gaze on screens for an extended period of time may compromise whole-body movement with dysfunction concentrated in the head, neck, thorax, shoulder girdle, arms and hands.

In *Freedom to Move*, Josephine Key observes, "Standing desks have become popular – yet if you cannot support your spine properly in sitting, you will not do so in standing" (p. 80).

This book offers an innovative rehabilitation model for spinal pain disorders. However, one need not have

spinal pain to benefit from the wisdom set forth in *Freedom to Move*. Josephine Key's clear map demonstrates how the spine, head, and proximal limb girdles form a functionally integrated system.

This book explains how to reinforce good movement habits and how to reeducate regions that lack movement clarity. The Key model is applicable across all disciplines of movement therapy. It reestablishes functionally important basic motor patterns in the early stage of recovery and also plays a role in improving elite performance.

Josephine Key takes a thorough, comprehensive approach to movement including "low load" movement for retraining patterns of the spine, head, shoulder girdle and pelvic girdle. The exercises progress to address proper sitting, sit to stand, proper standing, gluteal activation, squats, efficient walking and skills necessary for effective athletic performance.

Professionals whose practice already includes or could be enhanced by movement education may use this superb reference book throughout their careers. Practitioners may refine their own movement by practicing Key Moves. They may apply the detailed interrelationship of breathing, diaphragm movement, movement strategies, and pain to their own movement disciplines. The ability to redirect breathing and the internal pressure change mechanisms that enhance patterns of the axial deep myofascial system activity is at the core of the Key Moves approach.

Practitioners may customize Key Moves for their client's home or travel program. Or incorporate Key Moves that prepare their clients for efficient, pain free practice of their favorite activities.

Josephine Key succeeds in bringing research to the clinician by practically and accessibly placing the science within a functional movement context for movement therapists. Every movement educator may be assured that they can freely access the therapeutic wisdom generously offered in *Freedom to Move* while respecting scope of practice guidelines. With *Freedom to Move*, Josephine Key has created a masterful guide to improving quality of life through the freedom to be embodied.

Elizabeth Larkam
Author, *Fascia in Motion: Fascia-focused movement for Pilates (Handspring Publishing, 2017)*
California, USA
July 2018

Notes

1. James A. Levine, MD, PhD, *Get Up! Why Your Chair Is Killing You and What You Can Do About It* (New York: St Martin's Press, 2014), p. 103.

2. "Physical Inactivity: a global public health problem," World Health Organization, www.who.int/ncds/prevention/physical-activity/inactivity-global-health-problem/en/

3. Levine, *Get Up!*, pp. 70–71

FOREWORD *by Thomas Myers*

Josephine Key, in *Freedom to Move*, synthesizes contemporary practices from the movement arts, and builds them on a firm scaffolding of current understandings in physiotherapy.

Amidst the welter of information to which we are subject these days – some of it great, some more questionable – it is refreshing to find a book woven (like the fascia) into a tapestry that is stronger than any of its component parts.

The manual therapy practitioner will find application aplenty for introducing movement into their sessions and for homework. Rehabilitation workers will benefit from functional movement progressions for improved outcomes. For modern movement professionals, this book is a string in the labyrinth, leading through the spectrum of different practices available so that classic exercises and new adaptations and individual accommodations can be re-interpreted in light of sound principles.

Working out from the spine, Key identifies common postural strain patterns that may lead to pain patterns, working sequentially for clarity, but with the whole constantly in mind. Key looks for range and efficacy of movement more than range of motion for a particular joint. She looks at postural self-arrangement over strengthening or lengthening individual structures. She focuses on dynamic balance over static rigidity.

As an aside, I am also grateful that, rather than unattainably limber and fit models, she uses regular people for her illustrative photographs, giving the sense of how grounded Key's work is in the real world.

Thomas W Myers
Clarks Cove, ME, USA
July 2018

PREFACE

A successful clinical practice requires good therapy outcomes. This is easier said than done, but, to this end, for the past 35 or so years I have been on a self-directed learning path: postgraduate training; enquiring and reflective clinical practice; examining the research; exploring cross-disciplinary approaches; road-testing various treatment and exercise methodologies, and attempting to weed out the concepts that injure and harm. I needed to make sense of why so many people had spinal pain, and wanted my treatment interventions to yield more successful results. My "movement" journey began even earlier, when I worked in pediatrics helping facilitate the delayed neuromotor development of babies and infants. I also had the misfortune to "break my back" on three separate occasions (in the neck, low back, and coccyx) – hence I experienced firsthand how to find my way out of pain and dysfunction. The information proffered in this book is thus the synthesis of a dedicated clinician's journey.

Working with people in pain has taught me a great deal: how to see the missing links in their function, and how, when these are reestablished, there is not only an improvement in the quality of their posture, movement, and general performance but also a decrease in the level of pain they experience.

My purpose in writing this book, then, is to assist the cross-disciplinary movement therapist who seeks both to further their understanding of functional movement of the spine and torso and to fine tune their skills in prescribing and teaching exercises that restore movement function and help relieve pain.

At the same time, in the particular area of rehabilitation of spinal pain disorders, I am trying to bridge the gap between the physiotherapy-centered, evidence-informed "specific therapeutic exercise" approaches on the one hand and the more holistic, practical experiential approach of the various movement disciplines, such as Pilates and yoga, on the other.

I sincerely hope that you find this book helps you in your practice so you can observe the improved quality of movement and accompanying pain reduction that develops in your clients when important foundations of torso movement control are reestablished. In my experience, clients benefit physically both from rebuilding these patterns of control and from improved musculoskeletal fitness. Most clients appreciate and positively enjoy the challenge of exercising in a way that they are confident is safe for their spine and that promotes their general feeling of well-being.

The evolution of the material in this book rests upon multifarious influences. In general, I am particularly grateful to the work and ideas of many fine cross-disciplinary clinicians, researchers and thinkers in the field of movement therapy.

I would particularly like to acknowledge my partner, Andrea Clift, and long-time senior associate colleagues at Edgecliff Physiotherapy Sports and Spinal Centre, Fiona Condie, Caroline Harley, Micky Yim and Ajantha Suppiah, for being part of the long journey with me in the development of this work, which has gradually evolved from the shop floor and engine room of clinical practice. Theirs and the other associates' and staff's involvement in the work, and their questioning and input, have been invaluable.

Many thanks to our patients for giving our exercise program a go – enabling us to see them make significant changes – and for their positive feedback.

PREFACE *continued*

Next, I would like to thank Sarena Wolfaard from Handspring Publishing, not only for her belief that I had something to offer and her persistence in encouraging me to write this book, but also for her patience in waiting until I was ready to do so. And I would also like to thank the wonderful production team headed by Morven Dean for their patience and commitment to getting things right – with particular thanks to Ceinwen Sinclair, copyeditor, and Bruce Hogarth, illustrator/designer.

I am very appreciative to have had Belinda Meggitt, physiotherapist, Pilates practitioner, and patient on occasion, act as an initial editor of the manuscript, and I thank her for her comments and ideas about various aspects.

I would like to thank Tamar Kelly, Iyengar yoga teacher, for acting as the principal "ideal" model in many of the photos – and also Sherston Sheridan from Edgecliff Physiotherapy for modeling assistance. Thanks also to Mikey Leung for his great camera work.

And I especially thank Ian Breden, my dear husband, for his love, support, understanding and patience while I wrote another book, despite a particularly eventful year.

Josephine Key Dip Phys, PGD Manip Ther
Neuro-musculo-skeletal physiotherapist, Founder
of Edgecliff Physiotherapy Sports and Spinal Centre
and the Key Approach model for managing spinal
pain disorders,
Sydney, Australia
April 2018

INTRODUCTION

Spinal pain disorders are unfortunately an increasingly common problem in the community, in part attested to by the growing narcotic addiction which is burgeoning worldwide.

People with back pain and pains related to spinal dysfunction have special needs with regard to exercise. Specifically, exercise should help relieve their pain, restore missing basic elements in their movement function, and improve their quality of life.

This book offers an innovative rehabilitation model for spinal pain disorders. The model is particularly applicable in reestablishing functionally important basic motor patterns in the early stage of recovery but can also play a role in improving elite performance. It is a whole-person approach which addresses suboptimal control of posture and movement – the commonly apparent underlying feature of most spinal pain problems. The model is applicable across all disciplines of movement therapy.

There should not be any mystery about the prevalence of spinal pain – research and clinical evidence reveal that it is largely due to disuse and misuse of the spine. By developing faulty postural habits, people eventually lose adequate posturo-movement control, develop adaptive compensatory ways of moving, and become stiff. This is reflected in the body, and a practitioner with a trained eye and sensitive hands can discern why the client has a particular problem. This book focuses on appropriate exercise therapy to restore missing function.

The "Key Moves" approach involves looking at how a person moves, with the aim of changing any suboptimal movement behavior that creates abnormal tissue loading and injury. It is a unique system of movement for rehabilitating and liberating the spine

and optimizing its function. The method attempts to simplify movement and make it easier to see the common movement tendencies which underpin spinal pain disorders.

Re-establishing the "fundamental patterns" underpins the approach. These are components of functional movement that provide the foundations of the spinal movement control that are basic to its health and freedom to move. These are "low load" movement patterns, reliant on deep system control, which naturally activate muscles that are poorly active in timing, magnitude and sustained activity. The perceptuo-motor relearning of these basic phrases of natural spinal movement is aided by addressing function in "key parts" for the benefit of the whole movement system. As a house needs sound foundations, so too does the movement system.

Many in the sports industry commonly look at the big movements of the limbs without appreciating the vital role that torso control plays in effective functional movement. It is important that the movement practitioner appreciates the more specific, subtle control involved in these basic primary movement patterns – without which performance suffers.

Arguably, the strength of the Key Moves approach is that as well as identifying, "mapping," and describing the features of altered control, it directly addresses the alleviation of these by the prescription of therapeutic exercise more specific to the functional problems. Further, it offers an integrated-systems approach to therapeutic exercise/movement that is both practical and informed by evidence. One aim of this book is to bring the research to the clinician by practically and accessibly placing the science within a functional movement context for movement therapists.

This book is in two parts: Part A serves to enhance the practitioner's knowledge around the spine in health and dis/ease. It also examines research relating to spinal pain and exercise and serves as a comprehensive background reference to support the exercise therapy in Part B.

Chapter 3 deals with spinal movement "dysfunction," and Chapter 4 with "ideal function." Obviously, these two topics are interrelated, with knowledge of one feeding understanding of the other. Chapter 4 covers the "fundamental patterns of control" and gives a systematized perspective on the natural functional movement of the torso (the spine, head, and proximal limb girdles) and how this is altered in people with spinal and related pain disorders. It attempts to decode movement into a simpler framework in order to aid assessment and therapy.

Part B deals with the practical aspects of assessing, prescribing, and teaching therapeutic exercise to restore lost aspects of spinal function.

Chapter 7 contains 60 exercises and has been designed so that each reads rather like a recipe book, with step-by-step instructions for correctly performing each exercise. Provided that the instructions are followed correctly, the exercises are safe, effective, and enjoyable. Further aspects of movement therapy are covered in Chapters 8 and 9. Chapter 9 also includes embed codes to two videos and one audio recording of themed classes.

How to access the online videos

Chapter 9 includes QR codes that will take you to Instructional Videos / Audio that accompany the text. These QR codes can be scanned with a smart phone using an app, and many free apps are available to download. If you are using an iPad or iPhone running the latest software (iOS 11 or higher) then no additional app is required. Simply open your camera and point it at the code (no need to take a picture). A notification should pop down from the top and then tap that and you will be taken to the video.

GLOSSARY OF TERMS

ASLR test The active straight leg raise (ASLR) test tests the capacity and quality of spinal/axial stabilization when supine. A straight leg is raised off the bed 20 cm. Ideally, the pelvis remains stable and the center remains open, controlled with regular diaphragmatic breathing. There is no sensation of fatigue or pain.

Base of support Those parts of the body in contact with the ground or surface which support the spine in different ways. Movement emanates from the base of support. When the base of support (e.g., the sit bones) is poorly "centrated" and grounded, the spine has difficulty aligning itself and finding its "inner lift". The base will vary according to the postures and limb configurations chosen.

Bobath method An approach to neurological rehabilitation developed for children with cerebral palsy which can also be applied to adults after a stroke. The goal of the Bobath concept is to promote motor learning for efficient motor control in various environments, thereby improving function.

Bolster A firmly stuffed long pillow support used in yoga and usually found at yoga suppliers – mine is 85 cm long, 25 cm wide and about 13 cm high. Fig. 4.32 shows a bolster with other props.

Centration When the chosen base of support is "centrated", there is an even distribution of weight across it. This provides both stability and increased afferentation, which activates a physiological stabilization pattern; for example, correct foot centration will affect the alignment of the spine and the diaphragm's function. Joint centration refers to the concept that when joint surfaces are congruent or in maximal contact, with balanced activity between the agonists and antagonists working on either side of the joint/s, the forces on the joint are symmetrically distributed. The joint is in the mid range or neutral position, which allows ideal static or dynamic loading of the joint. The force will be a variable combination or gravity and those produced by neuromuscular activity. A global picture of centration is the standing "neutral" alignment where the spine holds the head, thorax, and pelvis centered directly over one another so that they are bisected by the gravitational line of force. Neuromuscular activity is minimal. Myofascial imbalance disturbs centration.

Compensations Habitual inferior movement strategies to make up for deficient deep system control, which jeopardise spinal health (see Chs 3, 4, 7).

Central nervous system (CNS) The part of the nervous system consisting of the brain and spinal cord – as distinct from the peripheral nervous system. It integrates information it receives from, and coordinates and influences the activity of, all parts of the body.

Functional movements Movements based on natural movements and their biomechanics. They are usually multi-planar, multi-joint movements which involve the spine and place demand on the body's axis and core musculature. The movements we learned as babies, during the developmental process, set up basic patterns of control integrated with the postural system. Through them we naturally possess flexibility, easy and free movement, motor skills and strength as needed.

Limbic system A collection of structures in the brain which support a variety of functions including motivation, emotion, learning, and memory. The limbic system is tightly connected to the prefrontal cortex. Some scientists contend that this connection is related to the pleasure obtained from solving problems, sensory processing, time perception, attention, consciousness, instincts, autonomic/vegetative control, and actions/motor behavior. Not a separate system as such.

Lower quadrant The lower half of the torso including the lower thorax, lumbar spine, pelvic/hip girdle, and the lower limbs.

Red flags A term used in musculoskeletal medicine to refer to signs and symptoms which may indicate another serious pathology, such as secondary bone cancer.

Triplanar Movement develops in essentially three planes: sagittal, frontal, and transverse, and this is useful to consider when analyzing movement. Triplanar movement involves all three movement planes.

Upper quadrant The upper half of the torso, which includes the upper spine and thorax, head and shoulder girdle, and arms.

GLOSSARY OF ABBREVIATIONS

ADIM	Abdominal drawing in maneuver
ALAW	Anterolateral abdominal wall
ANS	Autonomic nervous system
ASIS	Anterior superior iliac spine
ASLR	Active straight leg raise test
CAC	Central anterior cinch
CCC	Central conical cinch
CCP	Central cinch pattern
CPC	Central posterior cinch
FP	Fundamental pattern
GIRD	Glenohumeral internal rotation deficit
IAP	Intra-abdominal pressure mechanism
KPLWST	Key pelvic lateral weight shift test
LBP	Low back pain
LPT	Lower pole of the thorax
LPU	Lower pelvic unit
MCE	Motor control exercise
PFM	Pelvic floor muscles
PIIS	Posterior inferior iliac spine
PLG	Proximal limb girdle
PXS	Pelvic crossed syndrome
RCT	Randomized controlled trial
SIJ	Sacroiliac joint
3-D	Three dimensional

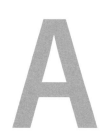

A

Laying the groundwork for an enhanced understanding of the spine in health and disease

The spine is one of the most complex structural and functional regions of our body and is involved in every activity and movement we do. When it functions well, we feel good, look good, and can perform well. On the other hand, it is also a major source of musculoskeletal pain, the increasing incidence of which represents a burgeoning and expensive problem.

The medical model has not been very successful in treating spinal pain, because it looks for structural pathologies in order to diagnose the cause. Yet we know that structural problems – "slipped disks," tears and the like – do not always occur, or, if they are found, may be incidental to the pain. Not being able to find a particular cause for a problem limits finding a solution. Most back pain is usually diagnosed as "nonspecific"; hence treatment has largely also been nonspecific, and had limited results.

A malfunctioning spine is not only the cause of most back pain, it can also be a major source of, or contributor to, many other musculoskeletal pains and injuries – both directly and indirectly.

If we are to better understand and more effectively treat spinal pain, we need to consider how well the spine functions – to appreciate the different qualities of its control in both health and disease. Simply looking at *how* the spine is supported and moves can indicate altered segmental loading patterns and likely repetitive tissue stress over time, and thus provide valuable insights into why the pain may have arisen.

The spine is commonly the victim in many exercise and fitness regimens

The quality of spinal control as we go about our daily lives determines both the state of the spine's health and the level of our general well-being. If our habitual movements are physiologically sound, we can perform well and participate in most exercise without pain or injury – but have you noticed how many people can't?

Undoubtedly, with the rise in obesity and our increasingly sedentary, technology-driven lifestyles, there is a need for many of us to become more active. Being a "couch potato" comes at a cost, and this message has been getting through (hence the flourishing fitness industry).

However, deciding to "get fit" can also be a problem, because there is an at-risk group in the community who simply do not have a sufficient level of function to support their fitness activity of choice – and so they "break down." Most spinal pain problems can be directly related to habitually inefficient patterns of control and/or poor advice and exercise prescription. For instance, the indirect effect of the exercise on the spine may not be well considered (e.g., lifting weights without being able to organize and stabilize the spine in a neutral posture), or exercises may be prescribed which adversely affect the spine, such as suggestions to "strengthen the core" by doing crunches and sit-ups, both of which harmfully compress the spine and, incidentally, do not properly work the core anyway.

A standard question I ask in taking my initial history with the client is: "what exercise do you do?" More often than not, I discover that elements of their training program, involving some – if not all – of their exercises (including stretches) are directly contributing to the development and/or perpetuation of the problem for which they are seeking help. Unfortunately, this can be particularly so in the case of elite athletes.

In this book, I hope to increase the understanding of what constitutes healthy torso movement – to support the functional demands on the spine – and how this is changed in people with pain. With a clearer picture of what is wrong, we are in a better position to prescribe exercise and movement that will restore function without pain.

How effective are exercise interventions for spinal pain?

It is generally accepted that if you have musculoskeletal pain, you should exercise. Maher (2004) pointed out that while exercise was considered to be one of the few evidence-based treatments for chronic back pain, there was uncertainty about which exercises were the most effective and how they should be prescribed. This is still the case, although there has been more relevant research in recent years.

The randomized controlled trial (RCT) is considered the gold standard for judging the benefits of treatments, without bias – and especially when the results from groups of trials are subjected to systematic review and meta-analysis (such as by Cochrane contributors) in order to answer a particular research question.

However, the exclusive use of quantitative approaches, such as RCTs, can risk a narrow understanding of the subject and there are progressively more calls to increase the number of *qualitative* research studies, which generate a different sort of knowledge (Petty et al 2012). The reductionism in research does not necessarily allow us to fully understand complex biological systems, particularly the movement system (see Wallden 2015). And bear in mind that most subjects in an exercise control group are classed as "normal" because they do not (yet) have pain, which does not necessarily mean that they function well or move optimally.

Physiotherapy-related research

Early research into back pain treated exercise as a generic intervention and the content of the exercises given was usually not described, and neither was the rationale for their inclusion. Unsurprisingly, the

results were disappointing. For studies to be useful and have clinical relevance, sufficient detail of the exercises is needed.

As spinal pain research is increasingly finding a substantial association between pain and altered control of posture and movement, there are an increasing number of studies testing the effectiveness of what are known as motor control exercises (MCEs). The results are equivocal.

In chronic low back pain (LBP), MCEs were found to be superior to minimal intervention (Macedo et al 2009), but compared with graded activity there were no significant differences (Macedo et al 2012). Two Cochrane systematic reviews (Saragiotto et al 2016; Macedo et al 2016) again found that MCEs were only "probably more effective than minimal intervention." More importantly, for both acute and chronic LBP patients, no clinically important difference was found between MCEs and other forms of exercise.

In the case of neck pain, Michaleff et al (2014) measured "comprehensive physiotherapy exercise" (specific MCEs and sensorimotor training, progressing to functional whole-body exercise) against simple advice for chronic whiplash disorders. Advice was found to be equally as effective as the exercise program.

A proposed solution to the poor treatment outcomes has been to attempt to identify patient subgroups and match them with more targeted exercise therapies. These studies have assigned patients to subgroups on the basis of observation, movement testing, and pain provocation. The most popular subgroups are the McKenzie method, Sahrmann's Movement System Impairment model and the O'Sullivan classification system. Both the Sahrmann and O'Sullivan models adopt an MCE approach to restoring functional movement.

Randomized trials on the McKenzie method have shown both favorable (Long et al 2004) and insignificant results (Machado et al 2010), and testing of the

Sahrmann model against education, exercise, and performance training (van Dillen et al 2016) showed no between-group differences.

To date the O'Sullivan model is showing more favorable outcomes. Vibe Fersum et al (2013) tested cognitive functional therapy (O'Sullivan's approach integrates both cognitive strategies and functional rehabilitation to change provocative movement and cognitive behaviors that provoke and maintain pain) against traditional manual therapy and exercise (either "general" exercise or MCE involving isolated contractions of the deep abdominal muscles). The cognitive functional therapy cohort demonstrated superior outcomes. However, one has to question *what proportion of the outcome was due to the functional movement/exercise as opposed to the cognitive behavioral therapy?* A further RCT on a particular O'Sullivan LBP subgroup compared a tailored MCE program with general exercise and found "no additional benefit of specific exercises targeting motor control impairment" (Saner et al 2015). A further study on the O'Sullivan system (Lehtola et al 2016) tested specific MCE and control of movement patterns against general exercise combined with manual therapy and only found that "MCE may be superior to general exercise."

In summary, patient subgrouping, where exercise therapy is more tailored to the needs of a specific patient group, could be leading to more positive outcomes. A recent systematic review, however, reveals that the credibility of subgroup claims in LBP trials was low (Saragiotto et al 2016a), which gives us food for thought.

More work is needed. In respect to posturo-movement dysfunction, it is clinically apparent that there is less heterogeneity than is generally understood. I have previously proposed (Key et al 2008; Key 2010) that two principal patient subgroup clusters are clinically apparent (albeit with common posturo-movement problems also), and that tailoring remedial exercise to these groups is clinically effective. These are described in Chapter 3.

Pilates

This popular fitness exercise program has been heavily adopted in clinical practice for treating LBP, and hence is attracting a lot more research.

Again, the results are equivocal. A systematic review (Lim et al 2011) comparing Pilates to other forms of exercise concluded that Pilates was better than no intervention but not superior to other exercise. The authors noted the relatively low quality of existing studies at that time. Although one RCT comparing Pilates to general exercise (Mostagi et al 2015) found no between-group differences for pain and functionality, when analyzed over time, the general exercise group showed increased functionality and flexibility. A Cochrane systematic review by Yamato et al (2015) found low-to-moderate quality evidence that Pilates is more effective than minimal intervention, but there was no conclusive evidence that it is superior to other forms of exercise.

Yoga

With its ancient traditions and focus upon physical postures, breathing techniques, relaxation, and meditation, yoga can be considered the forerunner of a biopsychosocial approach. Despite many people self-selecting yoga as a means of dealing with their back pain, it is not without its faults.

Eligible RCTs testing the effectiveness of yoga are far from numerous, thereby limiting the power of meta-analysis. Two allied RCTs, however, compared the results of practicing yoga against using a self-care book and conventional exercises (Sherman et al 2005) and stretching (Sherman et al 2011) for chronic LBP. There was no difference between the exercise groups, although yoga was shown to be superior to a self-care book.

A systematic review and meta-analysis of yoga for back pain (Cramer et al 2013) found strong evidence for short-term effectiveness and moderate evidence for long-term effectiveness of yoga for LBP, but none to suggest that yoga is more effective than other exercise programs. Another meta-analysis (Holtzman and Beggs 2013) found that post treatment, yoga had a medium-to-large effect on functional disability and pain. However, these authors cautioned against over-interpretation of these results, owing to the small number of RCTs, methodological concerns, and the need for further RCTs to compare yoga with an active control group. A Cochrane review of yoga treatment for chronic nonspecific LBP (Wieland et al 2017) suggested little or no difference between yoga and non-exercise with regard to back-related function.

Feldenkrais

A systematic review in 2015 (Hillier and Worley) analyzed 20 clinically based RCTs, but only three involved the musculoskeletal system and only one of these looked at LBP. While the majority of studies reported significant positive effects of Feldenkrais, methodological problems and the risk of bias was high in most studies, including the one on LBP.

Summary

There are no clear winners – no single form of exercise is superior to another (Saragiotto et al 2016). RCTs on each stream of exercise generally report some improvements against "usual care" but are not shown to be superior when compared to another form of exercise – indicating that keeping active by whatever means is better than doing nothing. The O'Sullivan model of patient subgrouping and cognitive functional therapy suggests more promising treatment outcomes for back pain, although this approach to exercise therapy alone was not necessarily superior.

Later in this book I attempt to shed further light upon patient subgroups and offer a more tailored approach to exercise therapy. The common movement faults are described in Chapter 3, and the remaining chapters offer a method of exercise which addresses these faults and restores meaningful function.

How can research results help us to improve spinal exercise prescription?

There has been a considerable shift in the focus of back pain research toward a more holistic functional approach since I wrote my previous book in 2008. Here, I will broadly summarize the research which directly pertains to therapeutic exercise, and significant individual studies will be further referenced throughout the text. A comprehensive overview of spinal research up to 2013 is provided in *Spinal control: The rehabilitation of back pain*, by Hodges, Cholewicki and Van Dieën.

The important take-home message: The deconditioning paradigm for LBP (loss of muscle strength and endurance, and reduced aerobic capacity) is obsolete (Smeets and Wittink 2007). Despite the common belief that "if you have back pain, you need to get strong," there is no conclusive evidence that weakness is related to back pain (Hamberg-van Reenan et al 2007), or that strengthening alleviates it.

There is, however, a proven *lack of neuromuscular ability*, with *altered adaptive control of movement* (Hodges and Smeets 2015) and *reduced postural endurance*. Following on from his article in 2003 that "relearning" more refined and skilled control and coordination appeared to be more important than strength and endurance training, Hodges (2013) also reported that the significance lay in *how* the nervous system controls posture and movement.

Research is increasingly looking at how motor control is altered in people with back pain and finding a redistribution of activity within and between muscles (Hodges 2011).

Essentially, there is evidence of atrophy (Hides et al 2007) and underactivity (Hides et al 2014) and/or delayed activity (McDonald et al 2009) in certain "deep" muscles. To compensate for this, some of the "superficial" or "global" muscles are overactive (Belavy et al 2007).

This imbalanced activity between the deep and superficial muscles impairs the person's ability to optimally control the basic functions which underlie all healthy movement – *posture* and *breathing*. Movement patterns and their quality suffer.

In general, movement quality deteriorates, becoming coarse and gross, and showing less variety. There is higher superficial muscle cocontraction, higher compressive loading on the spine, and impoverished sensory feedback; and this adaptive motor behavior becomes entrenched through reinforcement learning (Van Dieën et al 2017). The spine becomes stiff (Hodges et al 2009) – it does not move enough! It loses its "juice," flexibility, and the ability to fine-tune segmental movements, so postural stability suffers (Mok and Hodges 2013).

These findings challenge the hitherto popular spinal pain treatment paradigm that the spine is unstable and "needs to be stiffened" or strengthened. Importantly, undertaking a strengthening program can reinforce these compensatory movement patterns, negatively impacting the spine and other systems such as the "core."

Well connected: the role of fascia in movement

Sometimes described as the "Cinderella tissue," having been largely ignored until relatively recently, fascia provides the basic building blocks of functional anatomy, posture, and movement. It is affected by the nervous system and fluid dynamics, and it adapts to mechanical loading. In fact, fascia is changing our understanding of anatomy and how we move (see Schleip et al 2012).

A continuous, body-wide, three-dimensional, largely collagen matrix, the fascial system connects literally everything from head to toe. Fascial sheets of varying dimensions, layers, and thicknesses encase and give attachment to muscles and between the muscles – and give rise to the tendinous expansions which connect these to the bones. Hyaluronic acid, a water-loving mucous-like substance acts as a lubricant between the layers, allowing easy sliding or gliding of the various interfaces, layers, and different structures in movement.

I will use the term "myofascia," because the muscles are intimately connected with the fascial web – largely attaching into the fascia, but also existing within it and acting like contractile pockets which act to variably tension the system. In addition, fascial tissue itself has contractile cells within it, called myofibroblasts, which help modulate general resting muscle tone and the architecture of the fascial tissues (Schleip et al 2012).

The fascial system is a tensional network which has been likened to a tensegrity structure. This replaces the long-held Newtonian concept of the body as a bony skeletal frame on which the soft tissues are draped with one where an integrated fascial fabric has "floating" compression elements (the bones) enmeshed between the interstices of the tensioned (myofascial) elements (Levin and Martin 2012; Fig. 1.1).

Structural support, joint loading and movement are not only affected by the local myofascial tissues but by the whole tensegrity system. In a "biotensegrity" system, force transmission is nonlinear; in other words, forces applied to it are also transmitted tangentially and in all directions across the matrix.

Appreciating the functional body as a biotensegrity system helps the movement therapist understand how and why a movement initiated in one part of the body will create changes in tension (not only locally but also regionally and in other, often quite distant, parts) that contribute directly or indirectly to movement and/or stability.

This "whole system involvement" means the neuromuscular system does not need to work too hard to produce a given posture and movement, thus greatly reducing the energy and effort required in functional movement, yet enabling movement diversity.

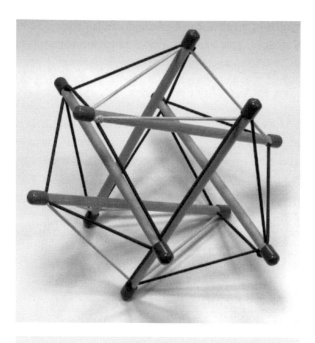

Figure 1.1

Simple model of a tensegrity icosahedron - a balanced tensegrity with three fold symmetry. Note that none of the struts or compression members touch one another. Shortening one tension member will unbalance the figure in all three dimensions. This model can show how local injury affects the entire body. The different colored tension members help one to understand the concept of "triangulation."

Copyright T. Flemons 2006: http://www.intensiondesigns.com/models. html

By initiating movements from key points of control we can influence the architecture of the whole tensegrity system, improving spinal flexibility and control while also accessing stiff regions and restrictions in the limb tissues. The effect is to promote better tissue elasticity and easier movement. This differs from the traditional approach of static stretching, which often does little to change the tensegrity of the fascial matrix.

Fascia possesses another important quality: its innate elasticity and energy storage capability allows for preparatory movements and "bounce," with the muscles acting intermittently to spring-load the system. The Australian kangaroo optimizes this spring-loaded system, where not only is the energy expenditure of movement minimized, but movement appears effortless and free.

The fascial system is constantly adapting to new stresses to meet the body's structural demands. Because of its viscoelastic properties, fascia deforms under repeated loading through creep and hysteresis, or it can show a plastic response and permanent deformation and dysfunction. If neuromuscular system activity is out of balance, this will disturb the tensional balance in the fascia and disturb the integrity of the whole biotensegrity system.

Fascia also serves as a body-wide mechanosensitive signaling system. It surprises many to learn just how richly innervated the fascial system is. With an exceptionally high density of mechanoreceptors and free nerve endings, it plays an important role in providing sensory information – including proprioception to support posture and movement. This also includes nociception if the fascia becomes "bound" and free nerve endings are activated.

Musculoskeletal pain and neuroplastic changes in the central nervous system

The brain is certainly "hot" at the moment within clinical research. The spinal segmental level of the nervous system, however, is yet to arouse such interest in back pain research.

The central nervous system (CNS) is like a computer: sorting "information in" and organizing "responses out." Like all our other body systems, it is constantly adapting in response to the information it receives; in other words, it has *plasticity*. Neuroplastic changes found in the CNS are increasingly being linked to musculoskeletal pain – whether looking at back pain science or tendinopathies (Rio et al 2015).

Neuroplasticity can underpin both negative and positive changes in sensorimotor aspects of lumbopelvic control. Altered movement, with loss of differential trunk muscle behavior and reduced activity from deep system muscles, such as transversus abdominis, results in their decreased representation in the motor cortex. This cortical reorganization is termed *cortical smudging* (Tsao et al 2011; Schabrun et al 2017). It is a case of "use it or lose it," with underused deep muscles losing their area and density of representation in the brain while the overactive global muscles heighten theirs. Cortical smudging is predictive of certain typical gross motor behaviors in LBP.

In addition, CNS hyperexcitability (also known as "central sensitization") and augmented CNS processing of peripheral noxious stimuli are also being increasingly reported in association with chronic musculoskeletal pain (Lim et al 2011a).

Wand et al (2011) provide an excellent review of other cortical changes found in LBP subjects and the implications for clinical practice.

On the positive side, this ability for CNS neuroplasticity can be exploited to our advantage in that we are actually able to *diminish the adverse input to the CNS* from the spinal segmental level by addressing the spinal and/or peripheral joint and myofascial problems with suitable manual therapy.

It is also possible for us to further change spinal movement behavior with tailored sensorimotor exercise therapy which tasks the brain to organize more physiological and skilled movement.

Specific or complex motor-skill learning, rather than mere motor activity, can lead to an increase in selective synaptic plasticity within the CNS and reorganization of movement representations within the motor cortex. It is the intensity of the focused attention that leads to plastic changes. Strength training or mere automatic motor activity, such as walking, does not achieve this (Kleim et al 1998; Remple et al 2001; Adkins et al 2007; Tsao et al 2010).

Injuries: the site of pain is not necessarily the source of pain: spinal segmental dysfunction and peripheral "symptom postcodes"

All regions of the body are functionally interdependent – biomechanically, myofascially, and neurophysiologically. The theory of regional interdependence (Sueki et al 2013) sees that seemingly unrelated impairments in a remote anatomical region may contribute to, or be associated with, the patient's primary complaint. The spine can be both culprit and victim (McCoss et al 2017); and in particular, the spinal joint itself can be a potent pain source.

The spinal column houses much of the nervous system, with the spinal cord and a dense matrix of nerves around each spinal segment helping to orchestrate the sensorimotor regulation of postural support and movement control of the spine itself. Supporting, stabilizing, and moving the spine, however, is a delicate balance that is easily disturbed by inefficient and poor patterns of postural and movement control, which can insidiously develop for many reasons. Gradually, the spine may *lose its ability to adapt* to the demands placed upon it, which results in altered spinal segmental loading and movement patterns, leading in turn to reactive joint and soft tissue stress, and local inflammation.

This inflammation may, to a greater or lesser extent, involve the local segmental nerves and those relaying information between the brain and spinal cord and the periphery. I call this segmental "*neural bother.*" Put simply, the nerves are unhappy, and information to and from the brain and the periphery, including the spine itself, becomes disturbed. Central nervous function is altered and dynamically maintained by the altered peripheral input. This is known as "central sensitization."

This segmental neural bother can be mild, where its effects are covert and subclinical (characterized by minor aches and pains which come and go), or marked, with overt symptoms which persist. These symptoms

9

Chapter 1

can be local (with pain in the spine itself), in the periphery (the limb girdles and limbs accounting for a varied array of peripheral pains) – or both (Fig. 1.2).

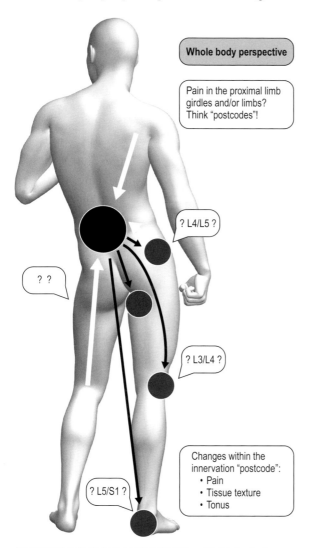

Figure 1.2
Biomechanically, the lumbar spine can be the victim of stiffness in the pelvis/hip and thorax/shoulder joints – and tight lower limb myofascia (represented by *thick white arrows* and *large black circle*). Conversely, the spine can be the cause of peripheral pains and stiffness (represented by the *smaller gray circles* and *thin black arrows*).

Clinically, it is common to find underlying spinal dysfunction in many seemingly unrelated repetitive strain and sporting injuries. Here, it is important to appreciate that although local spinal pain may be a feature, it usually is not. Many deny suffering from back pain, admitting upon questioning to "just stiffness." Usually this has been the situation for some time and feeling stiff has become a normal state.

Do not expect to necessarily reproduce the peripheral pain with general spinal movement testing. If you do, you have a flagrant problem!

While spinal movement testing is often equivocal, careful specific palpation of the likely spinal joint(s) and soft tissues will usually reveal significant dysfunction and extraordinarily tender and reactive tissues. Peripheral symptoms can be immediately reproduced – but often are not. However, this does not necessarily exclude the spine as a potential cause of peripheral symptoms ("where there's smoke, there's fire").

We need to consider what can be termed the *symptom postcode*. This is the peripheral symptom field resulting from spinal segmental dysfunction. When a particular nerve is bothered, it is likely that changes can be found within its innervation field or postcode.

Pain of varying quality, frequency, and severity is always a feature. Other changes in the tissues (spinal and/or peripheral) are also variably apparent, for example bogginess/swelling, allodynia, spontaneous pain, tenderness, trigger points, tightness, myofascial hypertonicity, lack of fascial slide, and joint dysfunction. Many recalcitrant conditions such as tendinopathies, hamstring problems, and hip bursitis are related to underlying lumbar and associated thoracic joint dysfunction. While there are usually underlying biomechanical problems, a sensitized nervous system is also commonly involved.

The thoracic spine is often a silent biomechanical and neurophysiological contributor to neck pain, LBP, and many musculoskeletal pain syndromes. The thorax houses the sympathetic nervous system which

10

is increasingly being implicated in tendinopathies (Jewson et al 2015) and other musculoskeletal pains. Yet to date, its contribution to dysfunctional movement and pain in the upper and lower quadrants has not been widely investigated.

Understanding this dysfunctional relationship between the spine and periphery can help the movement therapist address both the peripheral and spinal dysfunction more effectively.

To help map the symptom postcode, it is useful to be able to refer to dermatome (area of skin supplied by single posterior spinal nerve root) and myotome (the muscles and fascia supplied by that spinal nerve root) charts (Fig. 1.3). With practice, you become more

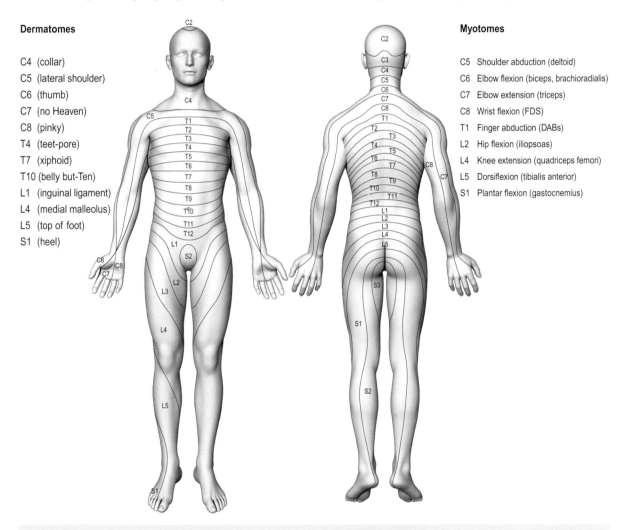

Dermatomes

C4 (collar)
C5 (lateral shoulder)
C6 (thumb)
C7 (no Heaven)
C8 (pinky)
T4 (teet-pore)
T7 (xiphoid)
T10 (belly but-Ten)
L1 (inguinal ligament)
L4 (medial malleolus)
L5 (top of foot)
S1 (heel)

Myotomes

C5 Shoulder abduction (deltoid)
C6 Elbow flexion (biceps, brachioradialis)
C7 Elbow extension (triceps)
C8 Wrist flexion (FDS)
T1 Finger abduction (DABs)
L2 Hip flexion (iliopsoas)
L4 Knee extension (quadriceps femori)
L5 Dorsiflexion (tibialis anterior)
S1 Plantar flexion (gastocnemius)

Figure 1.3

Dermatomes are not fixed anatomical or territorial entities but neurophysiological entities whose boundaries fluctuate according to the prevailing levels of spinal cord segment facilitation. Pain and other symptoms can occur within the dermatome and/or upregulation or weakness in the myotome.

familiar with these myofascial innervation fields, which indicate the spinal levels you should be checking. If you are a manual therapist and find problems at relevant levels, and treat these segments appropriately, you will usually find that the peripheral signs and symptoms change. This often occurs within the treatment session, or over a few treatments, depending upon the degree of dysfunction.

The postcode is also valuable for movement therapists to appreciate, because changing what happens in the spine may also help, for example, a client's hip pain.

An appreciation of functional interrelationships, not only between the spine and the limbs but between the nervous, myofascial, and joint systems, can help in understanding why the site of pain is not necessarily its source.

By appropriately addressing the spinal movement dysfunction, we can usually more effectively change back pain (and/or many injuries in the "pain postcode") and also dampen the central sensitization cycle, helping to bring people out of chronic pain.

The biopsychosocial model of care

This is now *the* accepted model of spinal pain care, replacing the hitherto unidimensional pathology-based model of Western medicine.

Spinal pain problems are a complex and variable mixture of biological, psychological, and social interactions which determine the cause, manifestation, and outcome of management. Research over recent decades has focused heavily on the psychosocial domain, possibly at the expense of biological factors. The risk with such a focus is that when the "bio" has not been well addressed, it becomes easy to shift the blame for poor treatment outcomes onto the client by saying it's a "psychosocial problem." Interestingly, a study by Steffens et al (2014) found that the majority of primary care clinicians considered biomechanical risk factors to be the most important triggers for sudden onset LBP.

For this reason, I am deliberately choosing to focus principally on the bio aspects – the bio- and myomechanics of spinal movement and functional control – as I consider that these are still not well enough understood or adequately redressed in spinal pain disorders, and this impedes effective rehabilitation.

The approach is founded on mindfulness in changing movement behavior, which contributes to changes in motor coordination and cortical reorganization (Kleim et al 1998; Remple et al 2001; Tsao et al 2010) – and has demonstrable cognitive benefits. Clients are frequently the victims of bad advice and succumb to disability. The client needs to understand how pain can become a vicious cycle and that habitual inferior patterns of posturo-movement usually underlie the genesis of most spinal pain and many injuries. They also need to be prepared to become actively involved in their rehabilitation.

While patients are a heterogeneous group, there are still common underlying physical traits which warrant further exploration, understanding and specific management. This will be covered in more detail in Chapter 3.

Recommended reading

Hodges PW (2011) Pain and motor control: From the laboratory to rehabilitation. J Electromyogr Kinesiol 21:220–228.

Hodges PW, Cholewicki J, Van Dieën J (eds) (2013) Spinal control: The rehabilitation of back pain; State of the art and science. Edinburgh: Churchill Livingstone Elsevier.

Myers T (2014) Anatomy Trains: Myofascial meridians for manual and movement therapists, 3rd edn. Edinburgh: Churchill Livingstone/Elsevier.

Schleip R, Findley TW, Chaitow L, Huijing P (eds) (2015) Fascia in sport and movement. Edinburgh: Handspring.

References

Adkins DL Boychuck J, Remple MS, Kleim J (2007) Motor training induces experience-specific patterns of plasticity across motor cortex and spinal cord. J Appl Physiol 101(6):1776–1782.

Belavy DL, Richardson CA, Wilson SJ et al (2007) Superficial lumbo-pelvic muscle activity and decreased co-contraction after 8 weeks of bedrest. Spine 32(1):E23–E29.

Cramer H, Lauche R, Haller H, Dobos G (2013) A systematic review and meta-analysis of yoga for low back pain. Clin J Pain 29(5):450–460.

Hamberg-van Reenen HH, Ariëns GA, Blatter BM et al (2007) A systematic review of the relation between physical capacity and future low back and neck/shoulder pain. Pain 130:93–107.

Hides JA, Belavý DL, Stanton W et al (2007) Magnetic resonance imaging assessment of trunk muscles during prolonged bedrest. Spine 32(15):1687–1692.

Hides JA, Stanton WR, Dilani Mendis M et al (2014) Small multifidus muscle size predicts football injuries. Orthop J Sports Med Jun; 2(6): 2325967114537588.

Hillier S, Worley A (2015) The effectiveness of the Feldenkrais method: A systematic review of the evidence. Evidence based complementary and alternative medicine. Article ID 752160-1-752160-12.

Hodges PW (2003) Core stability exercise in chronic low back pain. Orthop Clin North Am 34:245–254.

Hodges PW (2011) Pain and motor control: From the laboratory to rehabilitation. J Electromyogr Kinesiol 21:220–228.

Hodges PW (2013) Adaptation and rehabilitation: From motor neurones to motor cortex and behaviour. In: Hodges PW, Cholewicki J, Van Dieën JH (eds) Spinal control: The rehabilitation of back pain; State of the art and science. Edinburgh: Churchill Livingstone Elsevier.

Hodges PW, Smeets RJ (2015) Interaction between pain, movement, and physical activity: Short-term benefits, long-term consequences, and targets for treatment. Clin J Pain 31(2):97–107.

Hodges PW, Van den Hoorn W, Dawson A, Cholewicki J (2009) Changes in the mechanical properties of the trunk in low back pain may be associated with recurrence. J Biomech 42(1):61–66.

Hodges PW, Cholewicki J, Van Dieën JH (eds) (2013) Spinal control: The rehabilitation of back pain; State of the art and science. Edinburgh: Churchill Livingstone Elsevier.

Holtzman S, Beggs T (2013) Yoga for chronic low back pain: A meta-analysis of randomised controlled trials. Pain Res Manag 18(5):267–272.

Jewson JL, Lambert GW, Storr M, Gaida JE (2015) The sympathetic nervous system and tendinopathy: A systematic review. Sports Med 45(5):727–743.

Key J (2010) Back pain: A movement problem; A clinical approach incorporating relevant research and practice. Edinburgh: Churchill Livingstone Elsevier.

Key J, Clift A, Condie F, Harley C (2008) A model of movement dysfunction provides a classification system guiding diagnosis

and therapeutic care in spinal pain and related musculoskeletal syndromes: A paradigm shift—Part 2. J Bodyw Mov Ther 12(2):105–120.

Kleim JA, Swain RA, Armstrong KA et al (1998) Selective synaptic plasticity within the cerebellar cortex following complex motor skill learning. Neurobiology of Learning and Memory 69:274–289.

Lehtola V, Luomajoki H, Leinonen V et al (2016) Sub-classification based specific movement control exercises are superior to general exercise in subacute low back pain when both are combined with manual therapy: A randomised controlled trial. BMC Musculoskelet Disord 17:135.

Levin S, Martin DC (2012) Biotensegrity: The mechanics of fascia, in Schleip R, Findley T, Chaitow L, Huijing PA (eds) Fascia: The tensional network of the human body. Edinburgh: Churchill Livingstone Elsevier.

Lim ECW, Poh RL, Low AY, Wong WP (2011) Effects of Pilates based exercises on pain and disability in individuals with persistent nonspecific low back pain: A systematic review with meta-analysis. J Orthop Sports Phys Ther 41(2):70–79.

Lim ECW, Sterling M, Stone A, Vicenzino B (2011a) Central hyperexcitability as measured with nociceptive flexor reflex threshold in chronic musculoskeletal pain: A systematic review. Pain 152:1811–1820.

Long A, Donelson R, Fung T (2004) Does it matter what exercise?: A randomised controlled trial of exercise for low back pain. Spine 29(23):2593–2602.

McCoss CA, Johnston R, Edwards DJ et al (2017) Preliminary evidence of regional interdependent inhibition, using a "diaphragm release" to specifically induce an immediate hypoalgesic effect in the cervical spine. J Bodyw Mov Ther 21(2):362–374.

McDonald D, Moseley GL, Hodges PW (2009) Why do some patients keep hurting their back? Evidence of ongoing back muscle dysfunction during remission from recurrent back pain. Pain 142:183–188.

Macedo LG, Maher CG, Latimer J, McCauley J (2009) Motor control exercises for persistent nonspecific low back pain: A systematic review. Phys Ther 89(1):9–25.

Macedo LG, Latimer J, Maher CG et al (2012) Effect of motor control exercises versus graded activity in patients with chronic nonspecific LBP: A randomised controlled trial. Phys Ther 93(3):1–15.

Macedo LG, Saragiotto BT, Yamato TP et al (2016) Motor control exercise for acute non-specific low back pain(review). Cochrane Database of Systematic Reviews. Issue 2, CD012085.

Machado LAC, Maher CG, Herbert RD et al (2010) The effectiveness of the McKenzie method in addition to first-line care for acute low back pain: A randomised controlled trial. BMC Med 8:10.

Maher CG (2004) Effective physical treatment for chronic low back pain. Orthop Clin North Am 35:57–64.

Michaleff ZA, Maher CG, Lin CW et al (2014) Comprehensive physiotherapy exercise programme or advice for chronic whiplash (PROMISE): A pragmatic randomised controlled trial. Lancet April.

Mok N, Hodges PW (2013) Movement of the lumbar spine is critical for maintenance of postural recovery following support surface perturbation. Exp Brain Res 231:305–313.

Mostagi FQ, Dias JM, Pereira LM et al (2015) Pilates versus general exercise effectiveness on pain and functionality in non-specific chronic low back pain subjects. J Bodyw Mov Ther 19(4):636–645.

Petty NJ, Thomson OP, Stew G (2012) Ready for a paradigm shift? Part 1 introducing the philosophy of qualitative research. Man Ther 17(4):267–274.

Remple MS, Bruneau RM, VandenBerg PM et al (2001) Sensitivity of cortical movement representations to motor experience: Evidence that skill learning but not strength training induces cortical re-organisation. Behav Brain Res 123(2):133–141.

Rio E, Kidgell D, Moseley GL et al (2015) Tendon neuroplastic training: changing the way we think about tendon rehabilitation: A narrative review. Br J Sports Med 50(4):1–23.

Saner J, Kool J, Sieben JM et al (2015) A tailored exercise program versus general exercise for a subgroup of patients with low back pain and movement control impairment: A randomised controlled trial with one year follow up. Man Ther 20(5):672–679.

Saragiotto BT, Maher CG, Yamato TP et al (2016) Motor control exercise for non-specific low back pain: A Cochrane Collaboration review. Spine 41(16):1284–1295.

Saragiotto BT, Maher CG, Moseley AM et al (2016a) A systematic review reveals that the credibility of subgroup claims in low back pain trials was low. J Clin Epidemiol Nov; 79:3–9.

Schabrun S, Elgueta-Cancino EL, Hodges PW (2017) Smudging of the motor cortex is related to severity in low back pain. Spine 42(15):1172–1178.

Schleip R, Findley T, Chaitow L, Huijing P (eds) (2012) Fascia: The tensional network of the human body. Edinburgh: Churchill Livingstone Elsevier.

Schleip R, Jäger H, Klingler W (2012) Fascia is alive: How cells modulate the tonicity and architecture of fascial tissues. In: Schleip R, Findley T, Chaitow L, Huijing PA (eds) Fascia: The tensional network of the human body. Edinburgh: Churchill Livingstone Elsevier.

Sherman KJ, Cherkin DC, Erro J et al (2005) Comparing yoga, exercise and a self-care book for chronic low back pain: A randomized controlled trial. Ann Intern Med 143(12):849–856.

Sherman KJ, Cherkin DC, Wellman RD et al (2011) A randomised trial comparing yoga, stretching, and a self-care book for chronic LBP. Arch Inter Med 171(22):219–226.

Smeets RJEM, Wittink H (2007) The deconditioning paradigm for chronic low back pain unmasked? Pain 130:201–202.

Steffens D, Maher CG, Ferreira M et al (2014) Clinician's views on factors that trigger a sudden onset of low back pain. Eur Spine J 23(3):512–519.

Sueki DG, Cleland JA, Wainner RS (2013) Regional interdependence model of musculoskeletal dysfunction: Research, mechanisms and clinical implications. J Man Manip Ther 23:139–146.

Tsao H, Galea MP, Hodges PW (2010) Driving plasticity in the motor cortex in recurrent low back pain. Eur J Pain 14(8):832–839.

Tsao H, Danneels L, Hodges PW (2011) ISSLS Prize Winner: Smudging the motor brain in young adults with recurrent low back pain. Spine 36(21):1721–1727.

Van Dieën J, Flor H, Hodges PW (2017) Low back pain patients learn to adapt motor behaviour with adverse secondary consequences. Exerc Sport Sci Rev 45(4):223–229.

Van Dillen LR, Norton BJ, Sahrmann SA et al (2016) Efficacy of a classification-specific treatment and adherence on outcomes in people with chronic low back pain. A one year follow-up prospective, randomised, controlled clinical trial. Man Ther 24:52–64.

Vibe Fersum K, O'Sullivan P, Skouen JS et al (2013) Efficacy of classification-based cognitive functional therapy in patients with non-specific chronic low back pain: A randomized controlled trial. Eur J Pain 17(6):916–928.

Wallden M. (2015) "But we are infinitely more complex than a car": A systems approach to health and performance. J Bodyw Mov Ther 19(4):697–711.

Wand BM, Parkitny L, O'Connell NE et al (2011) Cortical changes in chronic low back pain: Current state of the art and implications for clinical practice. Man Ther 16(1):15–20.

Wieland LS, Skoetz N, Pilkington K et al (2017) Yoga treatment for chronic non-specific low back pain (Review) Cochrane Database of Systematic Reviews Issue 1 Art No. CD010671.

Yamato TP, Maher CG, Saragiotto BT et al (2015) Pilates for low back pain (review). Cochrane Database of Systematic Reviews Issue 7.

The vertebral axis:
A marriage between biotensegrity and neuromotor control

Gravity: establishing the axis and balancing the forces

Humans are born anatomically and functionally immature. It takes us 5 years to complete our motor development so that we can move effectively and independently; and we learn to move by learning to exploit the constant force of gravity.

The motor developmental process lays down important patterns of movement through which we develop our postural reflexes and sequentially achieve the motor milestones.

The spine is, of course, involved from the start. Control of the head and neck, and the ability to brace the core within the gravitational field, are the precursors to controlling the limbs (Kobesova and Kolar 2014). Control in the sagittal plane occurs first and is established by four and a half months. This allows for controlled weight shift and rotation to develop, as well as the gradual ability to counteract gravity through various postures, which increasingly bring the body axis upright and onto two legs.

At birth the spine and pelvis resemble a (floppy) kyphotic C curve in the sagittal plane (Fig. 2.1), known as the primary spinal curve. The secondary curves – the cervical and lumbar lordosis – develop gradually through the developmental process to create the S-shaped sagittal upright spine which affords flexibility, shock absorption, and resilience to the spine.

The development of pelvic control and the lumbar lordosis are particularly important to the integrity of the spinal curves and to the spine's antigravity "lift."

In a "neutral spine" the curves balance one another and there is minimal muscle activity in its maintenance (see Fig. 2.1). Note that the center of gravity of the body is just in front of the top of the sacrum and through the hip joints; also that the tailbone points back rather than being tucked under.

Our postural and movement systems are continually gravity dependent and gravity sensitive. We rely upon the support of the ground, engage with it, and utilize the ground reaction force to "push up" against gravity.

Microgravity studies have shown that the postural control system rapidly deteriorates without gravity and that this is associated with marked lumbopelvic muscle imbalance (Evetts et al 2014). Astronauts are known to have an increased risk of cervical and lumbar intervertebral disk herniation (Belavy et al 2015).

Essentially, the job of the spine, a highly articulated and flexible column, is to lengthen and operate against the forces of gravity, supporting the head and the proximal limb girdles in a diverse array of postures and movements. For most of our daily of activities it must sustain its function vertically without collapse or buckling. To do this there needs to be a balance between stiffness and mobility, to allow both stable antigravity support and movement.

Verticality and lengthening of the spine/torso is achieved by a combination of torso flexor and extensor muscle coactivation and the internal postural support afforded by the pressure-change mechanisms operating within the body cavity; that is, breathing and intra-abdominal pressure (IAP) (Hodges et al 2005).

Balanced torso flexor/extensor activity aligns the major units of mass – the head, thorax and pelvis, and the spine – in its natural curves, known as a "neutral spine." This is a point of reference: a "home base" that movement occurs away from and returns to.

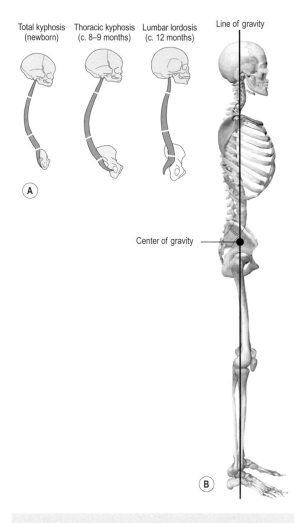

Total kyphosis (newborn) · Thoracic kyphosis (c. 8–9 months) · Lumbar lordosis (c. 12 months)

Line of gravity

Center of gravity

A

B

IAP is an automatic postural response which occurs prior to a movement occurring, in order to support and stabilize the spine. It can be likened to an internal air cushion in that by providing deep anterior support to the spine, it imparts a certain buoyancy, lightness, and ease to spinal postures. A child's party whistle nicely demonstrates the effect of IAP – up-righting of the whistle/axis is achieved by inflating the whistle/creating IAP (Fig. 2.2).

The contribution of IAP is important as it lessens the requirement for much superficial trunk muscle activity. Without optimal IAP, spinal support, and stability, verticality and movements requiring extension will involve excess coactivation of the spinal extensors – imparting a vertebral compressive stress, over-stiffening the spine and limiting movement.

Intrathoracic pressures also contribute to postural control and stability of the thorax. These are regulated by modulating the glottis (Massery et al 2013). This is also considered a diaphragm, and when spinal alignment is optimal, the three diaphragms (glottis, thoracic, and pelvic floor) are aligned over one another.

Figure 2.1

A) At birth the infant spine resembles a long C curve in the sagittal plane. Through the motor developmental process, the lumbar lordosis is apparent at about a year old, when the infant can achieve vertical postures on the feet. Spinopelvic control becomes further developed as motor skills become further refined. B) In the mature upright spine the head, thorax, and pelvis are balanced over one another and the gravitational line of force bisects the C0/1 joint and auditory canal, the shoulder, hip knee, and ankle joints – and neuromuscular activity is minimal. The center of gravity in standing is within the pelvis, just in front of the top of the sacrum.

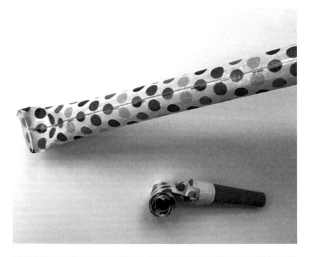

Figure 2.2

A paper party whistle is ordinarily collapsed, but when inflated changes its form.

Balance and stability are optimal when the glottis is engaged to modulate the airway, as in talking. In yoga, Ujjayi breathing is a glottal control technique which involves slightly contracting the throat/glottis while breathing through the nose. Closing the glottis and holding the breath helps increase both intrathoracic pressures and the IAP needed to stiffen the trunk for, say, a heavy lift. However, when this strategy is used for normal postural control it creates rigidity, and the "damping" movements needed to recover balance after perturbation are reduced.

Fascia, biotensegrity, and the axial architecture

The fascial system was introduced in Chapter 1 as a tensional network that has been likened to a tensegrity structure, which may help us better understand its musculoskeletal dynamics. Here, I deal with tensegrity in more detail.

True tensegrity structures balance tension and compression forces. They only transmit loads through tension and compression. As they are fully triangulated there are no bending moments or shear forces (see Fig. 1.1). They are lightweight, yet very strong and resilient, and can withstand considerable dynamic stress because any applied load is distributed to all parts of the structure simultaneously.

Tensegrities are self-stabilized, self-contained, and do not need external support. They are never, however, completely rigid, which means they have varying degrees of flexibility. The tension and compression vectors do not pass through the same point, but twist past each other, lending torque or rotation to the structure's geometry; hence tensegrities always possess clockwise and counter-clockwise rotations of compression and tension that additively cancel each other out to guarantee stability (Flemons 2007; see Fig. 1.1).

True tensegrities are said not to need the support of the ground, whereas our bodies clearly do. Nevertheless, modeling the torso as a biotensegrity structure helps illuminate its function. In this regard, I have previously described a construct that I described as the "body cylinder" (Key 2010). Conceptually, the compression elements of the torso (the spine, thorax, and pelvis), in association with a continuous tension network (the extensive "inner" and "outer" fascial matrix) form a roughly cylindrical architectural framework. This is stable, yet adaptable, being capable of deformation and shape change.

This occurs because of our ability to alter the volume and shape of the internal cavities via the breathing and IAP mechanisms, simultaneously changing tension in parts of the fascial matrix. These tensions are further distributed across the system in a nonlinear manner, such that axial postural adaptations and movements occur. Stability is paired with mobility.

The generated internal cavity pressures push out against the torso framework, helping to support it from inside as well as generating tension in the "outer fascia," such as the thoracolumbar fascia. For effective biotensegrity, this transverse internal expansion must have the capacity to match the level of outer myofascial activity. If that activity dominates (e.g., the thoracolumbar extensors), it constricts the torso, compresses the spine, limits movement, and further hampers effective internal support.

Optimal internal tensional support allows the outer tensional network to "let go," which means the neuromyofascial response can then be minimal without postural collapse. Movement is relaxed and free.

Levin and Martin (2012) point out that a tensegrity structure is stable with flexible joints: "Movement is not bending of hinges but expansion, repositioning and contraction of tensegrities." Their restrained expansion is what gives tensegrities their stability and ease.

The torso's tensegrity-like structure allows the spine to function well no matter how it is oriented in space, whether vertically, horizontally or in between.

Or upside down. It can accept load in any position; for example, we can stand on one arm or leg and reach out into space (Fig. 2.3).

Increased tension in one part of the body/tensegrity will be reflected through the whole structure. Changing the base of support and/or the point from

where the movement is initiated will bring about a redistribution of tension within the whole fascial system and a change in the whole axial architecture. In support and movement, tensions and counter-tensions are constantly fluctuating throughout the whole body.

However, sustained neuromuscular tension in one part (e.g., pelvic floor) leads to fascial "bind" and restriction, distorting the overall architecture and disturbing the synergy between balanced tension and compression components – and the ability for adaptable posturo-movement. Similarly, sustained underactivity of deep system myofascia and/or overextensibility of one part of the fascial matrix also disturbs the integrity of the whole structure and the body geometry, with ensuing collapse (Fig. 2.4).

Pre-tensioning of the fascial system and the hazards of excess tension

Optimal spinal stability and mobility is achieved when we can generate and balance tensional and compressive forces through the body tensegrity. First, we need to consider how the body pre-tensions the fascial system.

Healthy muscles at rest have tone but not tension. Fascia contains varying densities of smooth muscle-like fibroblasts or contractile cells in its

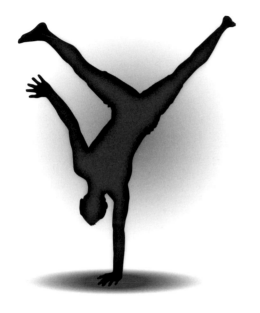

Figure 2.3
The body's structural and functional tensegrity allows us to reach into the space around us from varying bases of support.

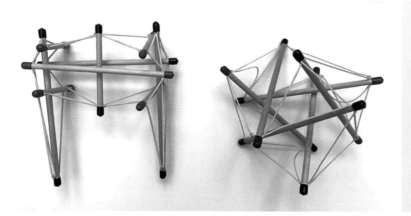

Figure 2.4
These tensegrity models help illustrate how imbalance in the tension elements distorts the whole system. Note how altered tension changes the geometry in the model of the pelvis on the *left*. And the collapse in the integrity of the whole structure when some elements are over slack in the model on the *right*. See the balanced tension model in Fig. 1.1.

matrix (Schleip et al 2005). These play a considerable role in modulating the tonicity or stiffness – and the architecture of the fascial envelope. The cells are also thought to be strongly influenced by the autonomic nervous system (ANS), where increased sympathetic activation may lead to increased cellular contraction within the fascial tissues (Schleip et al 2012).

The fascial network is also directly and indirectly tensioned via the muscular force transmission system (Turinna et al 2013). Fibers within a muscle have longitudinal, transverse, and oblique dispositions as they attach to both bone and fascia. Hence, during a contraction forces are distributed in multiple directions – not only directly moving the bone levers but simultaneously transmitting 30–40% of the generated force tangentially to the connective tissue outside the muscle. This extramuscular myofascial force transmission is the more important mechanism for muscular interaction, both between synergists and (particularly) between so-called antagonistic muscles located on the opposite side of the body or a limb (Huijing 2012).

The body tensegrity also appears to balance the tension/compression forces via the combination of vertical elongation and lift of the spine and the counter-tensions created by the horizontal widening of the core or "opening the center" (Fig. 2.5).

Monitoring and controlling the appropriate and shifting levels of myofascial tension that are needed for us to remain upright and move is largely the job of the nervous system. Like Goldilocks's porridge,

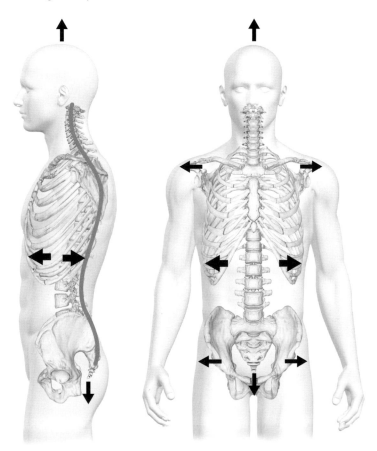

Figure 2.5

The task of the spine is to lengthen between the head and the tailbone, while that of the "core" is to provide inner tensional support to enable widening – particularly opening through the center but also to support widening in the proximal limb girdles.

myofascial tension needs to be just right for the prevailing conditions. In other words, although it is minimal when the body is at rest, at other times it requires sufficient tension to ensure effective antigravity support but not so much as to limit movement. Thanks to the fascial system, antigravity support can occur with very little neuromuscular activity.

The "pre-tension" to the fascial system goes hand in hand with the pre-movement responses of the inner postural system – in particular the IAP mechanism. Having said this, one of the defining attributes of our patients with spinal pain is that they "hold too much tension" and that "letting go" is commonly a problem, particularly in some regions of the torso: the buttocks and pelvic floor, around the center body, the neck and shoulders, and the jaw. Their neuromuscular systems are in relative overdrive, which is reflected in increased regional superficial (global) myofascial activity – and this is *always correlated with insufficient capacity of the internal tensional system or core*. This leads to excess compression, shortening, and restriction in the torso, thereby limiting free movement and disturbing the body's structural and functional tensegrity (see Ch. 3 for a more detailed examination).

One may also observe and/or palpate increased peripheral myofascial tone, particularly in the legs. This may be associated with pain in the major joints and is usually seen as a local problem of tight muscles which just need to be stretched. For the astute practitioner, however, it can be a valuable sign, indicative of significant spinal segmental dysfunction – a case of changes or symptoms in the "postcode" (see Ch. 1: Injuries).

Nervous system dysregulation: its effect on movement quality

Movement starts in the nervous system. Intention starts a voluntary movement and the nervous system regulates and monitors all movement. This is dependent upon the CNS receiving adequate sensory and environmental information, which it processes in order to formulate appropriate motor responses. In this process the CNS needs to integrate diverse sources of information – from the ANS (the sympathetic and parasympathetic nervous systems) and inputs from our emotional and intellectual selves.

Healthy biological systems are adaptable and self-regulating. The nervous system can prime our body to respond if our well-being is threatened, inducing the heightened state of arousal known as the "fight or flight" response. This involves a considerable amount of sympathetic nervous system activity. When the threat subsides, the nervous system adjusts, calms down and the parasympathetic or "rest and digest" system kicks in. Sympathetic activity is involved in "doing," whereas parasympathetic activity is involved in "being." Here, we can relax and replenish ourselves; we are calm, can take in our surroundings, are in tune with our senses, and able to experience and regulate ourselves – and we live well.

However, the busy, multitasking, high-stress, and stimulative 21st-century lifestyles can lead to nervous system dysregulation. The high end of the nervous activity spectrum dominates and the person is constantly anxious, tense, overreactive, and using unnecessary effort in simple movements. Experiencing the parasympathetic spectrum and restoring oneself becomes uncommon; chronic fatigue and burnout symptoms can appear. Nervous system imbalance will be reflected in motor system imbalance. The spine suffers.

Consider also that when the spine is poorly aligned, the head and pelvis are out of balance – which conceivably adversely influences both the craniosacral outflow of the parasympathetic nervous system and the sympathetic nervous system, which is located within the thorax.

It is important to recognize nervous system upregulation when prescribing therapeutic exercise.

In someone with an already pumped up nervous system, it does not make sense to prescribe hard and fast strengthening exercises which involve effort. This just leads to more tension and disturbed function. Remember, the research tells us that people with spinal pain are not weak! Their problem is more one of organizing coordination and control.

Rather, we should be exercising the parasympathetic "being" nervous system by prescribing the movements and actions they commonly find difficult – slow, gentle, discrete, well-controlled and differentiated responses. Good head and pelvic control will also help optimize function in the craniosacral outflow.

This is well understood by the yoga world from which the concepts of meditation and breath control emanated – activity working both spectrums of the nervous system between action, inaction, and restoration. However fine tuning the quality of the response is important in the poses because care must be taken not to over-challenge the clients beyond their abilities.

Similarly, Feldenkrais, Tai Chi Qigong and other meditative movement exercise systems have a long tradition of helping to reduce stress, calm the mind, and support balanced autonomic nervous activity.

The biopsychosocial model appreciates these complex interactions between our body, and our emotional and thinking selves: emotional stress creates changes in the body; altered bodily function such as poor postural control and altered breathing patterns can manifest as anxiety.

The key to refined movement control: balanced deep and superficial myofascial activity

Posture and movement go together. You cannot have healthy movement without appropriate postural sets to support it. They develop hand in hand during the neurodevelopmental process which lays down the functional connections between the head, proximal limb girdles, and spine. This ensures the shifting requirements for stability and movement through the axis and limbs are easily met. The tensions and counter-tensions imparted to the spine contribute to the development of its support and control mechanisms so that it can sustain verticality, support the limbs, and allow free and varied movement.

The myofascial system can be conceptually divided into a systemic "deep" or local muscle system and a superficial muscle system – each with differing structural and functional qualities (Key 2010).

The *deep system* is closely allied with the postural reflex mechanism. It provides core control (i.e., inner tensional postural support and stability of the spine against the effects of gravity) and counters the internal and external forces created by limb movement. The system is energy efficient and built for sustained low-grade activity and postural endurance.

It is also responsible for our intrinsic movements, fine-tuning spinal segmental control, and the discrete axial multisegmental adjustments needed for weight shift and balance.

As there are a large number of muscle spindles in the deep system myofascia, its activity is closely allied with interoception, proprioception and kinesthesia – the sense of our internal body, knowing where we are in space, and the ability to sense weight and modulate discrete movements with minimal muscular effort, respectively.

Deep system myofascia includes the intercostal web, the inner myofascial web of the torso – including the lower pelvic unit (LPU; Fig. 2.6) – the small spinal intersegmental muscles, the deep neck flexors, the deep hip rotators (particularly obturator internus), the lower scapular stabilizers, and the small muscles of the feet and hands.

What is known as the core could be described as the deep inner unit. Too often, it is confused with both an

Chapter 2

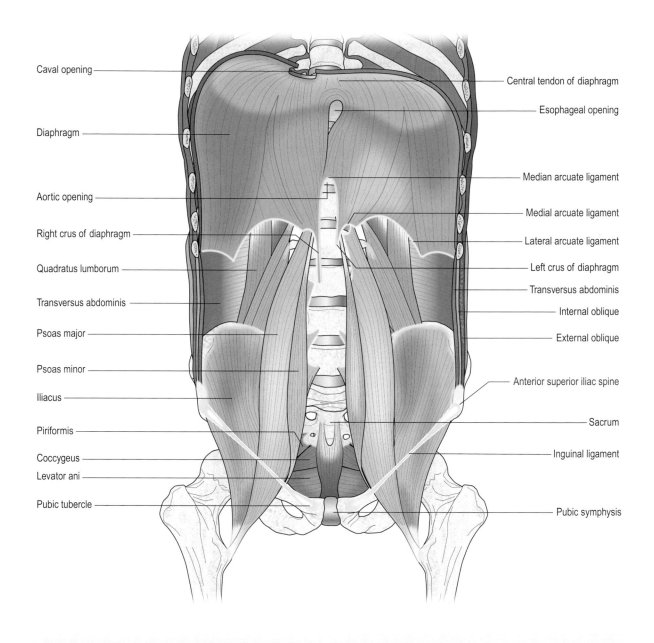

Caval opening
Diaphragm
Aortic opening
Right crus of diaphragm
Quadratus lumborum
Transversus abdominis
Psoas major
Psoas minor
Iliacus
Piriformis
Coccygeus
Levator ani
Pubic tubercle

Central tendon of diaphragm
Esophageal opening
Median arcuate ligament
Medial arcuate ligament
Lateral arcuate ligament
Left crus of diaphragm
Transversus abdominis
Internal oblique
External oblique
Anterior superior iliac spine
Sacrum
Inguinal ligament
Pubic symphysis

Figure 2.6

The lower pelvic unit acts to provide prevertebral and intrapelvic support and control.

Reproduced from Key (2010) with permission

instruction to pull your stomach in and overactivity of the upper abdominal wall. I deliberately make the distinction *lower* pelvic unit as it is the musculature of the

lower abdominal wall (and inner pelvis) which is important in both developing IAP for breathing and postural control *and* also for modulating pelvic myomechanics (see: "Opening the center" and Pelvic fulcrum). If you like, the LPU is responsible for both primary and pelvic core functions. In yoga, "engaging the mula bandha" (when correctly understood and actioned) is a technique aimed at improving activity in the LPU.

The deep system has an inherent tendency to inhibition, atrophy, weakness, and delayed activity – especially in conditions of pain, injury, fatigue, and emotional stress (Jull and Janda 1987). It is where we see the biopsychosocial aspects playing out.

On the other hand, the torso *superficial* or "global" muscle system is built for more phasic movement, where bursts of activity are required to control the limbs and the alignment of the major units of mass (the head, thorax, and pelvis). These large, usually polysegmental, trunk and limb muscles are involved in the more extrinsic movements, requiring strength, and in fast, ballistic "open-chain" limb movements. What they lack, however, is the fine motor control necessary for effective spinal stabilization. Effective deep system control is needed to generate the underlying mechanisms of inner tensional support and axial stability.

Long ago, Janda (1980) informed us that this system has an inherent tendency to be easily activated and strengthened and to dominate in movement patterns – particularly in states of pain, fatigue, injury, stress or effort, or when working out new or complex movement patterns. Their overactivity leads both to increased muscle tightness and shortness and to reduced fascial slide. Sensory perception is also diminished when these muscles dominate in movement patterns.

Healthy movement depends upon our ability to regulate the different inherent tendencies between the deep and superficial myofascial systems. There is a flexible balance of activity between them that enables a supple, adaptable uprightness together with grace, freedom, and lightness in movement – while maintaining the capacity to quickly adapt to any sudden strength demands without incident.

However, in people with spinal pain, balanced activity between the systems is lost: inadequate deep system control is accompanied by increased superficial activity and reduced cocontraction. The same imbalance has been found in inactivity, microgravity, and bedrest studies (Belavy et al 2007).

Increased superficial trunk muscle activity will have an inhibitory effect on the deep system, which likely becomes further underactive and wasted. Sustained underactivity in the deep system is always associated with compensatory overactivity in the superficial system. The inner tensional network providing postural support is lost and the person then has to hold themselves up via excess superficial trunk muscle activity and tension, with adverse consequences for the spine.

Therefore, if we are to help the client restore meaningful trunk function, we need to help redress the myofascial system imbalance and prescribe exercises that restore the deep system control deficits. This involves relearning basic motor skills which have been lost to everyday activity. The deep system is best activated via slow non-effortful movements which are finely modulated and tailored to reestablishing the important basic motor patterns necessary for spinal health and well-being.

It is important to appreciate that going to the gym and "working for strength" will likely further entrench superficial system dominance and the person's problems! Here are two important points to remember:

- You cannot build strength in muscles the brain has forgotten about.
- Strength relies upon adequate patterns of underlying deep system control.

Breathing: the most fundamental movement pattern

Breathing is the first and last action we do as we come into and leave this world. It happens automatically, and in either good or bad patterns. It is also the most basic motor pattern because it underlies *all* posture and movement.

Healthy breathing occurs if we allow it. A healthy axial tensegrity structure naturally makes space for the breath – it comes and goes like a gentle breeze wafting through a series of caves.

Breathing is also the link between emotion and motion. It is an important aspect of our ability to self-regulate between the extremes of doing and being. We breathe hard and fast when needing to really exert; minimally and slowly if meditating; and optimally in all states in between.

Our habitual breathing patterns are a window into our state of being – if you breathe well you are more likely to be happy and healthy. But the breath is often the victim in our hyped-up yet sedentary lives. With or without accompanying postural or movement dysfunction, persistent emotional arousal, tension, stress, and anxiety lead to habitual adverse changes in one's breathing, such that breathing pattern disorders are increasingly being recognized as a significant contributor to many mental, emotional, physical, and musculoskeletal health problems.

Recognizing and treating breathing pattern disorders is an extensive subject. If you would like a deeper understanding, see the recommended reading list at the end of the chapter. Here, I will briefly focus only on those aspects of breathing that are directly related to effective spinal control.

Essentially three principal aspects should be considered when assessing a client's breathing patterns:

- Where do they usually breathe?
- How do they usually breathe? (rate and volume)
- Can they breathe normally through sustained postures and during movement?

Normal breathing patterns: The diaphragm is the principal breathing muscle. It descends on contraction, creating a negative intrathoracic pressure which draws the air into the lungs. Its descent displaces the abdominal contents and, particularly if we are recumbent, we can see the belly move forward.

At rest, exhalation is considered to occur from passive recoil of the diaphragm. However, active exhalation involves the abdominal muscles, notably the deep transversus (Ishida and Watanabe 2013) and the pelvic floor (Hodges et al 2007).

When we are antigravity the postural system is active, and the breath more laterally expands the lower rib cage. (Given that a fish breathes through its gills, imagining gills over the lower lateral ribs is a helpful visualization when encouraging breathing here.) There is also a slight increase in the anteroposterior dimensions of the chest (Kolar et al 2014).

There should be no palpable tension or observable lift of the shoulders or upper chest, both being signs of an unhealthy breathing pattern which creates a vertical expansion. In contrast, a healthy breathing pattern creates a transverse expansion in the center body. This is where the breath should be during most activities of daily living, and it should be free to modulate in concert with variations in posture and movement.

Importantly, a healthy breathing pattern is always through the nose, which filters, warms, and humidifies the inhaled air. The diaphragm and nose are strongly reflexly linked – sniff and feel your diaphragm kick in.

The ideal breathing rate is considered to between 10 and 14 breaths per minute, the volume about 3–5 liters a minute (which is not much). The breath out should be longer than the breath in, and there should be a slight pause at the end of exhalation (Bradley 2014).

When there is a strong demand for the breath, the accessory breathing muscles come into play to augment air supply (scaleni, sternomastoids, pectorals, upper trapezii, levator scapulae). Their action lifts and expands the upper chest to increase air flow and capacity. The breathing rate and volume increase. This is a short-term response to a high demand. When the demand ceases, the breathing pattern and rate generally drop back to normal.

If we need extreme strength it is a normal reaction to momentarily hold the breath to augment postural support – known as the Valsalva maneuver. Otherwise breathing should be free to normally cycle during all movements.

A psychological shock can lead us to momentarily hold our breath. Fear and anxiety can increase the breathing rate and volume in preparation for fight and flight. These are usually short-lived responses.

However, many of our patients hyperventilate or over-breathe. Trapped by habit into "high-load" and stress-related breathing patterns, they suffer from poor diaphragmatic function, dominance of upper chest and mouth breathing, and a related increased rate and volume. Lifting the shoulders and gasping when talking are apparent. There is decreased lateral expansion of the lower rib cage and a tendency to asynchronous and paradoxical breathing (Courtney 2009). This suggests dominance of the crural over the costal diaphragm (De Troyer et al 1981). A tendency to breath holding in posture and movement is also common.

These disturbed breathing patterns create problems with the body's chemistry, feed anxiety and tension, and, most significantly, compromise effective core control and inner tensional support.

Slow, relaxed diaphragmatic breathing is an effective way to help reset ANS imbalance and amplify parasympathetic function.

When the gravity system is deficient, tension in the superficial trunk muscles increases in order "to hold ourselves up" – and this also includes the accessory breathing muscles. This excessive outer myofascial tension restricts the natural breath and distorts the axial tensegrity system. Excess tension and breath holding go together.

We need to help the client recreate space for the breath, and this is where relearning effective core control comes in.

"Opening the center": creating space for the breath and dispelling some myths around core control

I have written in some detail about the core (Key 2013); I proffer the most salient aspects here.

As touched on earlier, core control is the functional integration of breathing and the IAP mechanisms. Breathing and posture are inextricably intertwined: the breath supports posture, and posture supports the breath. They are mutually responsive and adaptable to the prevailing circumstances. Control of the core also provides the fundamentals of movement – the ability for a sustained, effortless uprightness while moving and breathing easily.

Breathing is a phasic activity in that it comes and it goes. When the principal breathing muscles – the diaphragm, deep transversus abdominis and the pelvic floor muscles (PFM) – are posturally active, they provide sustained tonic, yet adaptable, IAP to allow both breathing and movement.

In fact the IAP mechanism is common to both breathing and postural control. There is a fluctuating interplay between the diaphragm, transversus abdominis, and the PFM in coordinating shape and volume changes in the internal body cavities. These muscles therefore have a dual respiratory and postural role, which it is important to appreciate. IAP is the *simultaneous contraction* of the diaphragm, transversus abdominis, and PFM. It is worth noting that, while the oblique abdominals are important in controlling the alignment between the thorax and pelvis, they do not play a role in generating IAP (Hemborg and Moritz 1985).

The increase in IAP is a pre-movement response which prepares and stabilizes the spine against the forces created by gravity and movement, irrespective of the direction in which that will be. It is a key element of our postural system, helping to "stiffen" and internally support the spine against buckling. But there is no rigidity, and movement is free.

Paul Hodges and his group have carried out considerable research on postural control, looking at the IAP response. They have concentrated in particular on the transversus abdominis (Hodges 1999), whose activity he saw as a marker of how the whole mechanism was active. I believe his research has been somewhat misrepresented and misinterpreted, with the concept of core control being reduced to exhortations to "pull in your stomach" and/or "work those the abs." Importantly, he has also demonstrated the same pre-movement onsets occur at the same time in the diaphragm (Hodges et al 1997) and the pelvic floor (Hodges et al 2007) as part of generating and regulating IAP. Yet the transversus got all the attention and the diaphragm was largely ignored, despite it playing such a key role in IAP.

The breath and the core: Dissecting the breathing and IAP response is helpful in clearly comprehending them – the sequencing in vivo is in fact milliseconds apart:

1. As the diaphragm descends, the transversus stabilizes the lower rib cage through eccentric activity.

2. The diaphragm then sustains its descended position, while concentric activity in the lower transversus and pelvic floor builds up the IAP.

3. As the pressure rises, the lower rib cage expands laterally due to the effect of IAP pushing out through the zone of apposition in the lower thorax (Fig. 2.7).

This action also helps ensure that the thorax is aligned with the pelvis, whereby the thoracic and pelvic diaphragms are in optimal relationship and can functionally communicate.

4. We now have the postural support from IAP – which of course needs to be sustained while we also breathe and move. To do this, the tonic IAP activity also needs to vary: it is phasically modulated not only with breathing but also at the frequencies of limb movement in proportion to the reactive forces from the movement (Hodges and Gandevia 2000).

Understanding the dual phasic respiratory and tonic postural action of the diaphragm, transversus, and pelvic floor can be difficult at first, but this simple representation should make it clear (Fig. 2.8; Kolar 2009).

When we can integrate IAP for postural support and breathing, the inner tensional network is actively supporting the torso's tensegrity architecture. The *center is open* and, in effect, pushing outward to help tension the torso framework so that minimal superficial trunk muscle activity is required. The lower abdominal wall has the most activity, while the upper abdominal wall has the least, so as to allow the expansion of the lower pole of the thorax for IAP and breathing (Urquhart et al 2005).

The diaphragm descent is critical in IAP. In fact it has been shown to descend more in a postural challenge than during inhalation – particularly during lower limb activities (Kolar et al 2010) – and that this can be voluntarily controlled (Kolar et al 2009).

So if your client cannot breathe diaphragmatically, they will not be able to effectively control their core. If that is the case, you will have to be prepared to help them reestablish a normal diaphragmatic breathing pattern – and be patient! Entrenched maladaptive upper chest breathing patterns can be very difficult to inhibit.

Clients often do not want to know that there is something wrong with their breathing. However, if you sell it as a necessary part of core control, they will usually come on board.

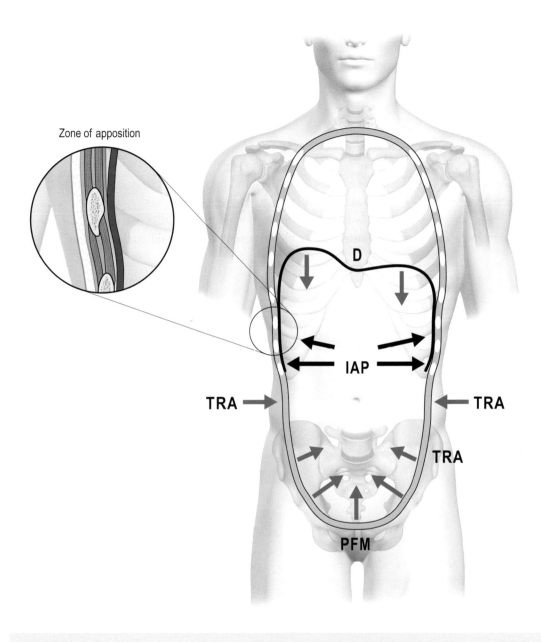

Zone of apposition

D

IAP

TRA

TRA

TRA

PFM

Figure 2.7

Diaphragm *(D)* descent reflexly activates the pelvic floor muscles *(PFM)* and transversus abdominis *(TRA)*, creating intra-abdominal pressure *(IAP)*. Acting through the zone of apposition, IAP expands the lower rib cage providing internal postural support and stability to the spine.

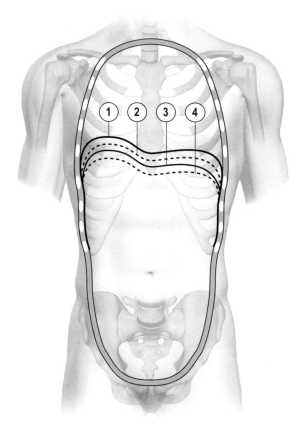

Figure 2.8

Conceptual schematic representation of the diaphragm's dual respiratory and postural role. 1 = diaphragm at rest; 2 = descent on inhalation; 3 = sustained descent in maintaining postural intra-abdominal pressure (IAP); 4 = combined sustained postural and respiratory activity. Similar activity conceivably occurs in the pelvic floor and transversus in their contribution to *IAP* and breathing.

Importantly, asking for isolated muscle actions of the transversus abdominis or pelvic floor can further disturb the IAP synergy, because the brain does not know about single muscles, only about actions and movements. Engaging the PFM or pulling in your stomach hampers the diaphragm's descent – as you will be able to confirm if you try it. In fact doing so

is likely to further reinforce maladaptive holding patterns and create further excess tension.

Rather, the ability to coordinate breathing and IAP in all posture and movement helps tone and strengthen all the inner core elements together, as nature intended them (McCook et al 2009).

To increase core capacity, "strengthening exercises" should ensure that the patterns of inner control can match the degree of superficial (global) myofascial activity.

Appreciating the reflex connections between the elements of IAP can be exploited in rehabilitation. Establishing better pelvic floor and lower transversus coactivation can improve diaphragm excursion and trunk stability against the imposed torque demands of a supine straight leg raise in people with pelvic girdle pain (O'Sullivan and Beales 2007). And diaphragmatic breathing can improve pelvic floor function and lessen incontinence (Hung et al 2010).

When core control and breathing are well integrated we can usually balance the potential competition between the respiratory and postural systems. However, when the core response is not well controlled and the respiratory system is really challenged (as in disease or demanding activity), respiration always wins – and the tonic postural function of IAP is lost (Hodges et al 2001). To compensate, splinting behavior of the superficial myofascial system occurs to try and support the spine.

Likewise, experimental inspiratory muscle fatigue (or weakness of the inner system) will result in a more rigid postural control strategy and decreased postural stability (Janssens et al 2010). The spine needs to move in order to be stable.

When the postural stabilization and breathing mechanisms are well integrated the abdominal wall is evenly toned and contoured, and the thorax infrasternal angle is approximately 90° (Clifton-Smith 2014) (Fig. 2.9). A well-functioning core opens out the lower

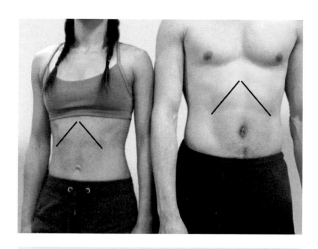

Figure 2.9

Both subjects are professional dancers. Note the even abdominal tone – and in particular the curve in the lateral waist – indicative of good transversus abdominis activity. The infrasternal angle (marked by the superimposed *lines*) forms an approximately 90° angle.

pole of the thorax, creating space for the breath, and also supports and stabilizes the spine. The lower thorax is stable but mobile. This is what I call opening the center. It is also *the* axial fundamental pattern (axial FP) that underlies free movement and a healthy spine (see Ch.4).

Pelvic fulcrum: the importance of the lower pelvic unit

The pelvis is a busy crossroads of function. It houses the body's center of gravity, so its small adjustments and movements can effect big changes through the spine and body as a whole. It is also the main agent of spinal support and the fulcrum for weight shift through the body. A functional decoupler, it transmits movement and load between the torso and legs.

Spinal movement cannot be understood without comprehending how the pelvis functions.

The pelvis, spine, and hips are biomechanically and functionally linked so that a change in one is always

reflected in the others. Compromised pelvic control is *always* at the heart of spinal and pelvic/hip pain disorders – and many lower limb pain syndromes. Yet in general, its dys/function is not well appreciated and hence is often overlooked. I have previously written on the pelvis in some detail (Key 2010).

Distilling the essence of pelvic movement control

The sacrum or "sacred bone" is indeed that, as it is both the base of the vertebral column and, nestled between the two pelvic bones (the innominates), forms part of the pelvic ring. Hence wherever the pelvis goes, the spine has to follow. The fact that much of the spine's movement is initiated in the pelvic girdle means that any pelvic movement dysfunction will be compensated for by maladaptive patterns of control in the spine above and in the hips and legs below.

The pelvis itself is very much a tensegrity-like structure. The bony ring formed by the sacrum and two innominates is stable yet deformable and capable of shape and volume change. To better understand this we need to review its unique functional anatomy.

First is the very important contribution made by the "deep system" continuous myofascial sheaths lining the pelvic and abdominal body cavities, which I have termed the lower pelvic unit (see Fig. 2.6).

The outer pelvic bones provide an extensive surface for many myofascial attachments – the glutei, the "deep 6" external hip rotators, and the other large pelvifemoral superficial muscles (i.e., the adductors, quadriceps, tensor fasciae latae, and hamstrings).

The myofascia of the anterolateral abdominal wall attaches to the superior pelvic rim; the spinal extensor system and associated fascial sheaths attach to the posterior rim and sacrum.

The pelvis is free to move in its full available repertoire when myofascial length/tension relationships are balanced, both between the inner and outer superficial myofascia attaching to it, and within each myofascial system.

The pelvic structure achieves its stability and its capability to change its dimensions via small but important intrapelvic movements which I have termed the pelvic fundamental patterns (pelvic FPs). These patterns are heavily reliant upon adequate deep system inner myofascial activity and tensional support to match the level of outer myofascial activity and tension.

To clearly understand the pelvic FPs we need to look further at pelvic/hip myomechanics and their influence on the spine.

Conceptually, the internal dimensions of the pelvis resemble two bowls. The superior pelvic bowl is wider and shallower and includes the iliac fossa (inner surface) of both ileums, the top part of the sacrum (S1–2) and the 5th lumbar vertebra. The deeper inferior pelvic bowl is formed by the lower sacrum and coccyx, the inner surfaces of the ischium and ischial tuberosities, the pubic rami, and the obturator foramen (Fig. 2.10). Note that the upper bowl faces forward, while the lower is inclined back.

These pelvic bowls can modulate their shape via the pelvic FPs, whereby narrowing the upper bowl widens the lower one, and vice versa. These pelvic actions simultaneously bring about changes in both the spine and hips.

The sacroiliac joint (SIJ) proper (from S1–3) lives in both bowls. It is very stable and only considered to have between 1° and 4° of actual movement – but it allows deformation of the pelvic ring via a series of complex intrapelvic motions: principally sacral nutation/counternutation and associated paired motion of the innominates, and sacral torsion via antagonistic motion of the innominates. The bowls change their shape in three dimensions and also twist.

In regard to SIJ function, it is important to appreciate the significant role played by the substantial

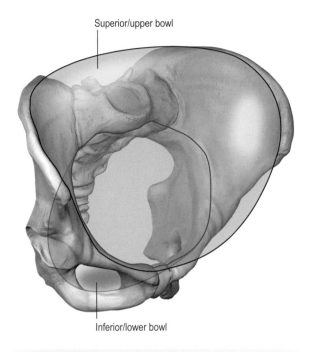

Superior/upper bowl

Inferior/lower bowl

Figure 2.10

Superior and inferior pelvic "bowls" – note that the upper bowl faces down and more forward; the lower faces down and backward.

syndesmosis within the inferior bowl – the dense soft tissue arrangement of fascia, muscles, and ligaments which not only contributes to pelvic myomechanics and shape change but also acts as an "elastic" shock absorber when we walk and jump etc.

The two pelvic innominate bones are like warped blades or flanges, with the plane of the ilia set almost at right angles to the plane of the ischium and pubis (Fig 2.11a).

The hip socket, or acetabulum, is at the intersection of these flanges. The acetabular roof is about level with the midpoint between of the upper and lower pelvic bowls (Fig. 2.11b), and its center is roughly level with the bottom of the SIJ proper. Note that the arcuate line defines the upper and lower of these pelvic bowls (Fig. 2.11c and see Fig. 2.10).

The center of gravity of the standing "anatomical body" falls approximately in front of the 2nd sacral vertebra and in line with the hip sockets (see Fig. 2.1).

The pelvic acetabular socket is supported on the femoral heads, i.e., the balls in the socket. The pelvis swings and swivels on the femoral heads in three dimensions, and all pelvic movements are always "closed-chain" hip movements, which in turn initiate movements of the trunk and affect the lower limbs.

In fact, all movements in the hip joint are multiaxial rotations – in the axes of the three cardinal planes and combinations thereof – whether closed-chain or open-chain movements.

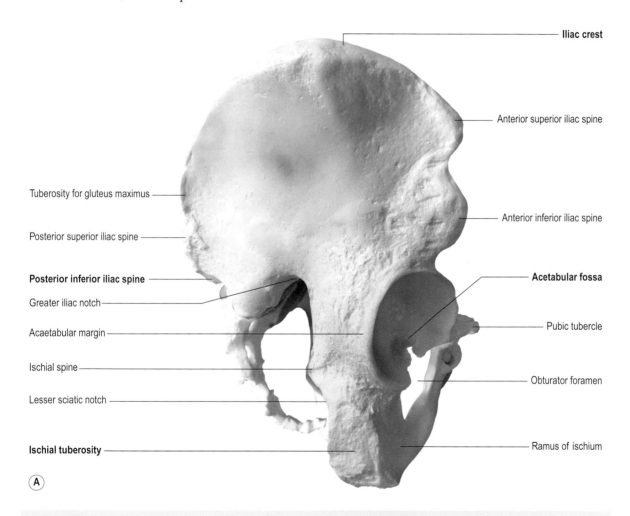

Iliac crest

Anterior superior iliac spine

Tuberosity for gluteus maximus

Anterior inferior iliac spine

Posterior superior iliac spine

Posterior inferior iliac spine

Acetabular fossa

Greater iliac notch

Acaetabular margin

Pubic tubercle

Ischial spine

Obturator foramen

Lesser sciatic notch

Ischial tuberosity

Ramus of ischium

(A)

Figure 2.11

The three-dimensional nature of the innominate anatomy in particular allows modulation of the pelvic ring around the fulcrum of the femoral head in the hip joint. The pelvic fundamental patterns are important in pelvic myomechanics and shape change. These movements essentially underlie control in the three planes of movement – and combinations thereof.

Chapter 2

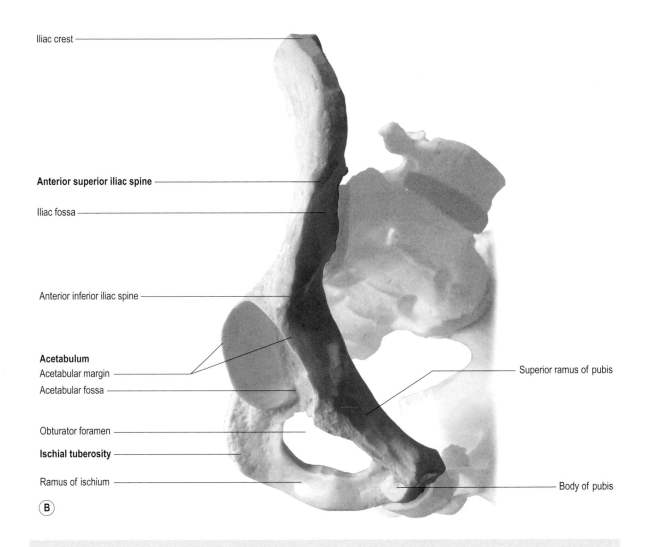

Iliac crest

Anterior superior iliac spine

Iliac fossa

Anterior inferior iliac spine

Acetabulum
Acetabular margin
Acetabular fossa

Superior ramus of pubis

Obturator foramen

Ischial tuberosity

Ramus of ischium

Body of pubis

(B)

Figure 2.11 *continued*

The hip joint can be thought of as the hub of a wheel as it is the axis about which the pelvis and/or leg swivels and rotates in the three cardinal planes of movement.

Either the socket rotates around the ball to modulate the pelvic shape (and create closed-chain hip movements, e.g., anterior pelvic rotation on a stable leg in forward bending) or the ball moves in the socket to create "open-chain" hip movements (e.g., lifting a leg into space on a stable pelvis).

Hence we see a shifting role of the pelvis in movement: being the stable part to support both the spine and lower limb function or the moving part that initiates weight shift and spinal movement. It can also fulfil both roles simultaneously. In any event, the hips and spine are also involved.

The warped shape of the innominates means that an anterior or posterior rotational movement in the sagittal plane produces a *simultaneous* coupled movement in the frontal plane (Fig. 2.12a).

32

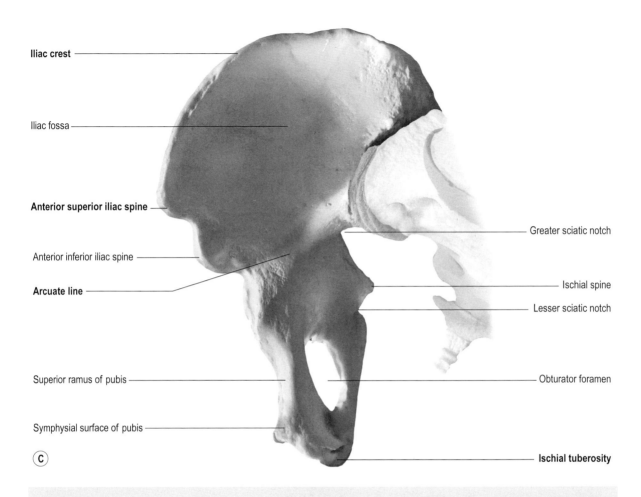

Iliac crest

Iliac fossa

Anterior superior iliac spine

Anterior inferior iliac spine

Arcuate line

Superior ramus of pubis

Symphysial surface of pubis

Greater sciatic notch

Ischial spine

Lesser sciatic notch

Obturator foramen

Ischial tuberosity

ⓒ

Figure 2.11 *continued*

Specifically: anterior innominate rotation is associated with ischial outflare and inflare of the ilia (Fig. 2.12b); posterior innominate rotation is associated with ischial inflare and outflare of the ilia. Thus altering the shape and volumes of the pelvic bowls creates rotations in the hip joint in two planes (Fig. 2.12c).

Importantly, whether the innominates are moving in a paired or antagonistic manner, they carry the sacrum, and hence the spine, with them.

- Closing the upper bowl brings the sacrum into nutation, and the lumbar spine into its neutral lordosis and into extension (see Fig. 2.12b).

- Opening the upper bowl brings the sacrum into counternutation and the lumbar spine into flexion (see Fig. 2.12c).

Overview of pelvic movement control

I focused upon intrapelvic control in the preceding pages as it is usually not well appreciated, even though it underlies all aspects of control.

Three main subsets of pelvic control are clinically apparent. It is helpful to consider each aspect to better comprehend the pelvis's motor abilities, although in functional movement all aspects will be active in various combinations and degrees.

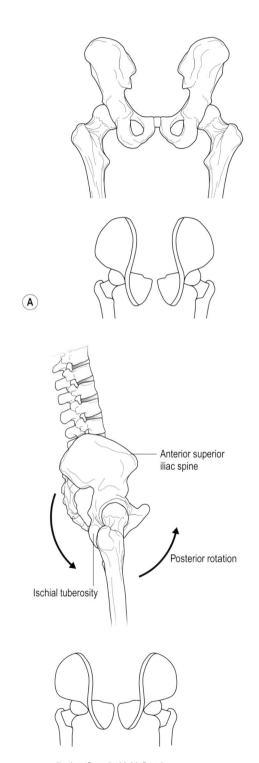

(A)

(C)

Ileal outflare, ischial inflare is
associated with posterior sagittal rotation

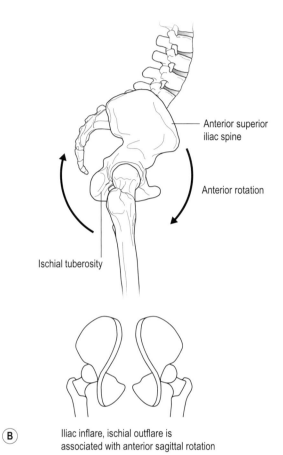

(B)

Iliac inflare, ischial outflare is
associated with anterior sagittal rotation

Figure 2.12

(A) Schematic posterior view of the innominates [sacrum
not shown]. (B) Due to their "twisted disc" shape, sagittal
innominate motion is also coupled with movement
in the frontal plane: an anterior innominate rotation
is coupled with ischial outflare, sacral nutation, and
lumbar extension; and (C) posterior innominate rotation
is associated with ischial inflare, sacral counternutation,
and lumbar flexion.

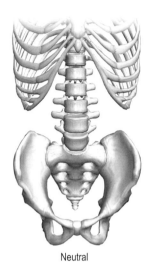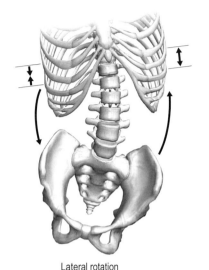

Neutral   Lateral rotation

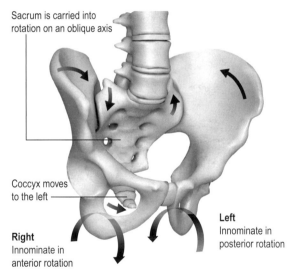

Figure 2.13

Lateral pelvic rotation on the femoral head in the frontal plane is associated with closed chain hip abduction (on the (L) here) and lateral flexion of the spine – including through the thorax.

Sacrum is carried into rotation on an oblique axis

Coccyx moves to the left

Right Innominate in anterior rotation

Left Innominate in posterior rotation

Figure 2.14

"Distorsion" of the pelvic ring initiates rotation in the transverse plane – in the pelvis, spine, and hip. The spine follows the sacrum and here moves into (R) rotation.

Intrapelvic control

This is the *foundation control* necessary if the pelvis is to behave as a healthy tensegrity structure – one which is both stable yet able to alter the relationships between the innominates and sacrum and thereby drive changes in the spine and hips.

Intrapelvic control is discrete, yet it is the basis of the pelvis being able to initiate and control its movement. Control is afforded by the pelvic FPs, of which there are four. These three-dimensional movements help control the rotary force couples of the pelvis in each plane of movement:

- The first and second pelvic patterns (pelvic FP1 and FP2) control anterior and posterior pelvic rotation or tilt in the sagittal plane. These are associated with lumbar extension and flexion, respectively (see Figs 2.12b and c).

- The third pelvic pattern (pelvic FP3) controls lateral pelvic rotation in the frontal plane. This is associated with lateral flexion of the spine (Fig. 2.13).

- The fourth pelvic pattern (pelvic FP4) controls intrapelvic rotation. It is a combination of pelvic

FP1 on one side and pelvic FP2 on the other, creating a torsion in the pelvic ring, which I have termed distorsion (Key 2010; Fig. 2.14). Through this the pelvis initiates and drives rotation in the horizontal plane – and through the spine and hips.

Spatial control

Ideally, when upright, the pelvis dynamically balances on the femoral heads and postures the spine above it close to the gravitational line of force or the "neutral" position (see Fig. 2.1).

In neutral, a degree of anterior pelvic tilt is typical (Herrington 2011), and there is balanced coactivation between the axial extensor and flexor myofascial systems. The habitual standing sagittal pelvic position directly affects spinal alignment above it. This means that posturing with an increased anterior tilt creates axial extensor system dominance, whereas posturing with an increased posterior tilt creates axial flexor dominance.

From neutral, the pelvis can well accommodate the fluctuating requirements between stability and mobility in space in order to support free trunk and leg movements. Three-dimensional spatial shifts forward, backward, sideways and into rotation and twist are possible.

Pelvic rotation on the femoral heads

The pelvis is the main agent of weight shift in the body. This requires control of the pelvic rotary force couples in the three planes of movement. These larger range, multidirectional, closed-chain hip movements build upon the intrapelvic control initiated by pelvic FPs, which continue to control the movement through range:

- Anterior pelvic rotation (or tilt) creates closed-chain hip flexion and lumbar extension. Posterior pelvic rotation (or tail tuck) creates closed-chain hip extension and lumbar flexion.

- Lateral pelvic rotation or tilt. Upward tilt creates closed-chain-hip abduction on the contralateral weight-bearing leg. It is the basis of weight shift onto one leg and creates a corresponding lateral shift of the spine to center it over the standing leg.

When lateral pelvic rotation control is poor the pelvis drops into downward tilt on unweighting the leg. The person cannot initiate weight shift through the pelvis and the spine is forced to compensate. This is known as the Trendelenburg effect.

- Horizontal plane control: forward and backward pelvic rotation. In standing, forward pelvic rotation creates closed-chain hip internal rotation on the contralateral weight-bearing side. Backward pelvic rotation creates hip external rotation on the contralateral weight-bearing side.

Spatial shifts and pelvic rotations are always coupled when standing and kneeling

- Posterior spatial shift is coupled with anterior pelvic rotation, which creates the important functional pattern of closed-chain hip flexion with a lumbar lordosis. This is usually missing in your clients (Fig. 2.15a).

- Anterior spatial shift is coupled with posterior pelvic rotation, which creates closed-chain hip extension and lumbar spine flexion. This is often overdeveloped in your clients (Fig. 2.15a).

- Mediolateral spatial shift is coupled with lateral pelvic rotation and lateral arcing of the spine and hip abduction/adduction (Fig. 2.15b).

- Forward and backward pelvic rotation initiates rotation in the spine and hips; this is usually associated with some lateral weight shift (Fig. 2.15c).

The largest shifts and rotations occur in the sagittal plane. Good sagittal plane control is a precursor to frontal plane control of lateral weight shift, which is a precursor for rotation and horizontal plane control. You need to be able to shift weight laterally in order to initiate rotation in your pelvis and hence through your spine, such as in walking.

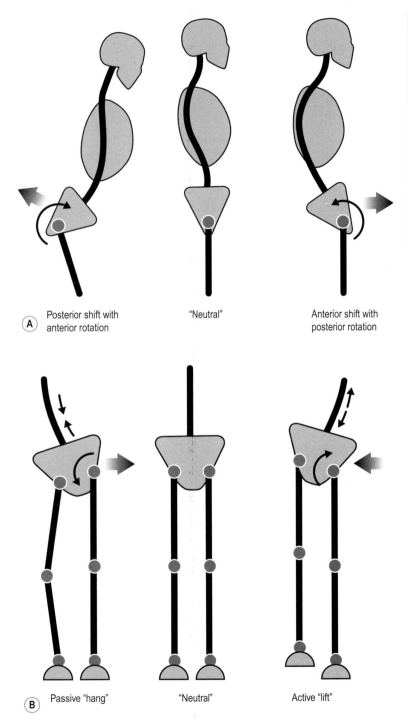

Figure 2.15
Pelvic shifts and rotations are coupled in each plane of movement: sagittal (a); frontal (b); transverse (c).

(A) Posterior shift with anterior rotation

"Neutral"

Anterior shift with posterior rotation

(B) Passive "hang"

"Neutral"

Active "lift"

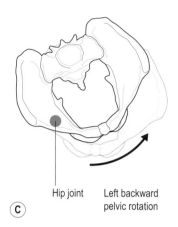

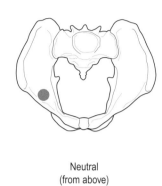

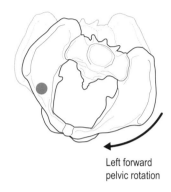

Hip joint Left backward pelvic rotation	Neutral (from above)	Left forward pelvic rotation

(c)

Figure 2.15 *continued*

Pelvic rotations, however, also bring about lateral weight shifts. Try lying down on your stomach and doing a backward pelvic rotation (see Ch. 7: Ex. 16).

Both the inner and outer pelvic myofascial collectives need to work synergistically in shifting patterns of eccentric and concentric control. This is necessary in order to control the pelvic rotary force couples, weight shifts, and various torques which occur in movement.

For example, this is particularly important in sagittal plane control of forward bending. The whole posterolateral myofascial chain of the lower limb attaches to the outer pelvis and sacrum. Known as the hip extensor mechanism, this allows us to suspend the trunk forward and return it to the vertical. In fact, the defining attribute of man over the apes is his buttocks, thanks to the development of the gluteus maximus for this purpose (Fig. 2.16).

However, if inner control – in particular the first pelvic pattern (pelvic FP1) – is deficient, the pattern does not occur as shown in Fig. 2.16a; instead, the outer, superficially dominant myofascia "wins" and the pelvis is predominantly postured and moved via anterior shift/posterior pelvic rotation strategies. The pelvis is habitually postured into posterior tilt or "tail

tuck" and becomes stiff here. This means that the lumbar spine cannot assume its neutral posture.

In forward bending, when control of the pelvic force couple into anterior rotation is lost (pelvic FP1) – the sit bones and tailbone cannot lead the movement (as shown in Fig. 2.16a). Hence active eccentric lengthening over the posterior aspect of the hip and thigh is reduced, and the lumbar spine is further pulled into end-range flexion, with predictable consequences for it over time (and also for the pelvis/hip).

The upper quadrant: thorax, shoulder girdle, head, and neck

We tend to view the spine as a column that is divorced from its place in the body. While it does, of course, form the backbone of the cylindrical-shaped body, its control is intimately related to what happens in the proximal limb girdles, thorax, and head.

Balanced three-dimensional length/tension relationships in the regional myofascia ensure both a neutral spine and spatial position of the thorax and proximal limb girdles, resulting in an efficient biotensegrity system which easily manages the shifting demands between stable support and mobility.

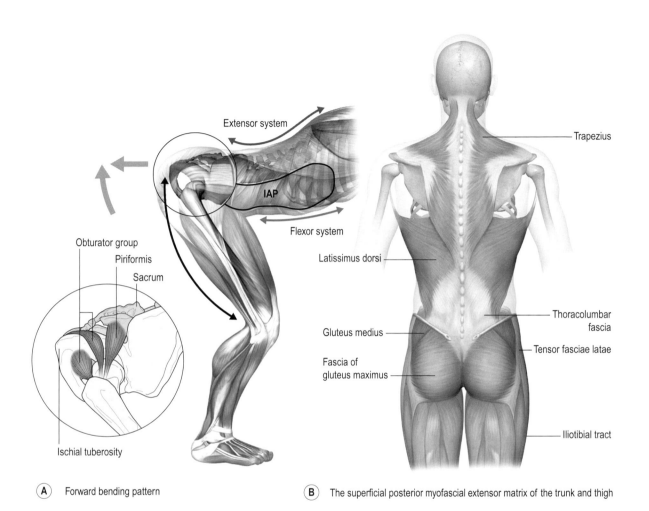

Extensor system

IAP

Flexor system

Obturator group

Piriformis

Sacrum

Ischial tuberosity

A Forward bending pattern

Trapezius

Latissimus dorsi

Gluteus medius

Fascia of gluteus maximus

Thoracolumbar fascia

Tensor fasciae latae

Iliotibial tract

B The superficial posterior myofascial extensor matrix of the trunk and thigh

Figure 2.16

(a) In forward bending, an effective extensor mechanism controls the pelvic "effort arm" in raising and lowering the torso. It is codependent upon adequate deep system control – particularly from the axial and 1st pelvic patterns in controlling the sagittal pelvic force couple to drive the ischia back and up. Eccentric activity is also necessary through the posterior pelvifemoral myofascial chain (principally the gluteus maximus, the deep external hip rotators and the hamstrings) to allow the ischia to reach back, widen and (most importantly) to lift (*arrows*). This also brakes the forward bending of the body. (b) Concentric activity in the posterior pelvifemoral myofascial chain pulls the ischia inferiorly to tip the pelvis back and allow lifting of the torso from forward bending.

All regions of the spine are functionally interdependent. In particular, the upper spine relies upon the quality of inner/core support and control in the lower half of the axis and pelvis. Anatomically and functionally the core extends up as far as the thoracic dorsal hinge around T6-T7. The upper quadrant can be considered as from the dorsal hinge to the crown of the head.

Thorax

Functionally, the dorsal hinge region divides the thorax into an upper and lower pole. Rib movements in the lower pole are principally like a bucket handle, to allow more widening, while those in the upper are more "pump handle" to allow increased anteroposterior dimensions (Fig. 2.17b).

The lower pole of the thorax (LPT) is more mobile than the upper. This allows both flexible breathing and core support mechanisms – which in themselves provide stability to the LPT. This flexible stability and mobility of the LPT allows 3-D adaptive translations of the spine in response to weight shift initiated in the pelvis. In the sagittal plane, during anterior/posterior translations of the thorax, 60% of the movement occurs between T8 and T12 (Harrison et al 2002). Similar movement is observed in the frontal (and less in the transverse) planes, to allow lateral weight shift and rotation.

The upper pole of the thorax is more stable, yet still mobile. It provides a stable foundation to support the shoulder girdle and adaptive postural support and movement control of the upper limb girdle, head, and neck (Fig. 2.17a,b).

Shoulder girdle

The shoulder girdle itself can also be considered as a tensegrity structure. Suspended in an adaptable tension network, the scapula moves around on the thorax and transfers energy and load between the arm, body axis, and spine through the soft tissues – irrespective of the direction of loading. There is no rigid compressive loading. Shoulder girdle stability, however, is reliant upon both balanced active control and flexibility.

Nearly every bone in the trunk, from the occiput to the pelvis, has myofascial attachment points from the shoulder girdle and upper humeral myofascia in one dimension or more. The wheel-like arrangement of the lines of muscle force through all planes gives enormous power to the arms and hands, not only in doing heavy work (in lifting, throwing, carrying, and pulling), but also in control of delicately centered movement of the hands and fingers. However, on the down-side, any imbalance in this extensive myofascial envelope of the shoulder girdle will alter the functioning of the whole torso.

Claviscapular unit

The claviscapular unit is the *key ingredient* in understanding upper quadrant function. The shoulder girdles (the clavicle and scapula unit plus the humeral head) are balanced on the top of the

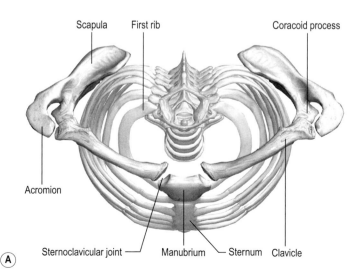

Scapula First rib Coracoid process

Acromion

Sternoclavicular joint — Manubrium — Sternum Clavicle

(A)

Figure 2.17

The manubrio-sternoclavicular joint is the only bony attachment of the shoulder girdle to the thorax; hence balanced length/tension in the shoulder girdle myofascia is important in its control.

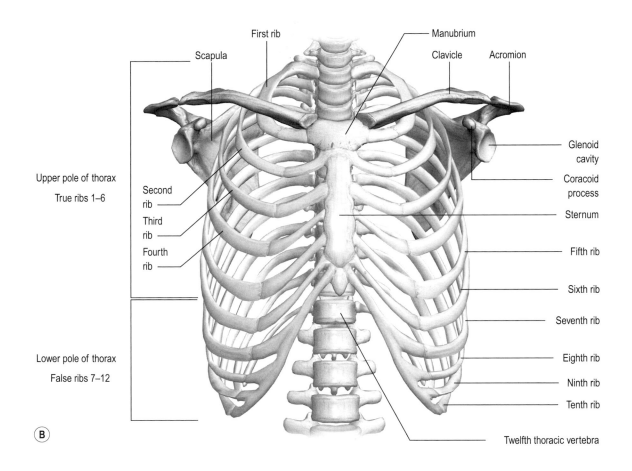

Upper pole of thorax
True ribs 1–6

Lower pole of thorax
False ribs 7–12

First rib

Scapula

Second rib

Third rib

Fourth rib

Manubrium

Clavicle

Acromion

Glenoid cavity

Coracoid process

Sternum

Fifth rib

Sixth rib

Seventh rib

Eighth rib

Ninth rib

Tenth rib

Twelfth thoracic vertebra

B

Figure 2.17 *continued*

bell-shaped thorax rather like a pair of epaulettes or shoulder pads (Fig 2.17a,b).

Their attachment to the torso is principally myofascial, except for the sternoclavicular joints. The crank-shaft-shaped clavicle acts as a strut that helps to guide claviscapular myomechanics in order to suitably support upper-limb function both in three-dimensional, wide-ranging spatial reach for hand function and adaptable weight bearing through the arms. The medial attachment of the clavicle to the manubrium of the sternum is important in transferring movement to the upper rib "rings" and to the spine (Fig 2.17b), as well as from the spine to the shoulder girdle.

Movements of the claviscapular unit

Claviscapular motion is a composite of three individual motions – whereby the scapula rotates in three dimensions and translates in two dimensions over the chest wall (Kibler et al 2008).

As in the pelvis these movements are coupled:

- Anterior and posterior rotation or tilt around a horizontal axis in the plane of the scapula. This is associated with both a superior/inferior and a protraction/retraction translation, respectively; i.e., posterior tilt is associated with an inferior and retraction translation (Fig. 2.18a,b).

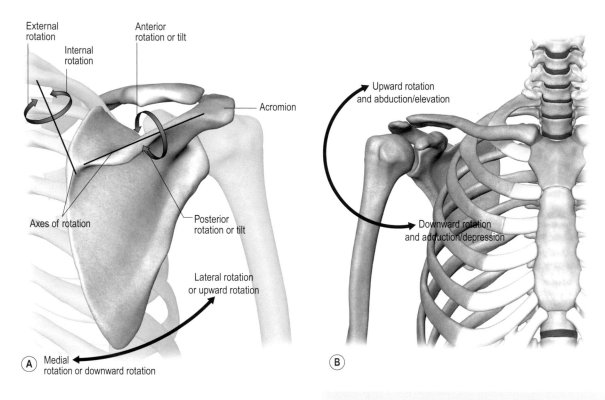

External
rotation

Internal
rotation

Anterior
rotation or tilt

Acromion

Axes of rotation

Posterior
rotation or tilt

Lateral rotation
or upward rotation

(A) Medial
rotation or downward rotation

Upward rotation
and abduction/elevation

Downward rotation
and adduction/depression

(B)

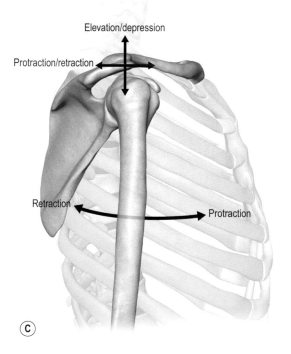

Elevation/depression

Protraction/retraction

Retraction

Protraction

(C)

Figure 2.18

Claviscapular motion is a composite of three individual
motions – whereby the scapula rotates in three planes and
translates in two dimensions over the chest wall.

- Upward and downward rotation around a horizontal axis perpendicular to the plane of the scapula. This is also coupled with superior and inferior translation, respectively (Fig. 2.18a,b).

- Internal and external rotation around a vertical axis through the plane of the scapula. This is coupled with protraction/retraction and superior/inferior translation, respectively (Fig. 2.18a,c).

All of these motions and translations are important in allowing the claviscapular unit to provide adaptive, spatially appropriate, and mobile yet stable support. This enables the rotator cuff to maintain congruence of the humeral head and optimal glenohumeral kinematics. To avoid subacromial impingement when the arm is elevated, the scapula must be able to posteriorly tilt, externally rotate, and upwardly rotate (Kibler et al 2008).

Movements of the shoulder girdle are closed kinetic chain, pre-movement postural responses which provide fluctuating support between either:

- closed kinetic chain arm movements, where the glenoid fossa of the scapula moves around the more stable humeral head – which creates movement in the upper spine, ribs, and shoulder (e.g., shoulder fundamental patterns; see Fig. 7.25) or weight shift initiated by the claviscapular unit while weight bearing through one arm in side sitting

or

- as open kinetic chain activities, where the claviscapular unit supports upper limb movement in space. Here, the humeral ball moves around in the glenoid socket, for example when raising an arm. This also involves some movement in the spine and thorax (Crosbie et al 2008). See Fig. 7.28.

Similar to the pelvis in lower-quadrant function, the claviscapular unit also acts as a functional decoupler between the spine and the upper limb (Fig. 2.19).

It is important to appreciate that by virtue of the manubrium/sternoclavicular, manubrial/sternocostal (rib), and costovertebral articulations (and extensive myofascial attachments) there is a *mutual functional interdependence* between the upper spine, thorax, and shoulder girdle. A change in one is reflected in the other. Moving the upper thoracic spine and the joints of the cervicothoracic junction involves shoulder girdle movements; shoulder girdle movements create movement in the upper thoracic spine and over the cervicothoracic junction. You cannot move one without the other (try it for yourself). We can exploit this in prescribing exercises for both upper spinal and shoulder problems.

The closed-chain movements of the claviscapular unit are therefore very important in both upper spinal movement control and that of the shoulder. I have called these the shoulder fundamental patterns (shoulder FPs), of which there are four. Similar to the pelvic FPs, these three-dimensional movements help control the rotary force couples of the claviscapular unit in each plane of movement.

- The first and second shoulder FPs control posterior and anterior rotation or tilt in the sagittal plane, respectively (Fig. 2.19a, and see Fig. 2.18). Shoulder FP1 is associated with cervicothoracic and upper thoracic spinal extension, shoulder FP2 with cervicothoracic and upper thoracic spinal flexion.

- The third shoulder FP controls lateral rotation in the frontal plane: upward and downward rotation of the scapula. An upward scapular rotation on one side is associated with a reciprocal downward rotation on the other side. Similar to the third pattern in the pelvis, shoulder FP3 is associated with lateral shift/side bending of the spine over the cervicothoracic junction and upper thoracic spine and thorax (see Figs 2.18 and 2.19b).

- The fourth shoulder FP controls shoulder girdle rotation in the horizontal plane – backward and forward rotation. Similar to the fourth pattern in the pelvis, these are contrarotations: backward shoulder rotation on one side induces a forward rotation on the other side. A backward shoulder rotation is associated with ipsilateral rotation over the cervicothoracic and upper thoracic regions of the spine and thorax (see Figs 2.18 and 2.19c).

Head and neck

As the pelvis dictates the quality of support and control in the lower spine, the upper thorax/shoulder girdle complex is the platform on which the head and neck find optimal support and function. A neutral thoracic spine and shoulder girdle are a

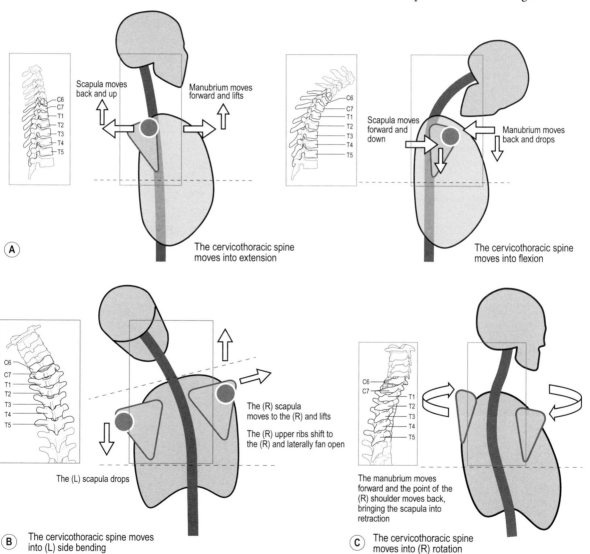

A

Scapula moves back and up

Manubrium moves forward and lifts

The cervicothoracic spine moves into extension

Scapula moves forward and down

Manubrium moves back and drops

The cervicothoracic spine moves into flexion

B The cervicothoracic spine moves into (L) side bending

The (R) scapula moves to the (R) and lifts

The (R) upper ribs shift to the (R) and laterally fan open

The (L) scapula drops

C The cervicothoracic spine moves into (R) rotation

The manubrium moves forward and the point of the (R) shoulder moves back, bringing the scapula into retraction

Figure 2.19

Claviscapular movements are directly associated with spinal and rib motions. For clarity these are shown in the three cardinal planes of movement: sagittal, frontal, and transverse.

prerequisite for achieving a neutral cervical spine and head position.

The head plays an important role in upper cervical spine biomechanics. The mid-cervical spine segments risk becoming the vulnerable, "weak," links when movement function over the cervicocranial joint complex above and the cervicothoracic junction below is impaired.

The head is the most significant sensory platform and agent of communication. It not only houses the brain but also the sensory organs which gather important information about our surroundings to ensure our survival; namely vision, hearing, smell, taste, speech, balance, and so on. The job of the spine is to lengthen and to support the head in such a way that it can easily and optimally orient to gather this information. The skull balances and rocks on the 1st cervical vertebra, C1 (Fig. 2.20).

The head is the driver and initiator of movement from the top part of the spine, largely driven by the senses – particularly the eyes and ears. In fact, our senses are deeply embedded in our evolutionary and developmental patterns of movement (Beach 2010).

Movements of the head are directly related to the upper cervical joint complex (C0–C3). These can also be distilled into four fundamental patterns which control rotations and associated translations in the three planes:

- The first and second head patterns provide sagittal control: the occipital condyles translate and rotate on the 1st cervical vertebra to produce flexion/nodding (head FP1) and head retraction and extension/reclination of the head and protraction (head FP2).

- The third head pattern controls frontal plane movements: lateral rotation or tilt up and down with slight lateral shift.

- The fourth head pattern controls rotation in the transverse plane. About 45%–50% of the available cervical movement into rotation occurs at C1–C2.

Dense receptive fields in the joints and suboccipital muscles influence muscle tone throughout the body. Also bear in mind that many of the cranial nerves exit the skull anterior to the C0–C1 joint; hence optimal spinal alignment and healthy patterns of head control or otherwise have the potential for wide-ranging effects throughout the body.

The head patterns are closely allied with eye movements in the same plane of movement, although this is not obligatory. Like the head, eye movements are multidirectional, but for simplicity it is useful to view their movements in the three planes. In fact, we can use eye movements to assist head pattern performance. We can also maintain a stable gaze while

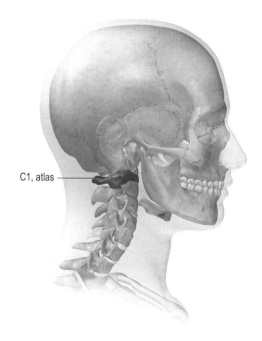

C1, atlas

Figure 2.20

The head is poised on the top of the spine and rocks and tilts in order to orient the sense organs – eyes, ears, nose – and for communication, expression, and alimentation.

the fourth pelvic pattern. He will then shift his weight onto the right ischium, repeating the sequence above. The better his sagittal-plane control of the lumbopelvic lordosis, the better he can manage this action.

A 1997 walking study found consequential trunk motion following pelvic displacements (Crosbie et al). Pelvic and shoulder girdle movements are functionally linked, and arm swing is coupled with pelvic rotation, which drives rotation in the upper spine.

When proximal limb girdle control is defective, movement starts to be initiated in the spine, and it is here where much of the problem of spinal pain lies. Excess superficial myofascial activity in some regions compresses and restricts those areas of the spine, disturbing segmental loading patterns and sequencing of movement through the spine. Efficient movement and energy transfer through the axial movement system is lost.

Biodiversity in movement

For many, the advent of school begins an increasingly sedentary lifestyle, which can cause physical development to plateau. Rather than optimizing our potential, we may develop a limited movement vocabulary, then aches and pains appear as we enter an insidious but habitual decline. Nevertheless, thanks to neuroplasticity, and through motivation, attention, exploration, and practice, we can learn to further develop our potential for mastering new motor abilities in many different ways.

Movement is supported by our postural system in a manner that is effortless, adaptable, and sustainable ad infinitum. Our posture tells a lot about the quality of our movement system. Natural movement is diverse, light, efficient, and free flowing. Elite athletes can maximize power, strength, and movement speed without compromising the fluidity of their performance. What is notable about healthy movement is that it has variety, is relaxed, and looks easy.

Well-organized neuromuscular systems allow any imaginable movement in three dimensions. A freely mobile spine is the foundation of movement freedom. Dancers use movement to express meaning as they carve shapes in space. Expressive and free movement gets its lightness when the pelvis and lower body can deal with gravity and support the spine, allowing the upper body to be liberated for gesture, manipulating the environment and manual skills.

Movement diversity relies on mastering the basic motor patterns during each stage of the developmental process. Successive patterns build on those already mastered and culminate in energy-efficient and effective torso control. At the heart of these patterns are important key movement phrases and sequences which are important for spinal control – the fundamental patterns.

Our patients with pain always have difficulty performing these, which accounts for many of their problems. Their movements become coarse, more primitive, and one dimensional. In due course this disturbs spinal function. When these fundamental patterns are adequately reestablished, the spine regains its freedom to move in three dimensions, and pain can become a thing of the past (see Ch. 4).

Recommended reading

Chaitow L, Bradley D, Gilbert C (2014) Recognizing and treating breathing pattern disorders: A multidisciplinary approach, 2nd edn. Edinburgh: Churchill Livingstone Elsevier.

Kobesova A, Kolar P (2014) Developmental kinesiology: Three levels of motor control in the assessment and treatment of the motor system. J Bodyw Mov Ther 18(1):23–33.

Myers T (2014) Anatomy Trains: Myofascial meridians for manual and movement therapists, 3rd edn. Edinburgh: Churchill Livingstone/Elsevier.

Schleip R, Findley T, Chaitow L, Huijing PA (2012) Fascia: The tensional network of the human body. Edinburgh: Churchill Livingstone Elsevier.

Todd ME (1937) The thinking body. A Dance Horizons Book. Princeton.

Wallden M (2017) The diaphragm - More than inspired design. J Bodyw Mov Ther 21(2):342–349.

References

Beach P (2010) Muscles and meridians: The manipulation of shape. Edinburgh: Churchill Livingstone Elsevier.

Belavy DL, Richardson CA, Wilson SJ et al. (2007) Superficial lumbo-pelvic muscle overactivity and decreased co contraction after 8 weeks of bed rest. Spine 32(1):E23–E29.

Belavy DL, Adams M, Brisby H et al (2015) Disc herniations in astronauts: What causes them, and what does it tell us about herniation on earth? Eur Spine J 25(1):144–154.

Bradley D (2014) Patterns of breathing dysfunction in hyperventilation and breathing patterns disorders. In: Chaitow L, Bradley D, Gilbert C. Recognising and treating breathing pattern disorders: A multidisciplinary approach, 2nd edn. Edinburgh: Churchill Livingstone Elsevier.

Clifton-Smith T (2014) Breathing pattern disorders and the athlete. In: Chaitow L, Bradley D, Gilbert C (eds), Recognising and treating breathing pattern disorders: A multidisciplinary approach, 2nd edn. Edinburgh: Churchill Livingstone Elsevier.

Crosbie J, Vachalathiti R, Smith R (1997) Patterns of spinal motion during walking. Gait Posture 5:6–12.

Crosbie J, Kilbreath SL, Hollman L, York S (2008) Scapulohumeral rhythm and associated spinal motion. Clin Biomech 23(2):184–192.

Courtney R (2009) The functions of breathing and its dysfunctions and their relationship to breathing therapy. Int J Osteopath Med 12(3):73–85.

De Troyer A, Sampson M, Sigrist S, Macklem PT (1981) The diaphragm: Two muscles. Science 213(4504):237–238.

Flemons T (2007) See: www.intensiondesigns.com.

Gracovetsky S (1997) Linking the spinal engine with the legs: A theory of human gait. In: Vleeming et al (eds) Movement, stability and low back pain: The essential role of the pelvis. Edinburgh: Churchill Livingstone.

Harrison DE, Cailliet R, Harrison D, Janik TJ (2002) How do anterior/posterior translations of the thoracic cage affect the sagittal lumbar spine, pelvic tilt and thoracic kyphosis? Eur Spine J 11:287–293.

Hemborg B, Moritz U (1985) Intra-abdominal pressure and trunk muscle activity during lifting II. Chronic low back pain patients. Scand J Rehab Med 17(1):5–13.

Herrington L (2011) Assessment of the degree of pelvic tilt within a normal asymptomatic population. Man Ther 16(6):646–648.

Hodges PW (1999) Is there a role for transversus abdominis in lumbo-pelvic stability? Man Ther 4(2):74–86.

Hodges PW, Gandevia SC (2000) Activation of the human diaphragm during a repetitive postural task. J Physiol 522(1):165–175.

Hodges PW, Butler JE, McKenzie DK, Gandevia SC (1997) Contraction of the human diaphragm during rapid postural adjustments. J Physiol 505(2):539–548.

Hodges PW, Heijnen I, Gandevia SC (2001) Postural activity of the diaphragm is reduced in humans when respiratory demand increases. J Physiol 537(3):999–1008.

Hodges PW, Eriksson AE, Shirley D, Gandevia SC (2005) Intra-abdominal pressure increases stiffness of the lumbar spine. J Biomech 38: 1873–1880.

Hodges PW, Sapsford R, Pengel LHM (2007) Postural and respiratory functions of the pelvic floor muscles. Neurourol Urodyn 26(3):362–371.

Huijing PA (2012) Myofascial force transmission: An introduction. In: Schleip R et al (eds) Fascia: The tensional network of the human body. Edinburgh: Churchill Livingstone Elsevier, Ch.3.2.

Hung HC, Hsiao SM, Chih SY et al. (2010) An alternative intervention for urinary incontinence: Retraining diaphragmatic, deep abdominal and pelvic floor coordinated function. Man Ther 15(3):273–279.

Ishida H, Watanabe S (2013) Changes in the lateral abdominal muscles' thickness immediately after the abdominal drawing in manoeuvre and maximum expiration. J Bodyw Mov Ther 17(2):254–258.

Janda V (1980) Muscles as a pathogenic factor in back pain. In: Proceedings of the IFOMT Conference, Christchurch, New Zealand, 1980.

Janssens L, Brumagne S, Polspoel K et al (2010) The effect of inspiratory muscle fatigue on postural control in people with and without recurrent low back pain. Spine 35(10):1088–1094.

Jull G, Janda V (1987) Muscles and motor control in low back pain: Assessment and management. In: Twomey L (ed.) Physical therapy of the low back. New York: Churchill Livingstone, pp.253–278.

Key J (2010) Back pain: A movement problem; A clinical approach incorporating relevant research and practice. Edinburgh: Churchill Livingstone Elsevier.

Key J (2013) "The core": Understanding it, and retraining its dysfunction. J Bodyw Mov Ther 17(4):541–559.

Kibler WB, Sciascia AD, Uhl TL et al (2008) Electromyographic analysis of specific exercises for scapular control in early phases of shoulder rehabilitation. Am J Sports Med 36(9):1789–1798.

Kobesova A, Kolar P (2014) Developmental kinesiology: Three levels of motor control in the assessment and treatment of the motor system. J Bodyw Mov Ther 18(1):23–33.

Kolar P, Neuwirth J, Sanda J et al (2009) Analysis of diaphragm movement during tidal breathing and during its activation while breath holding using MRI synchronised with spirometry. Physiol Res 58:383–392.

Kolar P, Sulc J, Kyncl M et al (2010) Stabilising function of the diaphragm: Dynamic MRI and synchronised spirometric assessment. J Appl Physiol 109(4):1064–1071.

Kolar P, Kobesova A, Valouchova P, Bitnar P (2014) Dynamic neuromuscular stabilisation: Developmental kinesiology: breathing stereotypes and postural-locomotion function. In: Chaitow L, Bradley D, Gilbert C Recognising and treating breathing pattern disorders: A multidisciplinary approach, 2nd edn. Edinburgh: Churchill Livingstone Elsevier.

Levin SM, Martin D-C (2012) Biotensegrity: The mechanics of fascia. In: Schleip R, Findley T, Chaitow L, Huijing PA. Fascia: The tensional network of the human body. Edinburgh: Churchill Livingstone Elsevier.

McCook DT, Vicenzino B, Hodges PW (2009) Activity of the deep abdominal muscles increases during submaximal flexion and extension efforts but antagonist co-contraction remains unchanged. J Electromyogr Kinesiol 19(5):754 –762.

Massery M, Hagins M, Stafford R et al (2013) Effect of airway control by glottal structures on postural stability. J Appl Physiol 115:483–490.

O'Sullivan PB, Beales DJ (2007) Changes in pelvic floor and diaphragm kinematics and respiratory patterns in subjects with sacroiliac joint pain following a motor learning intervention: A case series. Man Ther 12(3):209–218.

Persson P, Hirschfield H, Nilsson-Wikmar (2007) Associated sagittal spinal movements in performance of head pro- and retraction in healthy women: A kinematic analysis. Man Ther 12(2):119–125.

Schleip R, Klingler W, Lehmann-Horn F (2005) Active fascial contractility: Fascia may be able to contract in a smooth muscle-like manner and thereby influence musculoskeletal dynamics. Medical Hypotheses 65(2): 273–277.

Schleip R, Jäger H, Klingler W (2012) Fascia is alive: How cells modulate the tonicity and architecture of fascial tissues. In: Schleip R, Findley TW, Chaitow L, Huijing P (eds) Fascia: The tensional network of the human body. Edinburgh: Churchill Livingstone Elsevier pp. 157–164.

Tsang S, Szeto GPY, Lee RYW (2013) Normal kinematics of the neck: The interplay between the cervical and thoracic spines. Man Ther 18(5):431–437.

Tsao H, Galea MP, Hodges PW (2010) Driving plasticity in the motor cortex in recurrent low back pain. Eur J Pain 14(8):832–839.

Turinna A, Martinez-González, Stecco C (2013) The muscular force transmission system: Role of the intramuscular connective tissue. J Bodyw Mov Ther 17(1):95–102.

Urquhart DM, Hodges PW, Story IH (2005) Postural activity of the abdominal muscles varies between regions of these muscles and between body positions. Gait Posture 22(4):295–301.

Defining the problem:
What goes wrong in the spine that leads to pain?

3

Understanding the relationship between spinal pain and the common axial posturo-movement deficits directs appropriate exercise therapy. We therefore need to be clear about the nature of the problems we are trying to redress when prescribing movement.

Research amply shows that altered motor control is the underlying problem. It is apparent clinically that movements requiring "deep system" control deteriorate and are replaced by maladaptive movement responses employing excess activity of the superficial muscles (see Ch. 2, The key to refined movement control).

The changed myofascial activity patterns disturb the body's biotensegrity and alter the sagittal postural alignment and control of the torso, creating distinct clinical syndromes. What these all share is difficulty in naturally erecting the spine against gravity while breathing easily. This is readily seen in sitting, where spinal collapse is usual – or replaced by "holding one-self up" with excess tension.

Clinical syndromes

Previously described (Key 2010), the clinical syndromes are summarized here. Common to all is an underactive deep system and patchy hyperactivity of the superficial muscles.

Layer or stratification syndrome

Janda (1980) was the first to point out that the imbalanced myofascial activity generally occurs in regions – such that if we look at the front and (particularly) the back torso, we can see regional bands of myofascial hyperactivity and hypoactivity. He called this the layer or stratification syndrome (Figs 3.1 and 3.2).

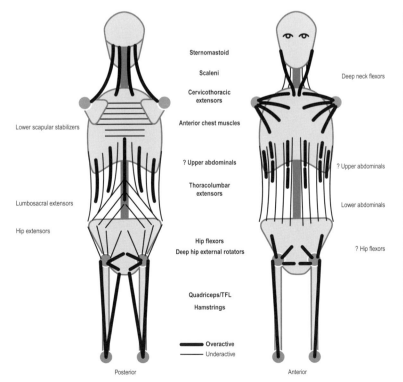

Figure 3.1

Schematic view of the layer or stratification syndrome; after Janda.

Sternomastoid

Scaleni

Cervicothoracic extensors

Anterior chest muscles

Deep neck flexors

Lower scapular stabilizers

? Upper abdominals

? Upper abdominals

Thoracolumbar extensors

Lumbosacral extensors

Lower abdominals

Hip extensors

Hip flexors

Deep hip external rotators

? Hip flexors

Quadriceps/TFL

Hamstrings

━━ Overactive
── Underactive

Posterior

Anterior

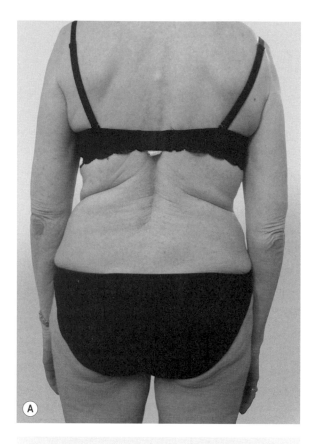

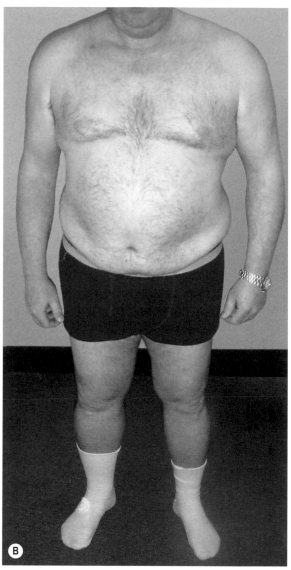

Figure 3.2

a) Posterior view of layer syndrome. Note the emptiness in the myofascia between the shoulder blades and over the lumbosacral area – and increased thoracolumbar activity – and incidentally the marked "Key sign." b) Anterior view of layer syndrome. Particularly note the underactivity of the whole abdominal wall.

As this syndrome is common in all patient populations to a greater or lesser extent, it offers a simple way to appreciate the altered myofascial activity in your clients.

Posteriorly, we see patchy extensor system activity with variable underactivity over the proximal limb girdles and hyperactivity around the neck/upper shoulders, the thoracolumbar region, and the posterior inferior myofascial chain of the lower limb.

Anteriorly, we see the same banding of activity in the flexor system, albeit not quite as clear cut. In the neck we generally see weakness of the deep neck flexors with hyperactivity of the sternomastoids and/or scaleni. Hyperactivity is also visible over the anterior shoulder girdle and commonly over the anterior hips and thighs, whereas the anterolateral abdominal wall shows either general underactivity or hyperactivity in the upper wall and hypoactivity in the lower.

It is important to appreciate that the imbalanced myofascial activity is not only apparent in posture but plays out in all movements in varying degree. This should be kept in mind when prescribing exercises – and during class situations, because understanding this tendency allows you to predict the likely responses and direct movement so as to redress the myofascial imbalance rather than reinforce it. We do so by facilitating deep system activity and using strategies which help to inhibit and encourage "letting go" of the excess superficial activity.

The variability in abdominal wall activity can be further understood by recognizing the pelvic crossed syndromes.

Pelvic crossed syndromes

In healthy sagittal control, the pelvis dynamically oscillates around the "neutral" zone – in slight anterior pelvic rotation. However, it is very common to see it postured at end range – either forward or back – and this directly affects how the spine above it is postured and controlled (Fig. 3.3).

This forms the basis for patient subgrouping. Two main clusters are apparent: those displaying posterior pelvic crossed syndrome (posterior PXS; Fig. 3.3b) and those with anterior pelvic crossed syndrome (anterior PXS; Fig. 3.3c).

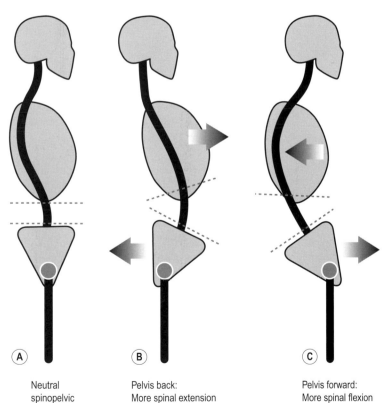

Figure 3.3
Pelvic position influences patterns of axial muscle activation and spinal curves. When the pelvis is postured "end range" it is also associated with an increased tilt. Note the oblique relationship between the thorax and pelvis. The thorax and pelvic misalignment impedes core control mechanisms.

(A)
Neutral
spinopelvic
alignment

(B)
Pelvis back:
More spinal extension

(C)
Pelvis forward:
More spinal flexion

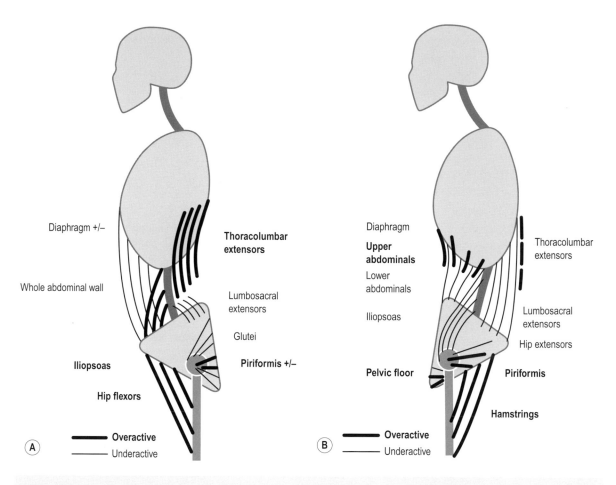

Figure 3.4

Schematic representation of imbalanced myofascial activity in the posterior PXS (a) and anterior PXS (b). Note the increased and decreased myofascial activity forms a "cross" pattern which disturbs thoracopelvic and hip-joint alignment.

These syndromes are illustrated further in Figures 3.4 and 3.5, and summarized in Table 3.1. These build upon Janda's original model of the pelvic crossed syndrome (1980, 2007), which I have renamed posterior (his original syndrome) and anterior, based upon the position of the pelvis.

Most patients are readily classifiable into either subgroup. However a mixed pelvic crossed syndrome (mixed PXS) can present. Here the client will display features of both crossed syndromes, but there will be

an underlying dominant tendency. Although this can occur for a number of reasons, it is often as a result of poorly conceived and administered exercise and fitness regimens. Appreciating each syndrome separately helps you absorb the composite presentation and see which is the relatively dominant one.

The anterolateral abdominal wall (ALAW) provides much insight into patient subgrouping. Underactivity of the whole ALAW is a defining feature of the posterior PXS group (Figs 3.2b, 3.4a, 3.5a, and 4.6). This group

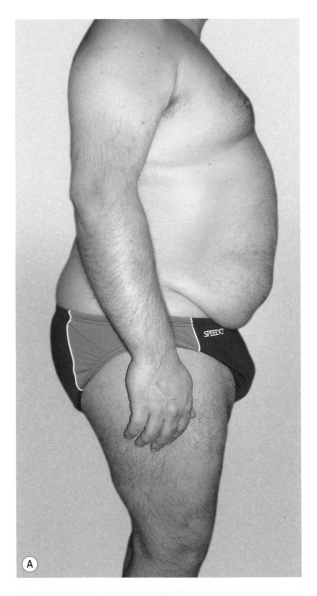

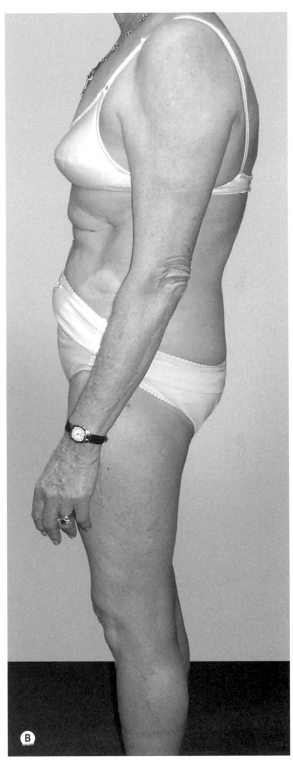

Figure 3.5

Sagittal view of a) posterior PXS – note the pelvis is back and the "open" abdominal wall; b) anterior PXS – note the marked hyperactivity in the upper abdominal wall, poor gluteal tone, and "tail-tuck." In both syndromes the pelvis and thorax are in a differing oblique relationship with each other.

Table 3.1
Key features of the pelvic crossed syndromes

Sagittal standing posture and related myofascial activity	Posterior pelvic crossed syndrome (PPXS)	Anterior pelvic crossed syndrome (APXS)
Pelvic position from neutral	Back in anterior tilt/rotation	Forward in posterior tilt/rotation
Thorax position from neutral	Forward – increased extensor system activity	Back – increased flexor system activity
Anterolateral abdominal wall (ALAW)	Underactivity of whole ALAW	Hyperactive upper ALAW; underactive lower ALAW
Hip posture	Flexion in "pure" case – may be compensated for by "butt clench"	Extension, abduction, external rotation
Defining body shape	Big belly, well-developed bottom and calves	Flabby lower belly, tail tuck and no bottom; poorly developed calves
Underactive myofascia: Lower pelvic unit is always underactive, with imbalance	**Transversus** ↓++, diaphragm, **iliacus, lumbar spine multifidus;** pelvic floor muscles ↓	**Diaphragm** ↓++; transversus, iliacus, lumbar **spine multifidus** ↓; pelvic floor muscles ↑/↓
Overactive and tight myofascia in the torso	**Thoracolumbar erector spinae;** lateral quadratus lumborum; serratus post inferior?; crural diaphragm?	**Upper oblique abdominals** and rectus abdominis, **pelvic floor muscles,** some intermittent thoracolumbar erector spinae
Overactive and tight myofascia in the pelvic girdle and lower limb	**Psoas, rectus femoris, tensor fasciae latae,** deep six external hip rotators? glutei? gastrocnemii?	**Hamstrings;** "deep 6" external hip rotators, **including pyriformis, glutei**

tend to have an otherwise overactive neuromuscular system with more obvious "holding patterns."

In the anterior PXS and mixed PXS groups there is hyperactivity of the upper ALAW and hypoactivity of the lower ALAW (Fig. 3.4b, 3.5b, and 3.6). This group tend to have low muscle tone and show more postural collapse. "Holding patterns" still prevail, however, though to a lesser degree.

In both groups the architecture of the core and its control are differently compromised. Kolar et al (2013) point out that when the alignment between the thorax and pelvis is altered they assume an oblique relationship to each other (see Fig. 3.3). This disturbs the reflex functional alliance between the thoracic and pelvic diaphragms with transversus. The shape and dimensions of the body cavity change, and

effective patterns of IAP to support and stabilize the spine are compromised (Fig. 3.7). This is important to appreciate because, when retraining the axial FP, each subgroup will require a different emphasis.

The pelvic crossed syndrome subgrouping also helps you predict likely patterns of restrictions and pain patterns in the hips/pelvis (see Table 3.1). For example, a person with posterior PXS will have quite good hip flexion but difficulty both in achieving good closed-chain hip extension and in controlling anterior rib thrust. Back pain and/or psoas and related groin pain syndromes are likely due to inadequate generation of IAP to support the anterior spine and provide proper stability for psoas' proximal attachments.

The anterior PXS subgroup find closed-chain hip extension easy, albeit in posterior pelvic rotation.

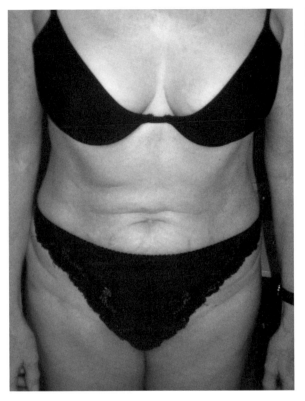

Figure 3.6

Note that the upper abdominal wall hyperactivity also known as a central anterior cinch both "draws in" the lower anterior rib cage and forms a supra-umbilical crease – and there is relative underactivity of the lower abdominal wall.

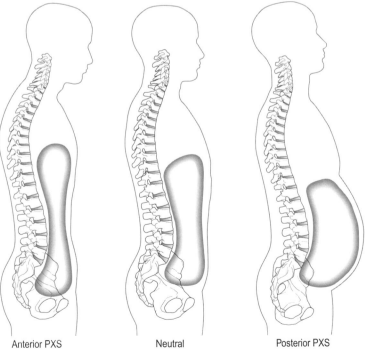

Anterior PXS   Neutral   Posterior PXS

Figure 3.7

Imbalanced myofascial activity and altered alignment changes the architecture of the body cavities and compromises internal pressure change mechanisms and effective "core control." Note the poor diaphragm descent in the anterior PXS with associated increased upper abdominal activity – and over-descent in the posterior PXS with poor abdominal activity.

However, owing to poor ability in the first pelvic pattern to control a neutral pelvic position, the quality of movement is jeopardized both in open-chain hip extension and flexion and in closed-chain hip flexion. Hip flexion becomes posterior pelvic tilt and lumbar flexion, which is detrimental to the functioning of the spine and/or pelvis. LBP, SIJ pain, gluteal tendinopathies hamstring problems, and so on, become more likely in time.

Shoulder (or upper) crossed syndrome

Also described by Janda (1980, 2007), this syndrome is always apparent in variable measure in *all* patients with upper quadrant pain disorders. It is partly a response to altered control of the pelvis and lower spine, but these days it is increasingly caused by our tendency to sit and work with our hands and head down and forward. Modern humans rarely raise their arms above their head. Technology has a lot to answer for!

The upper quadrant muscle imbalance further alters sagittal alignment thereby directly hampering patterns of control in the upper spine and shoulder girdle. This is shown in Figures 3.8 and 3.9, and summarized in Table 3.2.

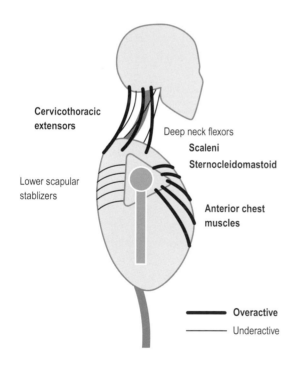

Cervicothoracic extensors

Deep neck flexors

Scaleni

Sternocleidomastoid

Lower scapular stablizers

Anterior chest muscles

—— Overactive
—— Underactive

Figure 3.8
Schematic view of the shoulder crossed syndrome; after Janda. Again, note the "cross pattern" of hypo- and hyper-myofascial activity alters alignment of the head, neck, thorax, and shoulder girdle.

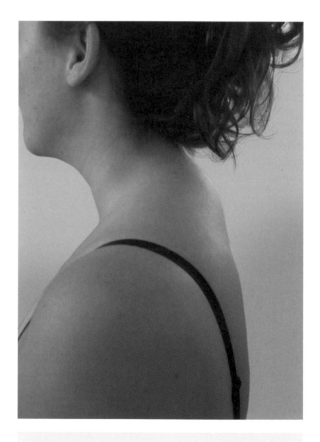

Figure 3.9
Shoulder crossed syndrome. Note the forward head posture and reactive tissues and "gibbous" over the joints of the cervicothoracic junction.

Table 3.2
Key features of the shoulder crossed syndrome

Sagittal alignment	Hyperactive/tight myofascia	Underactive/lengthened myofascia
Thoracic kyphosis including "gibbous" over cervicothoracic junction	**Anterior chest muscles** – pectoralis minor and major +, subclavius, serratus anterior	Spinal extensors C7-T7; **lower scapular stabilizers:** middle and lower trapezius +, rhomboids
Forward head posture with occipital reclination	**Sternomastoids, levator scapulae, cervical extensors, scaleni,** upper trapezius?	**Deep craniocervical neck flexors**
Round shoulders: "dome," anterior rotation of claviscapular unit	**Pectoralis minor and major,** S/H biceps, levator scapulae? rhomboids and serratus anterior	**Upper, middle and lower trapezius working with serratus** to stabilize scapula in retraction
Disturbed glenohumeral joint myomechanics	**Teres x2 and infraspinatus**	Subscapularis and supraspinatus

The shoulder crossed syndrome (SXS) is commonly associated with dysfunctional upper chest breathing patterns and a poor lumbopelvic base of support. The muscle hyperactivity and altered breathing patterns are apparent in all movement, particularly if trying too hard, being over-challenged, in pain, non-focused or tired.

Effects of the clinical syndromes on the spine itself The crossed syndromes show the altered sagittal alignment of the head, thorax, shoulder, and pelvic girdles. The spine is literally pulled into aberrant segmental loading patterns, resulting in the patient losing the natural spinal curves – the lumbar lordosis in particular. The sagittal spine can resemble the more primitive infant spine (see Fig. 2.1).

Notably, there is loss of spinal extension. The pelvis, shoulder girdle, and especially the thoracic region become stiff into flexion and the mid-lumbar and cervical spines compensate by becoming sites of "relative flexibility" (Sahrmann 2011) – and are more likely to become symptomatic.

The person becomes "sagittally stuck" in malalignment – and function in the junctional regions of the spine (where the major units of mass, i.e. the head, thorax, and pelvis meet the spine) also suffers, further stressing the mid-cervical and lumbar levels.

Altered spinal postures directly affect movement potential Sagittal fixation is associated with a predominant reliance on the second fundamental patterns of the head and proximal limb girdles in movement. This is co-associated with axial FP dysfunction – there is either collapse or "holding" around the center (see Ch. 4).

There is a corresponding lack of control in all the first FPs and their integration with effective axial FP control. This loss of effective sagittal spinal support and stabilization also limits the third and fourth axial and proximal limb girdle FPs, which give rise to the lateral and rotary spinal movements that are so important for spinal health and functional performance.

The inferior tethers

These are coarse superficial/global muscle dominant "lock-in" strategies adopted to support axial uprightness in the absence of effective deep system support and stable control during the simple movements required for ordinary daily function. When strength is required their activity is further reinforced.

The inferior tethers are active over the LPT and each proximal limb girdle. A reflex, crude, and generally bilateral response, they become the automatic postural set supporting movement. They cause or reinforce the abnormal axial "sagittal fixation" that contributes to the clinical syndromes and also lead to stiffness, adversely affecting movement function in the thorax, shoulders, and hips. (The cervical and lumbar spine regions are the victims; hence pain syndromes here are common.) They also tether, or hold, the proximal limb girdles and spine "centrally" in the frontal plane, limiting weight shift (particularly lateral) and rotation through the axis.

These tethers are frequently apparent in exercise classes, be they Pilates or yoga, when the focus becomes about people pushing beyond their functional limit to achieve a pose or feel their muscles "burn." One of the aims of this book is to support the exercise therapist to understand and enable their clients to inhibit and break up these holding patterns rather than promote their reinforcement.

Axial inferior tethers: the central cinch patterns

These describe the increased myofascial activity around the LPT which tether or limit movement and adaptable alignment and control of the LPT. Yet the LPT is in fact spatially unstable, which is evidenced when the ribs "pop forward" and/or lift.

Acting around the center, axial inferior tethers hold the spine centrally in the midline and create an "outer squeeze effect," thereby further limiting core control and sequential movements through the spine.

This excess activity varies according to the pelvic cross syndrome subgrouping:

- *Central posterior cinch* (CPC), a defining feature in the posterior PXS subgroup. We see dominant excess activity of the thoracolumbar erector spinae; serratus posterior inferior, and probably the crural diaphragm and psoas (Fig. 3.10). The hyperactivity is commonly apparent between about T7 and L3. There is corresponding underactivity of the abdominal wall.

- *Central anterior cinch* (CAC), seen in the anterior PXS subgroup. We see excess activity in the

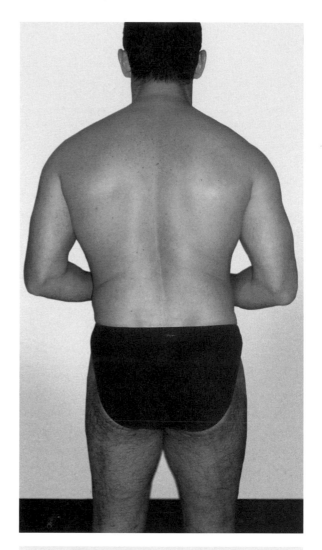

Figure 3.10

A central posterior cinch can vary from a prominent thoracolumbar erector spinae profile, resembling salami sausages, to less marked when myofascial cinch activity is milder. It is usually associated with poor myofascial activity and tone over the lumbosacral levels. Incidentally, also note the "butt clench" and leg "propping."

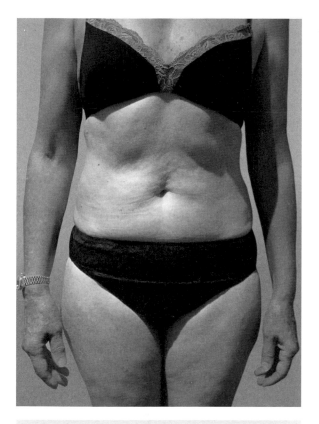

Figure 3.11

Central anterior cinch. Note the narrow infrasternal angle and increased upper abdominal tone relative to the lower abdominal wall.

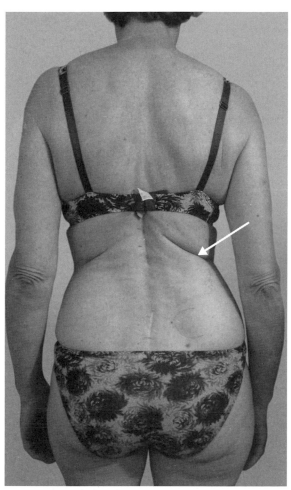

Figure 3.12

Central conical cinch. There is a layer syndrome including a central posterior cinch. Due to this and an active central anterior cinch, the lower pole of the thorax has been drawn in and forms a conical shape. Note the marked "Key sign" (*arrow*). Also note the subject has undergone surgery but will continue to experience spinal and related symptoms until her neuromuscular function improves.

upper abdominal wall (Fig. 3.11; see Fig. 3.6). Some CPC activity is also apparent, though more intermittent.

- *Central conical cinch*: Seen in the mixed PXS. This involves both CPC and CAC activity. The LPT is drawn into a conical shape (Fig. 3.12).

Some of these common disturbed patterns of central spinal support and stability have been demonstrated in limb load tests, such as the supine active straight leg raise (ASLR), which showed evident superficial upper abdominal bracing (i.e., CAC) and associated breath holding together with pelvic floor descent (O'Sullivan et al 2002). These subjects would have likely been anterior PXS dominant.

The central cinch patterns (CCPs) compensate for poor deep system internal support – yet as mentioned, their activity has an outer squeeze effect which further inhibits the internal axial FPs. If you reestablish the axial FP this lessens the central cinch activity.

The "Key sign" is indicative of CCP activity and related poor inner LPU core control (Fig. 3.13; also see Fig. 3.12). It is usually more prominent on the symptomatic side. The person is holding himself up trying to support and stabilize his spine from the outside. This imparts a compressive stress to the vertebrae, causing tissue reactivity and possibly neural system irritation

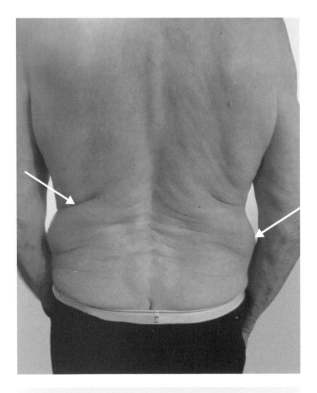

Figure 3.13

Bilateral "Key sign" more prominent on the left (*left arrow*). Note the "bulge" in the lateral waistline indicative of weak transversus abdominis and "core" activity (*right arrow*).

and symptoms in time. It may also be associated with observable transversus weakness (see Fig. 3.13). I should mention that a prominent unilateral Key sign can also be indicative of scoliosis.

Functional consequences of the CCPs

The following are the considerable effects of these patterns.

- They stiffen the spine in particular. "Fixing" the spine centrally, they block the axial FPs and limit the adaptive weight shifts and segmental adjustments through the spine and thorax needed for balance (Smith et al 2008) (Fig. 3.14; also see Figs 3.10, 3.12 and 3.13).

- They create "segmental lock down," disturbed spinal myomechanics and joint function, and likely "neural bother." Bear in mind that the sympathetic nervous system supply to the lower limb is T10–L2 (Williams and Warwick 1980) – and increased sympathetic drive to central and peripheral pain syndromes are increasingly being reported (Jewson et al 2015).

- The chronic tissue overloading leads to adaptive changes in the thoracolumbar perimuscular fascial tissues, which are thicker and more disorganized with reduced shear-strain transmission (Langevin et al 2009).

- They contribute to thoracic and rib cage stiffness – a common problem in all our clients!

- There is changed shape and function within the thorax. While it is difficult to get movement "into" the thorax (particularly in the "dome" and upper pole) the LPT loses spatial stability and adaptability because of poor inner control. *This needs to be borne in mind when devising exercises to improve thoracic mobility – otherwise the neck and low back suffer.*

- The changed thoracopelvic posture disturbs the functional relationship between the thoracic and

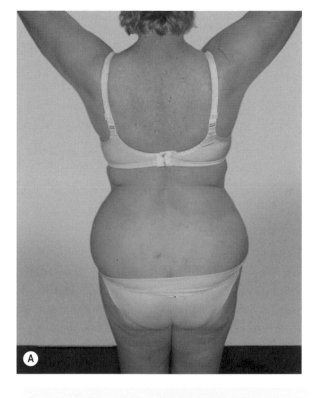

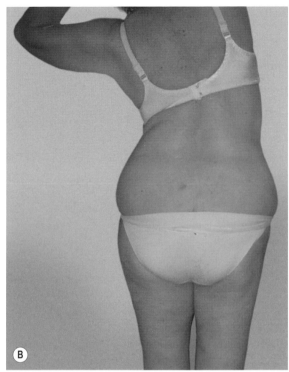

Figure 3.14

a) Central posterior cinch activity and pelvic "inferior tethers" are apparent in neutral standing with hands on the head. Also note the active "butt clench" and narrow inferior pelvis. b) This limits the initiation and control of lateral pelvic rotation when attempting the lateral weight transfer pattern – and the central posterior cinch activity remains. There is minimal lateral weight shift through the pelvis.

pelvic diaphragms – core-control mechanisms suffer, and this may even be apparent in elite sportspersons (Hides et al 2010).

• The resulting compression forces disturb breathing patterns (Roussel et al 2009), and postural diaphragmatic function is compromised (Kolar et al 2012).

• Altered breathing disturbs pelvic floor muscle myomechanics and continence (Smith et al 2007a).

• They create a central disconnect between the proximal limb girdles in movement, which limits segmental movement transmission through the spine, particularly in the thorax.

• They result in loss of rotation through the thorax, forcing the lumbar and cervical spine to compensate. This then further becomes one of the contributors to low back and/or neck pain.

The antidote to dominant CCPs is to reestablish control of the axial FP (see Ch.4: Controlling the center). Retraining this will require a different emphasis in each subgroup.

Postures and movements which require weight shift through the base of support and the need for the spine to go "off-center" – particularly in the frontal plane – help break up these central holding patterns (e.g., moving around from side-sitting postures; lateral weight shift pattern).

Chapter 3

It is important to realize that, *unless checked, the CCPs will automatically initiate and dominate all postures and movements – and become further reinforced in the CNS*, such as during a squat (Fig. 3.15).

Pelvic inferior tethers

Owing to inadequate LPU contribution in dynamic three-dimensional control of the pelvic rotary force couples (and sagittal control in particular), the person

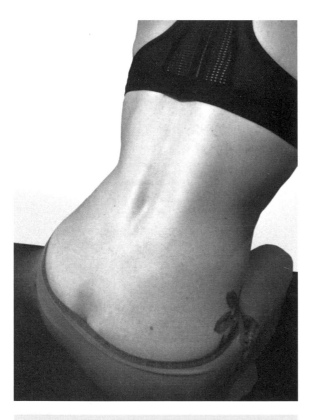

Figure 3.15
Because of inadequate intrapelvic and core control, the subject relies upon excess central posterior cinching during a squat. This creates excessive regional spinal compression which bothers the thoracolumbar segments. She presented with a history of chronic recurrent groin pain – the "postcode" for these segments. She had also received diagnoses of femoro-acetabular impingement and psoas tendonitis.

compensates by recruiting more superficial outer posterior/inferior pelvifemoral muscles.

They habitually adopt lock-in strategies of pelvic control, utilising a more primitive "total pattern" strategy of hip extension, abduction, external rotation, hyperextended knees, and foot pronation – which I call propping (Fig. 3.16). Alternatively, the client passively hangs on the iliofemoral ligaments in posterior pelvic tilt and tail tuck – particularly apparent in the anterior PXS client.

Either way, this leads to posterolateral myofascial dominance and tightness over the pelvis/hip and in the leg. The "deep six hip external rotators (obturators, piriformis, gemelli; quadratus femoris), posterior PFM, hamstrings, and gluteus maximus show increased resting tension, tenderness, shortness, tightness, "trigger points," and fascial "bind" due to their excessive contribution to movement. Clients often feel the need to constantly release and stretch these muscles.

Alternatively, the client may "hang" on one leg via the iliotibial band. Whichever the strategy, the lower limb kinetic chain loses its dynamism.

Clenching the buttocks and locking the knees in hyperextension "locks the ischial swing," which means the pelvis is held predominantly in the second pattern (pelvic FP2; Ch. 4). In time, it becomes tethered posteroinferiorly, with a corresponding lack of flexibility and "slide" within the posterior inferior pelvic/hip/leg myofascia, and a restricted ability in the ischia being free to swing back, wide, and up into pelvic FP1. Good closed-chain hip flexion is lost (e.g., in forward bending), which leads to the spine losing its alignment – in particular the lumbar lordosis (Fig. 3.17).

This is more marked, and a defining feature, in the anterior PXS subgroup.

Dominant activity of psoas and rectus femoris in the posterior PXS group can lead to tethering the pelvis anteroinferiorly. This is not as common

64

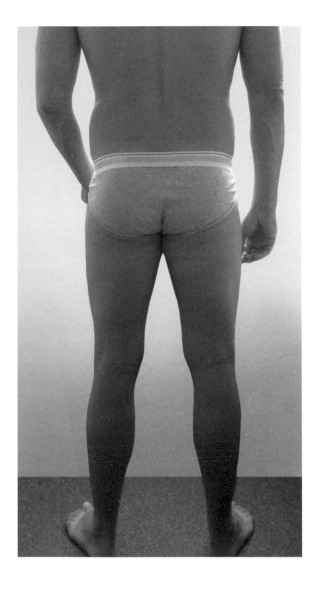

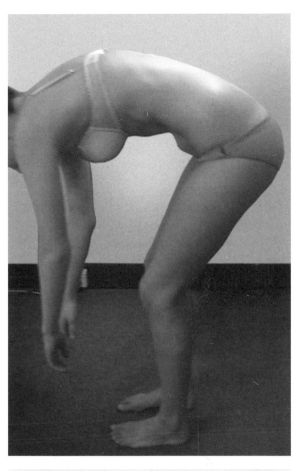

Figure 3.17

Dysfunctional forward bend pattern. The pelvic "inferior tethers" including tight hamstrings limit pelvic posterior shift and particularly anterior pelvic rotation. This is compensated for by flexing the whole spine. Note the engagement of the central anterior cinch and "folding" in the central torso. The subject suffered chronic sacroiliac and low back pain.

Figure 3.16

"Propping" involves dominance of the posterolateral inferior myofascial chain in a more "total pattern" of extension, abduction, and external rotation. It is usually more marked on the symptomatic side. The subject suffered chronic (L) recurrent hamstring and Achilles tendinopathy (see Ch. 5, Case study 1). Incidentally, note that despite going to the gym, he shows a "Key sign" and a waist bulge indicative of a weak transversus.

as the posteroinferior tether– but is seen especially in kneeling. It is associated with CPC activity and sagittal spinal malalignment (Fig. 3.18). This is the situation where better control of pelvic FP2 is really needed.

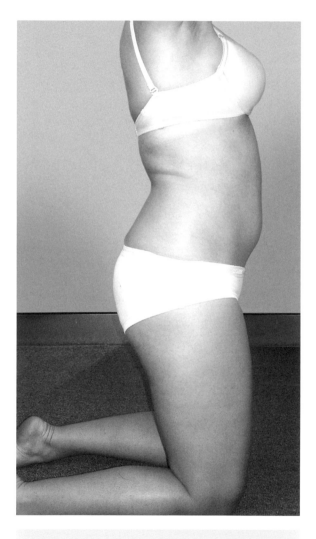

Figure 3.18

Effects of anterior inferior pelvic "inferior tethers" in kneeling. When the pelvis/hip cannot assume a neutral position the spine above is forced to compensate. Note the underactivity of the whole abdominal wall and dominance of posterior cinch activity – and the related "Key sign."

The functional consequences of the pelvic girdle inferior tethers

The effects of these tethers are wide-ranging. The lumbar spine is the area that suffers most, although the loss of pelvic alignment and control affects the whole spine.

The pelvic inferior tethers are operant in varying degree in *all* low back and pelvic pain disorders as well as in many lower quadrant pain syndromes, such as sciatica, tendinopathies, shin splints, and foot problems.

The imbalanced length/tension relationships between the inner and outer pelvifemoral myofascia not only limits the ability for control of pelvic FP1 but control of pelvic FPs 3 and 4 also suffers. The pelvis loses its ability to initiate three-dimensional movement – except into pelvic FP2. Intrapelvic movement and stability are lost, as is its freedom to swing and swivel on the femoral heads. This has further consequences:

- There is loss or decreased initiation of movement from the tailbone.

- Loss of pelvic FP1 control equates to *loss of lumbar lordosis* in posture and movement. The low lumbar spine and the SIJ are therefore vulnerable when loaded into end-range flexion and counternutation. Solomonow et al (2003) demonstrated how provocative this is for the lumbar joints, reporting that after just 20 minutes it could create local inflammation and neuromuscular spasm that took up to 24 hours to settle.

- There is a reduced range of hip movement and control – particularly of closed-chain hip flexion. Concentric acetabular wear and the increasing prevalence of hip replacements becomes predictable. Femoroacetabular impingement has been associated with active hip flexion in supine when the pelvis is posteriorly rotated (Van Houcke et al 2014).

- The low lumbar spine is required to compensate further by overflexing, on account of the reduced closed-chain hip flexion. This is particularly important in movements such as squatting and kicking. It is the weak link in the kinetic movement chain. As the innervation of the whole lower limb posterior myofascial chain emanates from the lumbosacral levels, when these segments are "bothered," increased neural irritation and myofascial tightness will result. A vicious cycle sets in (see Ch. 1, On injuries). This is usually the underlying dysfunction in many recurrent hamstring problems (including tears) and tendinopathies within the posterior myofascial chain.

- An asymmetrical pelvic inferior tethering can lead to a fixed pelvic "distorsion" or asymmetry of the innominates (see Fig. 2.14). This is common in low back and SIJ pain (Adhia et al 2016) and in many lower limb pain syndromes. Clinically, there is increased posterior rotation and abduction of the ilia on the symptomatic side, together with adduction of the ischial tuberosity.

- The loss of lumbopelvic control into neutral and extension is also directly related to the excess maladaptive CCP behavior – the person finds it difficult to disassociate attempted lumbopelvic motion from thoracolumbar motion (Elgueta-Cancino et al 2014) – the tailbone cannot go back, so the ribs go forward (see Fig. 3.15, 3.19 and Fig. 4.13b).

- In sitting, habitual pelvic collapse into posterior tilt (pelvic FP2) means the spine is repeatedly loaded in end-range flexion (see Fig. 3.32). The lack of good hip flexion via pelvic FP1 means attempting a "neutral spine" results in a CPC strategy instead, which is usually short lived, and collapse ensues (see Sitting and Fig. 4.13b).

- The *lumbosacral* spine becomes flexed. This is caused by reliance upon the pelvic inferior tethers and co-related CPC activity and can lead to the mistaken belief that there is an increased lumbar lordosis – leading to prescribing exercises to "flatten the back." Rather, this is a pseudo lordosis due

to excess thoracolumbar erector spinae activity (Fig. 3.19a). Note the normal alignment of the lumbosacral spine in the skeleton (Fig. 3.19b).

- In standing, the extension/abduction/external rotation synergy commonly dominates (see Fig. 3.16). The posterolateral myofascial chain becomes tight and the feet will tend to pronate. This compromises the ability for adaptable "grounding" and weight shift through the feet. It is important to recognize that this pattern plays out in various upright exercises, such as squats, and in the standing poses in yoga. Unless the

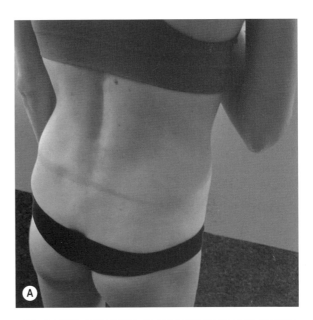

Figure 3.19

a) Central posterior cinch hyperactivity usually begins at around L3 (upwards to the dorsal hinge region) and can lead one to think that there is an "excess lordosis." Even if it is so, it is important to appreciate that it is high lumbar and not over the L4/5–S1/2 levels; hence I term it a "pseudo-lordosis." Manual palpation of the thoracolumbar levels usually demonstrates reduced segmental movement into extension, and the low lumbar levels are often particularly quite flexed. Note the poor lumbosacral lordosis and scant multifidus tone.

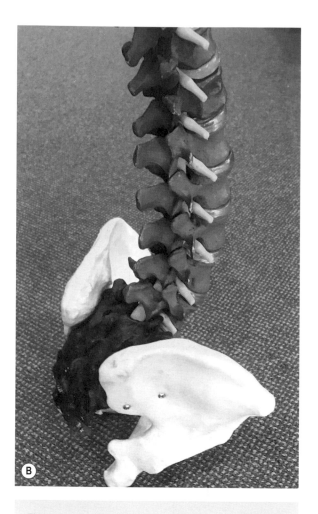

Figure 3.19 *continued*
b) In the model of a spine/pelvis, note the relatively acute lumbosacral angle between the sacrum (*black*) and the lumbar vertebrae (*gray*).

client can initiate and drive the movement from the pelvis via the pelvic FPs, spinal alignment is lost (see Fig. 3.15) with predictable increased tension in the upper body inferior tethers and central cinch activity (Fig. 3.20a). "Breaking up the holding patterns" becomes one of the therapeutic exercise goals. Working for pelvic control in various postures with the legs in flexion not only helps gain better control but mobilizes the lower limb

myofascia. The ability to ground the foot well and engage the heel/sit bone connection (see Ch. 8) enables the pelvis to lead the movement and the spine to maintain "the line" (Fig. 3.20b).

- The pelvic inferior tethers disturb control of the three-dimensional rotary force couples needed when standing on one leg. The pelvis not only drops on the contralateral side but is often pulled into posterior tilt and, probably, rotation. The mistake many clinicians make is in presuming this is due solely to weak gluteal muscles. Posterior pelvic pain has been associated with poor or delayed internal pelvic stability on active hip flexion in standing. Associated with a greater degree of posterior innominate rotation, this is caused by increased use of the hamstrings and external obliques in an attempt to stabilize the pelvis (Bussey and Milosavljevic 2015). The deep hip external rotators are also implicated.

- This "total pattern" synergy will be recruited when the client is challenged. For example, during hip extension in standing, or on all fours, the hip joint is also locked into external rotation, rotating the pelvis back on the leg-lifting side. This results in the spine being pulled into rotation and, particularly, flexion (Fig. 3.21).

- Dominant pelvic inferior tether activity (see Fig. 3.14a) and poor control of pelvic FP1 has a knock-on effect in pelvic FP3 resulting in a difficulty in initiating the lateral weight shift pattern through the pelvis, which is prerequisite in allowing axial FP3 to follow (see Fig. 3.14b).

I draw attention to the current common practice of prescribing isolated "glutes" training as a potential solution to a wide variety of lower quadrant pain disorders. Often based upon an inadequate understanding of healthy function, *many of these exercises actually increase the dominance of the pelvic inferior tether pattern.* (For example, the Clam exercise can create even more problems!)

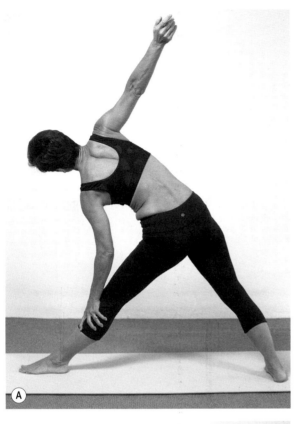

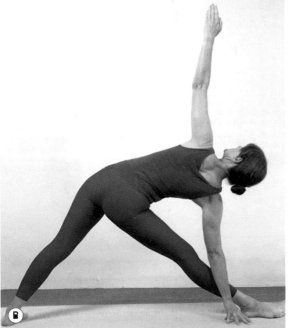

Figure 3.20

a) Reliance upon the pelvic "inferior tether" synergy when intrapelvic control is poor, means that during Trikonasana pose the pelvis cannot initiate and drive the movement and spinal alignment is lost. b) Good pelvic control allows it to lead the movement and the spine is free to elongate.

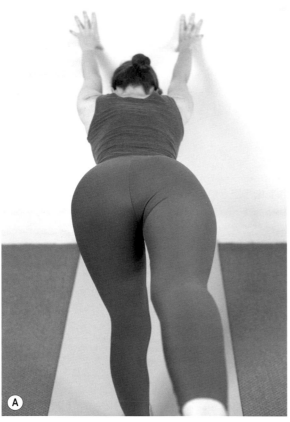

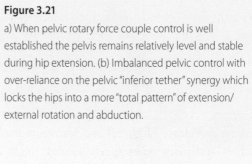

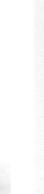

Figure 3.21

a) When pelvic rotary force couple control is well established the pelvis remains relatively level and stable during hip extension. (b) Imbalanced pelvic control with over-reliance on the pelvic "inferior tether" synergy which locks the hips into a more "total pattern" of extension/ external rotation and abduction.

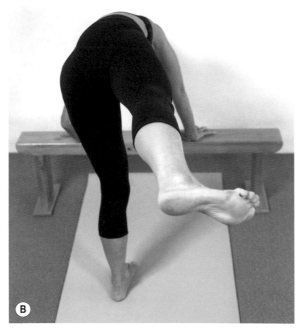

Unless control of the three-dimensional pelvic rotary force couples is understood and reestablished – notably control of pelvic FP1 – common exercises such as squats will be attempted via the dominant inferior tether synergy with consequent adverse effects on the spine (see Fig. 3.15).

You may wish to consider the extent to which the increasing prevalence of gluteal and hamstring tendinopathies, and many other sports injuries, might be relatable to excessive, poorly conceived strengthening exercises targeted at a single muscle. While hip abductor weakness has been shown in gluteal tendinopathy (Allison, Vicenzino, Wrigley et al 2016) this study tested static isometric strength in supine without regard for actively engaging the frontal plane rotary force couple needed for functional control (i.e., pelvic FP3). When this was tested in standing on one leg (Allison, Bennell, Grimaldi et al 2016) and walking (Allison, Vicenzino, Bennell et al 2016), weakness and altered kinematics of the whole frontal plane pelvic force couple were apparent with contralateral pelvic drop and excess ipsilateral pelvic shift and hip adduction (see Fig. 4.18a). In fact gluteus medius may be overactive in people with back pain (Bussey et al 2016) and in those with hamstring injuries (Franettovich Smith et al 2017) as it strives to stabilize the pelvis in the absence of good LPU coactivity.

I suggest that restoring control of pelvic FP1 and FP3 during a variety of movement-specific exercises is a more effective way of restoring lateral pelvic control and healthy lumbo/pelvic/hip function and of settling symptoms in a shorter time frame (see Fig. 4.19a,b).

The antidote to the adverse effects of the pelvic inferior tethers on the spine is mastery of the fundamental pelvic patterns through movement.

The shoulder inferior tethers: synonymous with the shoulder crossed syndrome

The shoulder tethers are a significant cause of loss of neutral alignment and function in the upper quadrant. This is especially the case in the thorax and shoulder girdle. The cervical spine also becomes the victim as it is unable to position itself in neutral and thus its control is affected (Helgadottir et al 2011).

The shoulder inferior tethers underlie all neck, shoulder, and upper limb pain disorders to a greater or lesser degree. They are also associated with dysfunctional upper chest breathing patterns.

The poor contribution of the upper thoracic spinal extensors and posterior lower scapula stabilizers disturbs balance and control of the three-dimensional scapula rotary force couples, particularly sagittal control.

This is related to an over-reliance upon the anterior shoulder girdle muscles for upper limb function. There is overactivity of the anterior shoulder girdle (depressors and protractors) and the upper limb flexors. This is associated with a dominance and reliance upon the more primitive total pattern synergy of flexion, adduction, and internal rotation for shoulder girdle stabilization and arm use. It is where they are "strong." The arms are infrequently used above the head, the result of which is that the extension/abduction/external rotation synergy of the upper limb is diminished in range and control.

This dominant pattern of upper limb activity and postural collapse leads to active and adaptive shortening and impeded slide of the related myofascia (the pectorals – major and, particularly, minor; subclavius; serratus anterior; and, probably, short head of biceps), which tethers the claviscapular unit anteroinferiorly, compromising its three-dimensional function:

- In the sagittal plane, the clavicle is held in downward or anterior rotation and the scapula is in anterior rotation. Upward clavicular rotation and posterior scapular rotation or tilt are reduced.

- In the frontal plane, clavicular depression and downward rotation of the scapula dominate, with clavicular elevation and upward rotation of the scapula being correspondingly reduced.

- In the transverse plane, the claviscapular unit is held in protraction and internal rotation, with retraction and external rotation being correspondingly reduced.

The functional consequences of the shoulder girdle inferior tethers

Again, these are considerable. While they undoubtedly compromise shoulder girdle function, the most underappreciated yet probably most significant effects are on the upper spine.

When the claviscapular unit is held in shoulder FP2, it brings the head into FP2. Try it for yourself. Upper quadrant postural and activity patterns become 2nd pattern dominant, and the spine suffers.

The anterior drift of the shoulder girdle pulls the upper thoracic spine and cervicothoracic junctional levels into flexion. Segmental stiffness ensues in time, which has two major effects:

- The person develops a "dome." This refers to an increased thoracic kyphosis and segmental stiffness into extension, side bending, and rotation through the upper thorax between T1 and the dorsal hinge at around T6–7. This limits adaptive postures and movement through the upper thorax to support neck and shoulder mobility and control (Fig. 3.22).

- The altered segmental loading between C1 and T7 can lead to chronic inflammation and neural bother, with accompanying variable changes in the tone and texture of the myofascia innervated by those irritable segments. Such changes are apparent over the chest wall and shoulder girdle, both anteriorly and posteriorly (see Ch. 1, On injuries). For instance, pectoral innervation is C5–T1; teres is C5–7 (Kendall et al 1993). The chest wall myofascia has thoracic segmental innervation. The myofascial hyperactivity can be due to segmental dysfunction and/or

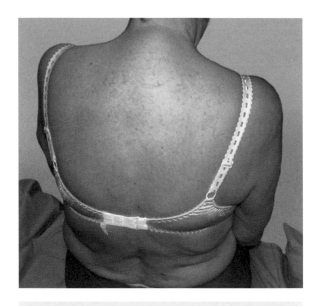

Figure 3.22
Thoracic "dome." Note the increased segmental flexion continues through the cervicothoracic junction; the upper thoracic spine and shoulder girdle provide poor postural support for the head and neck.

adaptive changes in habitual CNS neuromuscular patterning.

The poor posterior inferior scapular stability and the altered claviscapular myomechanics can lead to an adaptive syndesmosis or thickening of (probably) the upper fibers of serratus anterior myofascia, which binds the superior-medial scapula to the upper ribs (in particular ribs 2–5). This further reduces free three-dimensional slide and mobility between the under surface of the scapula and the chest wall.

An upper Key sign is indicative of this (Fig. 3.23). Here, competent palpatory testing of the spinal and related rib joints will usually reveal marked allodynia and restriction. It also frequently reproduces shoulder or arm pain. When thoracic joint function is compromised, the sympathetic nervous system is also affected. When this is really significant, a puffy, glassy

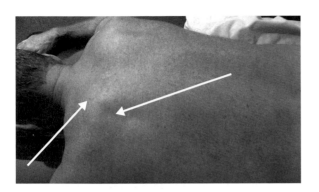

Figure 3.23
An "upper Key sign": comprises a band of increased myofascial activity from the supero-medial border of the scapula to the spine (*left arrow*) which is usually associated with reactive soft tissues between the medial border of the scapula and the spine (*right arrow*). The subject was lying prone and suffered from bilateral shoulder pain worse on the (L).

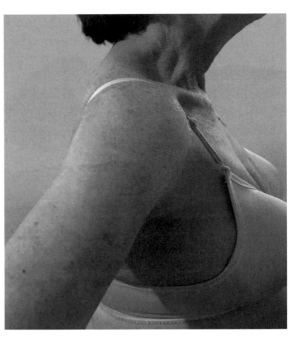

Figure 3.24
Sternoclavicular drop creates difficulty with shoulder FP1 – and is compensated for with neck tension and the elbows pulling back instead of the points of the shoulders.

quality of the myofascia is also apparent; and welts may appear in response to palpation. The sympathetic nervous system is increasingly implicated in distal pain syndromes (Jewson et al 2015) as levels T1–5 supply the head and neck, and T2–5 supply the upper limb (Williams and Warwick 1980).

- The upper thoracic extension and the sternal lift and protraction necessary to support claviscapular activity in performing shoulder FP1 becomes more difficult. Shoulder FP3 and FP4 also suffer. The client is likely to compensate by tensing the neck and arms instead (Fig. 3.24; see also Figs 4.23c and 4.26c). If this is not mastered, the dysfunction remains and recurrent neck and shoulder problems become likely.

The altered center of gravity in the shoulder girdle and upper thorax creates a forward head posture and associated reclination or extension of the occiput (head FP2). The head may be also postured in a degree of tilt or rotation. There is overactivity of the sterno-mastoids and usually the scalenes, with underactivity

in the deep neck flexors. Cervical alignment, stability and control suffers further (Fig. 3.25).

- The dominance of head FP2 leads to difficulty with head FP1, and by association, with patterns 3 and 4.

- The loss of three-dimensional movement within the cervicocranial joint complex leads to compensatory movement over the mid-cervical levels – creating overstress and reactive changes, which increase the likelihood of degenerative changes.

- Cervical and head pain disorders are predictable, as are those referred to the upper limb. Remember that neural bother can also facilitate or inhibit the upper limb girdle myofascia and change control of joint function (e.g., rotator cuff muscle innervation is primarily C5–6).

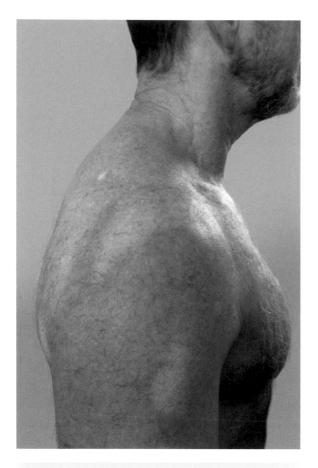

Figure 3.25
Shoulder crossed syndrome. Note the increased pectoral tone which pulls the shoulder girdle forward and increases the upper thoracic and cervicothoracic curve, bringing the head forward. Note also the loss of cervical alignment with increased tone in the sternomastoid, scalenes, and upper trapezius. The skin creases in the mid-cervical region indicate these segments are forced to overly compensate in posturo-movement.

- Clinically, head FP2 dominance and related C0/1/2 dysfunction is associated with jaw (and ear) problems and can also conceivably interfere with cranial nerve function because many of them exit via foramen around the base of the skull which are just anterolateral to the C0–1 joints.

The claviscapular inferior myofascial tethering commonly underpins scapular dyskinesis (the alteration of its kinematics), which hampers its ability to spatially position in a way that provides stable control to support arm function. Scapular dyskinesis is present in a high percentage of shoulder injuries with a common, though variable, three-dimensional functional deficit of reduced upward rotation, posterior tilt, and external rotation (Struyf et al 2011; Kibler et al 2013) (Fig. 3.26).

When functioning optimally, the upper, middle and lower parts of trapezius work with serratus as a force couple to upwardly rotate the scapula in the frontal plane for arm elevation. Middle and lower trapezius resist the lateral pull from serratus and help stabilize the scapula on the chest wall in some retraction. Mottram (1997) also proposes that the upper and middle trapezius draw the clavicle and scapula backward while raising the lateral end of the clavicle, causing upward rotation of the scapula.

When the middle and lower trapezius are underactive, the force couple control and scapular stability is lost. Compensatory abnormal elevation is accomplished by hyperactivity of levator scapulae, which acts to downwardly rotate the scapula, also creating neck tension.

Changes in timing may also occur with both early and excessive activation of upper trapezius (and an associated delay and inadequate activity in lower trapezius), resulting in excessive elevation of the shoulder girdle during arm elevation (Cools et al 2013).

Scapular winging is commonly assumed to be related to weakness of the serratus anterior. However, clinically, there is usually strong protraction – and somewhat short serratus myofascia, with commonly decreased passive mobility of the scapula on the chest wall in a principally posterosuperior direction. Serratus is not a homogenous muscle: three distinct subdivisions have been identified, with two distinct fascicles attaching to the superior and inferior aspects of rib 2 (Webb et al 2016) (Fig. 3.27).

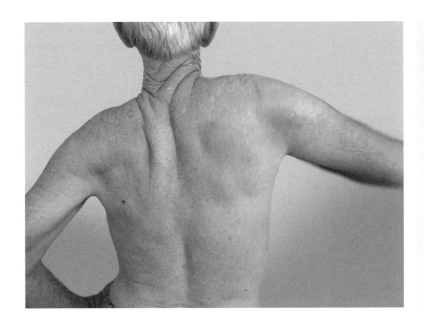

Figure 3.26
Arm elevation with loss of scapular force couple control from serratus and middle and lower trapezius results in scapular hitching from rhomboids/levator scapulae and upper trapezius. There is poor upward rotation, posterior tilt and retraction, and excessive activity in the neck and the posterior rotator cuff/infraspinatus to try and control the humeral head.

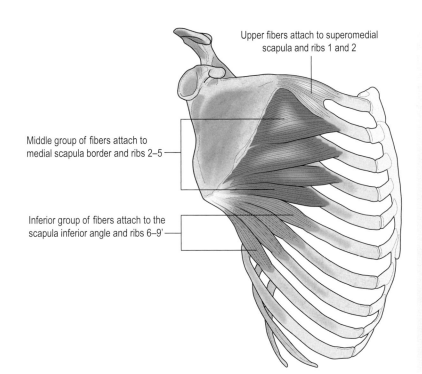

Upper fibers attach to superomedial scapula and ribs 1 and 2

Middle group of fibers attach to medial scapula border and ribs 2–5

Inferior group of fibers attach to the scapula inferior angle and ribs 6–9'

Figure 3.27
Serratus anterior has three distinct groups of fibres which are more apparent when the scapula is peeled back of the chest wall. Note that the fibres from the superomedial and medial scapular borders attach to the first three ribs – particularly the 2nd rib. Rib dysfunctions frequently underlie shoulder pain syndromes – and the 2nd rib in particular is always involved (and usually the 3rd).

Clinically, the upper fascicles attaching to ribs 1–3 (and often down to the 5th rib) are commonly short and form an apparent syndesmosis, seemingly the result of an attempt to stabilize the scapula on the chest wall in the absence of adequate posteroinferior stability. With pectoralis minor, these upper fibers can hold the scapula in anterior tilt, internal rotation, and depression. A depressed scapula is also likely to lead to upper limb neural tissue mechanosensitivity (Martínez-Merinero et al 2017).

This anteroinferior tethering passively restricts both claviscapular elevation and retraction (a combination of posterior tilt and external rotation). Control is further compromised due to poor middle and lower trapezius coactivity with serratus inappropriately positioning and stabilizing the scapula in some retraction.

The anteroinferior claviscapular tethering leads to a prominence of the inferior angle, termed pseudo winging of the scapula (Mottram 1997) (Fig. 3.28). This is likely to engender increased claviscapular anterior tilt and depression when attempting the first,

third and fourth shoulder patterns, unless checked. It will also lead to attempting scapula retraction by using excess rhomboid and levator scapulae activity, which further elevates (yet downwardly rotates) the scapula (Fig. 3.29). The posterior rotator cuff is also overactive.

A further common compensation is to attempt retraction by fixing or tensing the arm and over-engaging the humeroscapular muscles – particularly the posterior rotator cuff and teres – which in fact further abducts or protracts the scapula (see Figs 4.23c and 4.26c).

The aberrant claviscapular control leads to disturbed "centration" of the humeral head in the socket and altered glenohumeral joint myomechanics (Ludewig and Reynolds 2009). It becomes the "victim,"

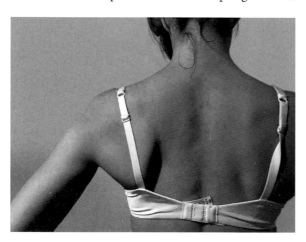

Figure 3.28
"Pseudo winging" of the scapula with associated anterior claviscapular tethering and poor posterior lower scapular stabilizer activity. Note the increased activity in the rhomboids, upper trapezius, and levator scapulae.

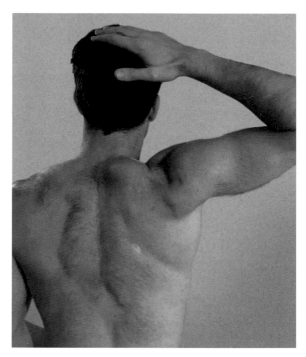

Figure 3.29
Attempting scapular retraction with the arm up. Note the excess levator scapulae, rhomboid and posterior rotator cuff activity. Performed correctly this exercise lengthens the posterior cuff and improves lower scapular stabilizer activity.

while the "criminal" is the reduced upper spinal and claviscapular control.

Glenohumeral internal rotation deficit (GIRD) is a common finding in shoulder pain. The claviscapular tethering and related protraction bring the humeral head spatially forward and off center in the glenoid, thereby disturbing balance in the rotator cuff and resulting in increased activity in infraspinatus, teres and, possibly, supraspinatus in attempting to stabilize the glenohumeral joint. Their subsequent myofascial bind/shortening limits glenohumeral abduction, horizontal flexion, and especially internal rotation – particularly when the arm is abducted or elevated.

Associated underactivity in the medial scapular stabilizers means that the scapula is pulled into abduction or protraction and anterior tilt during abduction or elevation of the arm. Subacromial impingement and related syndromes are likely (Fig. 3.30).

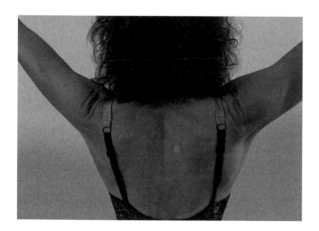

Figure 3.30
Overactivity of the posterior rotator cuff leads to GIRD. This limits glenohumeral abduction, horizontal flexion, and internal rotation Note that on elevation, the (R) posterior and inferior axilla myofascia does not open out well and that the scapula is pulled laterally around the chest wall with overactivity of the upper trapezius and underactivity of lower trapezius. The subject suffered chronic (R) shoulder pain.

A problem for therapists is that they tend to see the shoulders and spine as having independent problems, whereas they are functionally interrelated: one affects the other.

Drilling the shoulder fundamental patterns in varying postures and arm positions wakes up cervicothoracic spinal movement to enable the appropriate postural sets to support upper limb function. They also encourage lengthening of the shoulder inferior tethers and help to "re-groove" the trapezius force couples. This enables better coactivity between the middle and lower trapezius and the serratus, which is needed for effective control and stability of the scapula in all three dimensions.

Unless good sagittal alignment through control of shoulder FP1 is established, neither shoulder FP3 nor FP4 can be performed without compensation. Control of both the spine and shoulder is suboptimal.

Together, shoulder FP1 and FP3 help mobilize the cervicothoracic junction and upper thoracic spine into extension and side bending. This also brings about improved upward scapular rotation in the frontal plane and retraction/posterior tilt. If these patterns are conducted with one hand on the head, for instance, there is the added bonus of inhibiting and lengthening the posterior rotator cuff and related myofascia (see Fig. 7.27a,b) while also improving retraction.

Shoulder FP1 and FP4 together mobilize the cervicothoracic junction and upper thoracic spine into extension and rotation, thus improving posterior tilt and external rotation (retraction) of the scapula (see Fig. 7.25c).

Reestablishment of shoulder FP1 improves thoracic alignment and allows the cervical spine to align more optimally. This is by no means automatic, however, as control of the head on the neck (specifically head FP1) usually needs to be addressed (Fig. 3.31a).

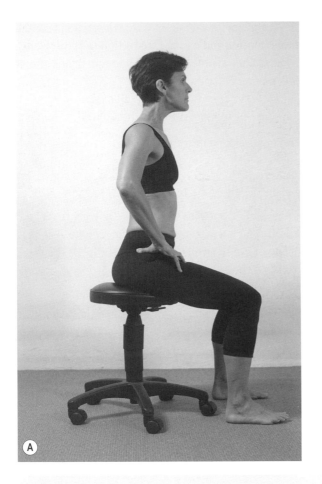
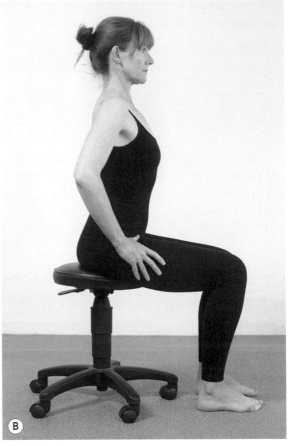

Figure 3.31

a) Engaging shoulder FP1 does not automatically bring the head into a neutral alignment but is a prerequisite to being able to posteriorly shift and anteriorly tilt the occiput to achieve elongation of the neck and a neutral cervical and head posture seen in b).

The craniocervical flexion test (head FP1) has been shown to reduce chronic neck pain (Falla et al 2012). Clients need careful cueing and manual guidance to correctly isolate this head pattern, owing to a tendency toward gross movements dominated by sternomastoid and anterior scalene activity in people with neck pain (O'Leary et al 2011).

When head FP1 is adequately mastered in supine, the client is coached in head retraction with head FP1 when upright. Here, it is important that there is pre-activation of shoulder FP1 (Fig. 3.31b) to avoid shearing and overworking the mid-cervical segments. However, with attention to detail in coactivating head FP1 with shoulder FP1, it is a great way to simultaneously train both the "lazy" deep neck flexors and lower scapular stabilizers, and achieve lift in the head and neck together with healthier patterns of upper spinal control.

Anyone sitting at a computer should not only be mindful of how they sit (see Sitting) but also perform shoulder and head FPs as "pause gymnastics" throughout the day to reawaken the upper spine.

Being mindful of the predictable compensations described above makes the practitioner alert to the likelihood of these when attempting the shoulder FPs (see Ch. 4). The most common fault when trying shoulder FP1 is inadequate protraction and lift of the manubrium, with associated clavicular posterior rotation and retraction, to optimally support the scapula – and sustaining this in shoulder FP3 and FP4.

This underlies the second most common fault: abnormal anterior depression when attempting to retract the scapulae (see Figs 3.24, 4.23c and 4.26c). The posterior tilt and external rotation need to be emphasized.

The shoulder FPs are initially taught with the hands on the iliac crests, which unloads the clavicle off the upper rib rings, making it easier to bring the manubrium up and forward without clavicular depression. If the shoulder FPs are correct, the arms remain relaxed and the elbows remain wide. When the arm rather than the claviscapular unit tries to lead the movement, there is no manubrial movement, the elbows pull back and in while the point of the shoulder moves forward and probably down, indicating that unwanted inferior tether patterning is dominant (see Fig. 3.24). Performed correctly, the shoulder FPs specifically activate the "lazy" upper thoracic spinal extensors and posterior lower scapular stabilizers.

While working the shoulder FPs it is particularly important to stay mindful of "control of the center." Collapse of the center – or fixing it via CCPs – is common.

The client needs to learn to control and stabilize the center against the actions of the proximal limb girdles.

Other common features of altered movement in people with spinal and related pains

Altered movement behavior can be hard for the novice to detect. The changes can be covert or overt; either way, even subtle alterations can significantly affect spinal control.

Movement becomes coarser and is accompanied by excess tension and effort. A reduction in tactile acuity (Luomajoki and Moseley 2011), proprioception, and other sensory modalities means that the client often has a poor idea not only of spatial relationships but of the sense of weight and finely modulated movement (O'Sullivan et al 2003). Competence in performing specific sensorimotor tests is diminished (Elsig et al 2014), and it can be difficult to isolate and dissociate movement (e.g., performing pelvic FP1 without CPC activity).

There is impairment and a functional disconnection between the FPs. In particular, movement initiated from the pelvis suffers most, with forward weight shifts being initiated more from the second patterns in the head and shoulder girdle than from the first pattern in the pelvis.

Because of poor pelvic control, there is often a reliance upon the shoulder inferior tethers for stability and level change, such as pushing down with the arms to stand up. The ability to control the center via the axial FP while activating the FPs in the limb girdles is diminished.

In addition, there is a general and regional loss of extension. Stiffness in the thorax and a disturbed functional relationship between it and the head and pelvis/tailbone are likely to influence autonomic nervous system dysregulation. This is because the thorax houses the sympathetic nervous system while the craniosacral outflow of the parasympathetic nervous system is located in the head and pelvis.

The combination of postural collapse and excessive regional superficial neuromuscular activity means movement is, by and large, confined to poorly aligned primary sagittal plane activity. Lateral and rotary movements are diminished. The spine becomes stiff (Hodges et al 2009), losing its "juicy" segmental flexibility and elasticity. Righting and equilibrium reactions, and balance all suffer (Mok et al 2011).

In consequence, the person attempts to maintain stability in the gravitational field by means of tensing, or "locking in," the limbs and related axial fixing postures – with excess grasping in the upper limb and stiffening of the legs.

When working to sustain postures and to move, such clients will frequently "hold themselves up and away from the ground" rather than yielding to it and finding the ground reaction force through the base of support, which would naturally activate the postural system. The poor patterns of proximal stabilization in spatially appropriate positions means that movement is initiated distally in the limbs rather than proximally via the FPs.

Movements of the torso and proximal limb girdles "going back" in space are unfamiliar (e.g., reaching the tailbone back in the forward bend pattern; open-chain hip extension; head retraction).

Uneven movement transmission through the spinal segments is apparent with regional blocks (e.g., thoracic spine) and the consequent need for some segments to act like a relative hinge in movement (e.g., L4–5); alternatively, there may be loss of directional control and range (e.g., lumbosacral extension).

The spine is not the only victim of disturbed regulation of the inner pressure change mechanisms. Associated problems with breathing and continence have also been well documented (Smith et al 2014). Breathing pattern disorders are common: upper chest breathing, hyperventilation, and breath holding when moving are the most prevalent (see Ch. 2, Breathing).

Always ask about incontinence in your female clients – you will be very surprised how widespread it is! And unfortunately many will have been doing isolated PFM exercises which can compound "core dysfunction" (see Ch. 2, "Opening the center").

Research by Smith and colleagues (2007a) challenges the assumption that incontinence is associated with reduced pelvic floor activity. They found increased pelvic floor and abdominal activity (likely upper) associated with postural perturbations in incontinent women. A related study (2007b) found delayed pelvic floor postural activity but increased contraction amplitude. Importantly, an RCT involving retraining coordinated function of diaphragmatic, deep abdominal, and PFM in incontinent subjects (Hung et al 2010) achieved a 90% cure or improvement. However, a later Cochrane systematic review (Hay-Smith et al 2012) of treatment for incontinence was unable to make any strong recommendations as to the best approach to pelvic floor muscle training.

Sitting

Dysfunctional sitting postures are probably the major driver of spinal dysfunction. Believe it or not, most people do not know how to sit properly (or without support); hence sustaining a physiological sitting posture is difficult and uncommon – and this is even true in a room full of yogis!

With the increasing pattern of sedentary leisure pursuits, and work practices involving long periods of sitting, the intellect is at work but not the body. Prolonged sitting has become the "new smoking epidemic" affecting public health.

Given that contemporary furniture by and large encourages lying back in sitting, relaxing is becoming synonymous with collapsing. Slumping is almost universal (see Fig. 3.32; also see Fig. 7.23a)

Standing desks have become popular – yet if you cannot support your spine properly in sitting, you will not do so in standing. Learning to sit well is basic to a healthy spine. And pelvic control is prime.

Sitting with the pelvis and spine in neutral naturally activates the LPU and core (Andersson E et al 1995;

O'Sullivan et al 2002a; Park et al 2013), and it is basic to upper spine neutral postures (Caneiro et al 2010). Being mindful of *how* you choose to sit, and learning to move via the pelvic fundamental patterns can be a great core workout.

Habitual "slump sitting" is usual in patient populations (O'Sullivan, Mitchell et al 2006). This switches off the LPU or core stabilizing systems (O'Sullivan, Dankaerts, Burnett, Chen et al 2006). The core muscles become weak and forget their role, so attempts to sit up invariably involve poor pelvic control and compensatory central cinch superficial muscle activity (O'Sullivan, Dankaerts, Burnett, Farrell et al 2006) – and increased upper body tension (Fig. 3.33).

Sitting with crossed thighs or putting your feet up invariably creates posterior pelvic tilt and end-range spinal flexion. The same goes for watching television or reading in bed – or spending time in hospital in the semi- or high Fowler's position. Unfortunately, half sitting/lying is very common. Pain can occur as a result of both collapsed sitting and when using superficial tension to "hold oneself up."

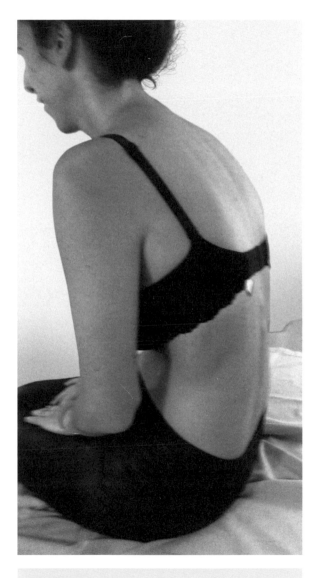

Figure 3.32
Slump sitting is highly prevalent. The spine is eccentrically loaded and core mechanisms are hampered.

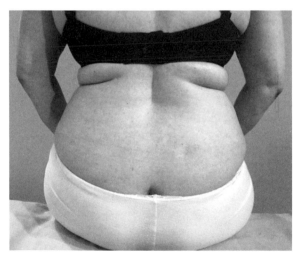

Figure 3.33
Without effective core support "sitting up" invariably involves central posterior cinching. Note the poor pelvic base of support and myofascial tone over the lower lumbar spine and sacrum, and the evident "Key signs"

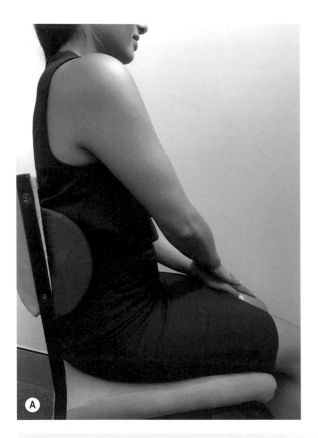
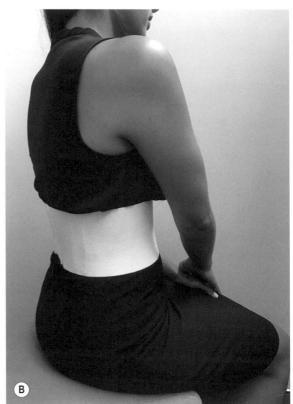

Figure 3.34

a) Sitting on flat-top chair with a "D lumbar roll" support. b) Self-supported sitting is aided when using the Key Moves Core Retrainer Belt.

Retraining effective patterns of core control can take a while to become adequate for sustained anti-gravity support and function. Hence in the early stages of retraining to sit correctly, it is advisable to provide back support so that the spine is in the upright neutral position with the hips and knees as close to a right angle as possible. A pillow placed in the lordosis can further support the spine (Fig. 3.34a). This will help to reduce the need for superficial muscle holding patterns (Curran et al 2015). Clients should be encouraged to coactivate pelvic FP1 and the axial FP – and also spend periods of time sitting without the back support while doing the same. The Key Moves Core

Retrainer Belt (see Ch. 8) can be a valuable aid here and is useful in helping gain active inner support while working at a desk (Fig. 3.34b).

The feet are also a problem

The feet are valuable windows as to what is happening in the pelvis. When lower limb inferior tether strategies are relied upon, the legs stiffly "prop" and are habitually postured in abduction and external rotation. Seeing a client with externally rotated feet (duck feet) immediately makes you suspect pelvic inferior tethers. Here, the body weight is taken more on the medial foot and there is collapse of the transverse and longitudinal arches together with poor intrinsic activity (Fig. 3.35a). A hallux valgus deformity is common. In time, the feet begin to "break down" and commonly resemble paddles as they lose malleability, adaptability and spring. Their dexterity in connecting well with the ground is lost, and, as the ankles lose dorsiflexion range, centering the talus over the calcaneum becomes less likely.

When the feet are poorly grounded the client will find it harder to soften the legs and find the point of initiation in the pelvic patterns (especially pelvic FP1). Well centrated and grounded feet (Fig. 3.35b) facilitate the reflex chain where the client can better connect with the pelvic FPs and diaphragm via the heel/sit-bone connection (see Fig. 3.20b). This requires a flexible ankle and pliable distribution of weight through the "tripod" of the foot, with a particular focus on taking the weight through the outer heel and the balls of the big and little toe. A small Blackroll can not only help mobilize the foot and ankle, it can improve sensory awareness and dexterity of the feet (see Ch. 2, The feet and Ch. 7, Ex. 58).

The hands: Similarly, when weight bearing through the hands, locking the anterior shoulder and elbows and the common myofascial restrictions in the upper limb make it difficult for the client to properly ground and center the hand – weight falls to its outer edge, and the second metacarpal lifts (Fig. 3.36a,b). This makes it difficult to find the reflex connection with the shoulder blades – in particular shoulder FP1, which is important in weight bearing and yoga (e.g., in dog pose).

Walking

When deep system control is deficient, and the spine is stiff and lacks extension, locomotion suffers. Inadequate pelvic/hip flexibility and control is fundamental to this, so when it becomes marked then a more rigid, heavy-footed loping style of walking commonly develops.

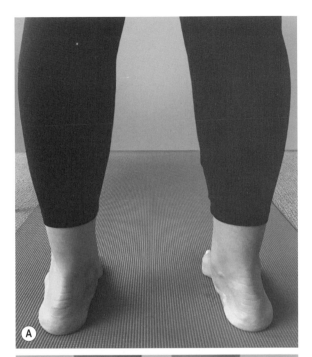

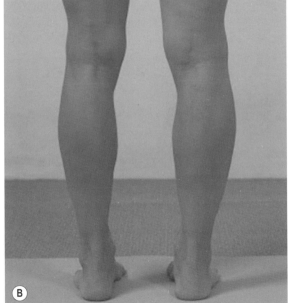

Figure 3.35

a) Poorly centrated and aligned feet with medial collapse and pronation. b) Well aligned and grounded feet allow the knees to center over the mid foot.

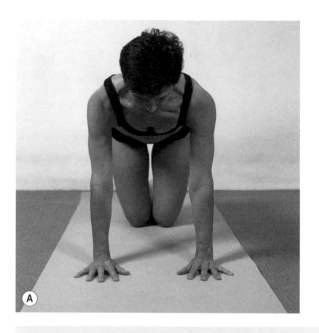 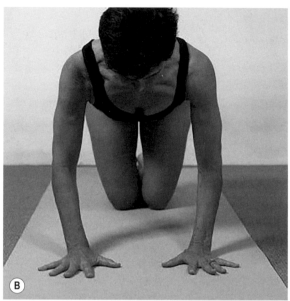

Figure 3.36

a) Locking the anterior shoulders and stiffening the arms leads to poor centration and grounding of the hands. Note the lift of the 2nd metacarpal and that the weight falls to the lateral hand. b) Engaging a more neutral position of the shoulder girdle and softening the arms helps facilitate a more centered hand position. Note that the weight is now more evenly distributed through the metacarpal heads.

Central fixing of the pelvis and spine through inferior tether activity results in poor weight shift and load transfer through the pelvis, which is compensated for by trunk side bending and thoracolumbar rigidity to bring the body weight over the standing leg (Trendelenburg effect). Single leg stance and propulsion suffer. Rotation through the pelvis and axis is also diminished, accompanied by reduced contralateral rotation of the limbs (Müller et al 2015). The benefits of the fascial matrix in spring-loading the system are lost and walking loses its ease, elasticity, and energy efficiency. Stride length is reduced. Rather than being propelled forward by the feet, some almost pull themselves along by the arms (see Ch.8: Walking well).

References

Adhia DB, Milosavljevic S, Tumilty S, Bussey M (2016) Innominate movement patterns, rotation trends and range of motion in individuals with low back pain of sacroiliac joint origin. Man Ther 21:100–108.

Allison K, Bennell KL, Grimaldi A et al (2016) Single leg stance control in individuals with symptomatic gluteal tendinopathy. Gait Posture 49:108–113.

Allison K, Vicenzino B, Wrigley TV et al (2016) Hip abductor muscle weakness in individuals with gluteal tendinopathy. Med Sci Sports Exerc 48(3):346–352.

Allison K, Vicenzino B, Bennell KL et al (2016) Kinematics and kinetics during walking in individuals with gluteal tendinopathy. Clin Biomech 32:56–63.

Andersson E, Oddsson L, Grundström H, Thorstesson A (1995) The role of psoas and iliacus muscles for stability and movement of the lumbar spine, pelvis and hip. Scand J Med Sci Sports 5:10–16.

Bussey MD, Milosavljevic S (2015) Asymmetric pelvic bracing and altered kinematics in patients with posterior pelvic pain who present with postural muscle delay. Clin Biomech (Bristol, Avon) 30(1):71–77.

Bussey MD, Kennedy JE, Kennedy G (2016) Gluteus medius coactivation response in field hockey players with and without low back pain. Phys Ther Sport 17:24–29.

Caneiro JP, O'Sullivan P, Burnett A et al (2010) The influence of different sitting postures on head/neck posture and muscle activity. Man Ther 15:54–60.

Cools AMJ, Struyf F, De Mey K et al (2013) Rehabilitation of scapular dyskinesis: From the office worker to the elite overhead athlete. Br J Sports Med. doi: 10.1136/bjsports-2013-092148.

Curran M, O'Sullivan L, O'Sullivan P et al (2015) Does using a chair backrest or reducing seated hip flexion influence trunk muscle activity and discomfort? A systematic review. Hum Factors 57(7):1115–1148.

Elgueta-Cancino E, Schabrun S, Danneels L, Hodges P (2014) A clinical test of lumbopelvic control: Development and reliability of a clinical test of dissociation of lumbo-pelvic and thoracolumbar motion. Man Ther 19(5):418–424.

Elsig S, Luomajoki H, Sattelmayer M et al (2014) Sensori-motor tests, such as movement control and laterality judgement accuracy in persons with recurrent neck pain and controls. A case control study. Man Ther 19(6):555–561.

Falla D, O'Leary S, Farina D, Jull G (2012) The change in deep cervical flexor activity after training is associated with the degree of pain reduction in patients with chronic neck pain. Clin J Pain 28(7):620–634.

Franettovich Smith MM, Bonacci J, Mendis MD et al (2017) Gluteus medius activation during running is a risk factor for season hamstring injuries in elite footballers. J Sci Med Sport Feb 20(2):159–163.

Hay-Smith J, Herderschee R, Dumoulin C, Herbison P (2012) Comparisons of approaches to pelvic floor muscle training for urinary incontinence in women: An abridged Cochrane Systematic review. Eur J Physiol Rehabil Med 2012 48:689–705.

Helgadottir H, Kristjansson, Mottram S et al (2011) Altered alignment of the shoulder girdle and cervical spine in patients with insidious onset neck pain and whiplash associated disorder. J Appl Biomech 27:181–191.

Hides JA, Boughen CL, Stanton W (2010) A magnetic resonance imaging investigation of the transversus abdominis muscle during drawing in of the abdominal wall in elite Australian Football League players with and without low back pain. J Orthop Sports Phys Ther 40 (1):4–10.

Hodges P, van den Hoorn W, Dawson A, Cholewicki J (2009) Changes in the mechanical properties of the trunk in low back pain may be associated with recurrence. J Biomech 42:61–66.

Hung H-C, Hsiao SM, Chih SY et al (2010) An alternative intervention for urinary incontinence: Retraining diaphragmatic, deep abdominal and pelvic floor co-ordinated function. Man Ther 15(3):273–279.

Janda V (1980) Muscles as a pathogenic factor in back pain. In: International Federation of Orthopaedic Manipulative Therapists. Fourth conference, New Zealand, pp.17–18.

Janda V, Frank C, Liebenson C (2007) Evaluation of muscular imbalance. In: Liebenson C (ed.) Rehabilitation of the spine: A practitioner's manual, 2nd edn. Philadelphia: Lippincott Williams and Wilkins.

Jewson JL, Lambert GW, Storr M, Gaida JE (2015) The sympathetic nervous system and tendinopathy: A systematic review. Sports Med 45:727–743.

Kendall FP, McCreary EK, Provance PG (1993) Muscles: Testing and function with posture and pain, 4th edn. Baltimore: Williams and Wilkins.

Key J (2010) Back pain: A movement problem. A clinical approach incorporating relevant research and practice. Edinburgh: Churchill Livingstone Elsevier.

Kibler WB, Sciascia AD, Uhl TL et al (2008) Electromyographic analysis of specific exercises for scapular control in early phases of shoulder rehabilitation. Am J Sports Med 36(9):1789–1798.

Kibler WB, Ludewig PM, McClure P et al (2013) Clinical implications of scapular dyskinesis in shoulder injury: The 2013 consensus statement from the "scapular summit". Br J Sports Med10.1136/bjsports-2013_092425.

Kolar P, Sulc J, Kyncl M et al (2012) Postural function of the diaphragm in persons with and without chronic low back pain. J Orthop Sports Phys Ther 42(4):352–362.

Kolar P, Lewit K, Dyrhonová O (2013) Assessment approaches focused on the function of the movement system. In: Pavel Kolar et al Clinical rehabilitation. Prague: Rehabilitation Prague School.

Langevin HM, Stevens-Tuttle D, Fox JR et al (2009) Ultrasound evidence of altered lumbar connective tissue structure in human subjects with chronic low back pain. BMC Musculoskelet Disord 10:151.

Ludewig PM, Reynolds JF (2009) The association of scapular kinematics and glenohumeral joint pathologies. J Orthop Sports Phys Ther 39(2):90–104.

Luomajoki H, Moseley GL (2011) Tactile acuity and lumbopelvic motor control in patients with back pain and healthy controls. Br J Sports Med 45:437–440.

Martínez-Merinero P, Lluch E, Gallezo-Izquierdo T et al (2017) The influence of depressed scapular alignment on upper limb neural tissue mechanosensitivity and local pressure pain sensitivity. Musculoskelet Sci Prac 29:60–65.

Mok NW, Brauer S, Hodges PW (2011) Changes in lumbar movement in people with low back pain are related to compromised balance. Spine 36(1):E45–E52.

Mottram SL (1997) Dynamic stability of the scapula. Man Ther 2(3):123–131.

Müller R, Ertelt T, Blickhan R (2015) Low back pain affects trunk as well as lower limb movements during walking and running. J Biomech 48(6):1009–1014.

O'Leary S, Falla D, Jull G (2011) The relationship between superficial muscle activity during the cranio-cervical flexion test and clinical features in patients with chronic neck pain. Man Ther Oct 16(5):452–455.

O'Sullivan PB, Grahamslaw KM, Kendell M et al (2000) The effect of different standing and sitting postures on trunk muscle activity in a pain free population. Spine 27(11):1238–1244.

O'Sullivan PB, Beales DJ, Beetham JA et al (2002) Altered motor control strategies in subjects with sacroiliac pain during active straight leg raise test. Spine 27(1):E1–E8.

O'Sullivan PB, Burnett A, Floyd AN et al (2003) Lumbar repositioning defect in a specific low back pain population. Spine 28(10): 1074–1079.

O'Sullivan PB, Dankaerts W, Burnett A, Chen et al (2006) Evaluation of the flexion relaxation phenomenon of the trunk muscles in sitting. Spine 31(17):2009–2016.

O'Sullivan PB, Dankaerts W, Burnett A, Farrell et al (2006) Effect of different upright sitting postures on spinal-pelvic curvature and trunk muscle activation in a pain-free population. Spine 31(19):E707– E712.

O'Sullivan PB, Mitchell T, Bulich P et al (2006) The relationship between posture and back muscle endurance in industrial workers with flexion related back pain. Man Ther 11:264–271.

Park RJ, Tsao H, Claus A et al (2013) Changes in the regional activity of the psoas major and quadratus lumborum with voluntary trunk and hip tasks and different spinal curvatures in sitting. J Orthop and Sports Phys Ther 43(2):74–82.

Roussel N, Nijs J, Truijen S et al (2009) Altered breathing patterns during lumbopelvic motor control tests in chronic low back pain: A case control study. Eur Spine J 18(7): 1066–1073.

Sahrmann S and Associates (2011) Movement system impairment syndromes of the extremities, cervical and thoracic spines – considerations for acute and long-term management. St Louis, MO: Elsevier Mosby.

Smith MD, Coppieters MW, Hodges PW (2007a) Postural response of the pelvic floor and abdominal muscles in women with and without incontinence. Neurourol Urodyn 26(3):377–385.

Smith MD, Coppieters MW, Hodges PW (2007b) Postural activity of the pelvic floor muscles is delayed during rapid arm movements in women with stress urinary incontinence. Int Urogynecol J Pelvic Floor Dysfunction 18(8):901–911.

Smith MD, Coppieters MW, Hodges PW (2008) Is balance different in women with and without stress urinary incontinence? Neurourol Urodyn 27(1):71–78.

Smith MD, Russell A, Hodges PW (2014) The relationship between incontinence, breathing disorders, gastrointestinal symptoms and back pain in women – a longitudinal cohort study. Clin J Pain 30(2):162–167.

Solomonow M, Hatipkarasulu S, Zhou BH et al (2003) Biomechanics and electromyography of a common idiopathic low back disorder. Spine 28(12):1235–1248.

Struyf F, Nijs J, Baeyens JP et al (2011) Scapular positioning and movement in unimpaired shoulders, shoulder impingement syndrome, and glenohumeral instability. Scand J Med Sci Sports 21(3):352–358.

Van Houke J, Pattyn C, Vanden Bossche L et al (2014) The pelvifemoral rhythm in cam-type femoroacetabular impingement. Clin Biomech 29(1):63–67.

Webb AL, O'Sullivan E, Stokes M, Mottram S (2016) A novel cadaveric study of the morphometry of serratus anterior muscle: One part, two parts, three parts, four? Anat Sci Int doi: 10.1007/s12565-016-0379-1.

Williams and Warwick (1980) Gray's Anatomy, 36th edn. Edinburgh: Churchill Livingstone, p.1138.

Moving from the "deep" sensorimotor system

Although the distinction between the "deep" and "superficial" myofascial systems is somewhat conceptual, it is useful when comprehending their differing inherent qualities in movement.

Research and clinical evidence shows that people with spinal pain syndromes share a common (though variable) difficulty with deep system control in that it is underactive, delayed and poorly sustained. As far as movement is concerned, what is not used is forgotten. Adaptive motor patterns which are overly reliant on superficial trunk muscle activity become apparent – and eventually entrenched – at a cost to spinal control and health. In due course, habitual dysfunctional posturo-movement control feels normal.

Clinically, spinal pain syndromes and altered movement are always found together. Motor dysfunction leads to pain. Pain further changes motor control (Hodges et al 2015). Hence to change the pain we need to change movement behavior.

If therapeutic movement and exercise is to be effective, it needs to restore the client's function. To do this we need to help the client reexperience and, to a degree, relearn to move in such a way as to reestablish the important patterns of control that are dependent on the deep system. Specific training of "lazy" deep-system muscles has shown positive neuroplastic changes in the brain (Tsao et al 2010).

So what are the ideal features of movement that is more deep system dominant?

Important features of healthy movement

Looking at how babies and young children develop informs a lot about movement. New movements are initially effortful but with practice and repetition (and determination!) become free and easy. Gross motor skills develop first, becoming more complex and refined.

Mature motor behavior is distinguished by the great variety of available movement and feasible possibilities. A lot of your patients, however, have lost various aspects and qualities of fine motor control of the torso. The following list identifies the natural qualities of healthy movement.

- The ability to easily gain and sustain a posture while breathing naturally. Being able to align the spine in the "neutral" upright posture is of particular importance. The deep system provides enduring yet flexible postural support without tension.

- Adaptable control, meaning that the body is freely responsive to a change in loading conditions (either a change in where the gravitational line of force affects the body tensegrity or an imposed external load).

  This in part involves shifting control between the fluctuating demands for stability and mobility: stabilizing or moving one part (e.g., pelvis) and moving another (e.g., hip).

- Balance and stability underpinned by the ability to perform intrinsic, discrete micro-movements and adjustments (in contrast to large, more extrinsic gross or coarse movements).

- An effective core that supports and stabilizes the spine – and connects movement between the upper and lower body.

- Spinal movement can ensue from varying points of initiation (i.e., either of the proximal limb girdles and/or the head) and then sequences freely through the rest of the spine.

- Movement always involves weight shifts over the base of support and is possible in all directions, which is particularly important when initiated from the pelvis.

- There is effective control of sagittal support and lateral weight shift – the precondition for rotation. Rotation is involved in: transitioning between postures and level change; simple activities of daily living (e.g., walking); all skilled body movements; and most sporting activities.

- The ability to dissociate movement of one part from another (e.g., hip from lumbar spine).

- The ability to explore the kinesphere (the space around the body).

- Movement is free and light, with minimal effort and no unnecessary tension.

- Movements are smooth and flowing rather than explosive, staccato, and jerky.

- The speed of movement is adjustable. It is easier to move quickly than slowly, but as we refine our motor skills we can better sustain and slow actions. This is necessary for the development of fine motor skills.

- Proprioception is good. Healthy movement is reliant on this. It conventionally involves four components: kinesthesia, or sense of position and movement sense; sense of tension or force; sense of balance; sense of effort and heaviness (Brumagne et al 2013, p.219).

The ability to sense our body weight and both yield and push away from gravity through the support surface is an important element in facilitating better deep system control.

Movement is multidimensional; its deconstruction into the three cardinal movement planes, however, helps us to decode it and understand how movement is built. Healthy, mature antigravity movement relies upon effective sagittal plane control, which is the precursor to accomplished frontal plane control. These are the precursors to effective transverse plane control (see Fig. 4.1).

Diaphragmatic breathing: *the fundamental pattern*

Breathing is the link between emotion and motion. Stress and anxiety engender tension and alter the breathing pattern – which will then be reflected in the body. Altered posture changes breathing. You cannot claim to adopt a biopsychosocial approach unless you address *how* your client breathes (see Ch. 2, Breathing).

Diaphragmatic breathing is the natural way to breathe. The diaphragm is both a breathing and a postural muscle. Newborn babies breathe with the diaphragm but have no postural control. During our development the "breathing" diaphragm becomes integrated with the postural system via its contribution to IAP - the point of initiation of deep system control (see Ch.2, "Opening the center").

Diaphragmatic breathing is the forerunner to it being effective in postural control. Hence ensuring that your client has a proper diaphragmatic breathing pattern is fundamental to all other exercise.

Fundamental patterns: specific movement phrases providing "key" points of control

The fundamental patterns (FPs) provide the foundations of spinal support and control. They not only reinstate freedom of spinal movement but are also an essential part of protecting the spine while accessing restrictions in the fascial and joint systems in order to improve flexibility and function.

My understanding of the FPs has evolved through empirical evidence derived from clinical practice, informed by the research and wide-ranging enquiry.

I recognized common patterns of joint and soft tissue dysfunction in people with spinal and related pain disorders, and that these were directly related to altered patterns of movement in the central axis. It also became apparent that the FPs were always a common missing ingredient in their movements.

Clinical evidence indicates that the FPs underlie all natural movement.

These important specific patterns of movement are reliant upon adequate deep myofascial system activity. In fact, their correct activation naturally activates the deep system. They act as a point of initiation of a movement which the spine continues. Operant in the three cardinal movement planes, they are responsible for the initiation and control of:

- antigravity "lift," maintenance of the spinal "neutral curves," and the alignment of the major units of mass (i.e., the head, thorax, and pelvis) in the sagittal plane

- weight shift over the base of support and through the spine

- rotation (which underlies all functional movement, especially sporting prowess).

These key points of control also act to redistribute tension throughout the three-dimensional axial tensegrity matrix, controlling shape change, and contributing to both spinal stabilization and movement.

They enable opening of the body and working into stiff regions of the spine and their related myofascial restrictions. Through them we can also access joint and fascial restrictions in the proximal limb girdles and limbs, while at the same time protecting the well-being of the spine.

Incorporating the FPs in a movement-class setting is an effective way of helping your client both move out of pain and move a lot better. Through them we can contribute to neurological reprogramming of the brain's substandard movement habits: "we train the brain to ease the pain."

Understanding the role of FPs in spinal movement helps simplify movement science and aids the assessment of movement in: the clinic, therapeutic exercise class situations (e.g., yoga, Pilates) or the fitness industry. Apart from their therapeutic value, reestablishing them and reincorporating them into movement enhances well-being, the practice of yoga (etc.), and improves sports performance.

General features of the fundamental patterns

The FPs are subtle, specific, well-isolated phrases or components of movement which appear to be key in basic patterns of control. Compared to your client's habitual tension-dominant movement behavior, they could be described as discrete micro-movements that test neuromotor control – an exercise in perception and sensorimotor ability.

Their correct performance requires focused attention in order to feel the correct action and fine tune the desired response. Effort and excess superficial tension in movement dulls the senses.

Your client will need reminding to "let go" and find the "soft movement." The use of imagery, appropriate verbal cues, and sensitive feedback via touch and/or different verbal instruction will be important.

There are four sets or groups of FPs – each group specifically governing either "the center," pelvic girdle, shoulder girdle or head. (Background information supporting an understanding of these is provided in Chapter 2 – see Opening the center, The pelvic fulcrum, and The upper quadrant.) Collective functional balance in the FPs allows the main units of mass (the head, thorax, and pelvis) to align over one another to support the spine in posture and movement. The groups contribute to the spine's freedom to move, and they have four numbered subdivisions, each principally controlling movement in one of the three cardinal planes (see Fig. 4.1):

- Patterns 1 and 2 in each group control:
  - alignment and flexion/extension movements in the sagittal plane
  - anterior and posterior rotation in the proximal limb girdles and head
- Pattern 3 in each group controls:
  - movements in the frontal plane – lateral weight shift, side bending, lengthening the side body
  - lateral rotation in the proximal limb girdles and head
- Pattern 4 in each group controls:
  - rotation in the transverse plane initiated in the proximal limb girdles/head and sequencing through the torso.

For ease of description, each set is described as an abbreviation for its region plus the relevant number. For example, pelvic fundamental pattern 1 becomes pelvic FP1.

Except for those governing the head, the fundamental patterns are closed-chain movements initiated in the axis and proximal limb girdles. They serve the dual roles of appropriate spatial postural positioning and support, providing both stability and mobility of the axis to support limb function.

As proximal initiation of movement in the limb girdles is usually deficient, the client will generally try to compensate by tensing the limb instead – hence cueing them to yield their weight to the support surface and consciously relax the limbs helps achieve the correct pattern.

It is important to appreciate that while each fundamental pattern principally controls the force couples in one plane, they are in fact three-dimensional movements with subtle coupled movements also occurring in the other two planes. This will be elaborated under each pattern.

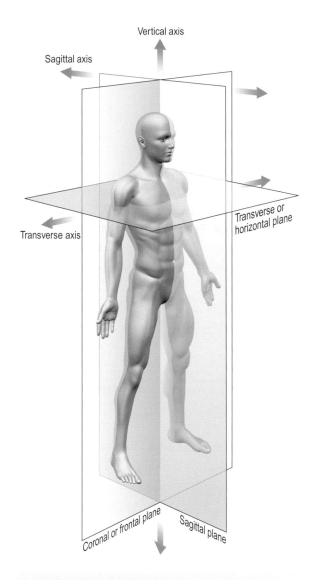

Figure 4.1

The three cardinal axes and planes of movement. The vertical axis equates to the gravitational line of force. Ideally the body segments are centered over one another and closely aligned within this – creating a "neutral" posture.

In the case of the head and limb girdle patterns: they work in synergy. Movement will be initiated in one and follow in the others. The spine is the conduit in movement sequencing through the axis. The timing and sequencing of movement from the point of initiation is subtle but significant.

There is a functional relationship between all the FPs – and between each group within the primary movements in the same cardinal plane in both posture and movement. For example, a neutral spinal posture is achieved by controlling the axial FP and coactivating all the first patterns, i.e., in the pelvis, shoulder girdle, and head (Fig. 4.2).

Functional movement, however, also involves combinations of FP control in additional planes of movement. As an example: maintaining a neutral spine, as described above, while adding pelvic FP3 to unweight one sit bone will then also slightly involve the third patterns in the shoulder girdle and head.

The four groups of fundamental movement patterns

The FPs are initially taught in supine or side lying (i.e., gravity is effectively eliminated) in order to reduce or bypass the habitual neuromuscular responses of the postural system. This makes it

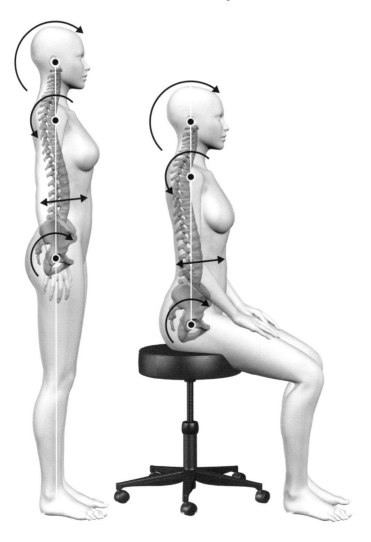

Figure 4.2

A "neutral" spine is achieved with minimal muscle tension when the sagittal force couples are balanced and there is integrated control between the axial fundamental pattern and the 1st patterns in the proximal limb girdles and head. The gravitational line of force passes through the atlanto-occipital, shoulder, and hip joints.

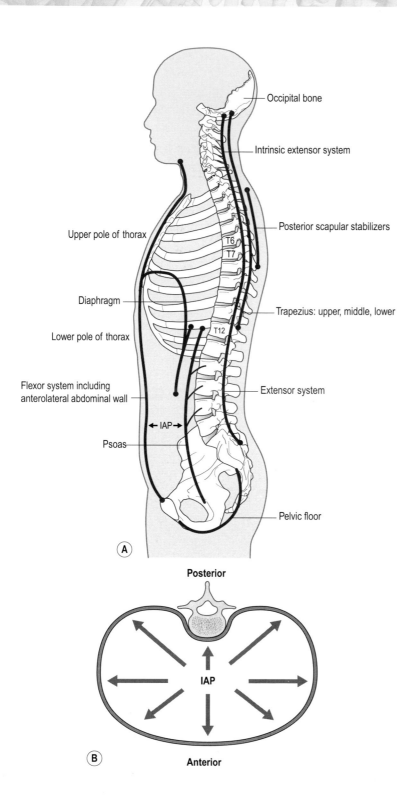

Occipital bone

Intrinsic extensor system

Upper pole of thorax

Posterior scapular stabilizers

T6
T7

Diaphragm

Trapezius: upper, middle, lower

Lower pole of thorax

T12

Flexor system including
anterolateral abdominal wall

Extensor system

← IAP →

Psoas

Pelvic floor

(A)

Posterior

IAP

(B)

Anterior

Figure 4.3

a) A well-aligned spine optimizes "core" control mechanisms. Flexor and extensor system activity is balanced and intra-abdominal pressure (IAP) supports the anterior spine. It also expands the lower rib cage and central torso three dimensionally – in particular laterally. b) Thus it "opens the center" body, helping to maintain the optimal spatial alignment between the thorax and pelvis, and helping preserve the body's longitudinal integrity. Through it we can readily change the volumes of the body cavities, contributing also to changes in body shape in posturo-movement.

easier for the client to achieve and sense the required "unfamiliar" movement.

Initially, some clients really struggle with being able to organize and feel the movement due to poor perceptuo-motor awareness. Explain to them that the FPs are in fact micro-movements and adjustments, as they will invariably attempt the movement from superficial-muscle "overkill." Giving them the movement passively can facilitate the correct response and help them to experience its feel. Practice, repetition, and feedback are important in learning – hence small group classes are ideal.

The axial FP needs to be sufficiently established to maintain spinal alignment and stability and an open center when working for control in the head and proximal limb girdle patterns.

The first patterns in the head and proximal limb girdles will be predictably deficient in your clients and it is important to reestablish them in order to gain control of sagittal alignment before expecting good control of the third and fourth patterns.

When established, all the patterns are combined in various ways and incorporated into a great variety of other postures and movements which incorporate increasing gravitational load and movement complexity.

Active quick tests for each can be done in sitting. Formal testing for the axial FP, the pelvic FPs and the head FP1 is done in lying.

Controlling the center: the axial fundamental pattern

The central torso is, ideally, shaped like a cylinder, which assists the body's tensegrity both in supporting the spine and limbs and in withstanding the stresses they create in movement. For this to be effective, the thorax and pelvis need to be aligned in the neutral spinal curves and with adequate core support (Fig. 4.3; and see Figs 2.1, 2.5 and 2.7).

I call this the center: it controls the thoracopelvic relationship and internal support (see Fig. 4.3).

The breath and IAP work together via modulated activity in the LPU to stabilize the lower pole of the thorax three dimensionally and provide counter-tension against the potential constrictions created by the outer trunk myofascial activity and the torques imposed by gravity and moving the limbs (see Fig. 4.3).

This is the axial fundamental pattern. I am indebted to Professor Paul Hodges' large body of research and that of Dr Pavel Kolar in helping me clarify this pattern. (See these sections in Ch. 2: Breathing; "Opening the center.")

There is deep anterior support for the lower half of the spine, and the upper and lower body are functionally connected through control of the center.

Axial FP quick test movement

a) The ability to firm the inguinal fossa medial to the anterior superior iliac spine (ASIS; Fig. 4.4).

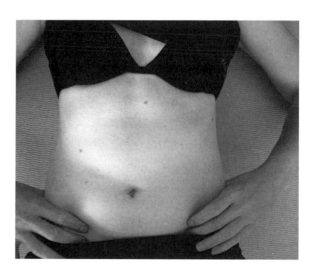

Figure 4.4

The subject's middle fingers are palpating for lower pelvic unit activity just medial to the anterior iliac spines. Note the open center, the even abdominal tone and that the infrasternal angle is approximately 90°.

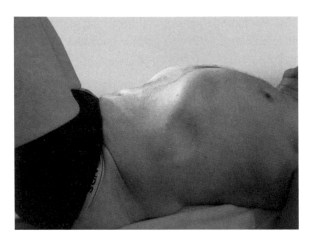

Figure 4.6

In supine, when there is poor tone in the anterolateral abdominal wall the rib cage is lifted and there is a wide infrasternal angle.

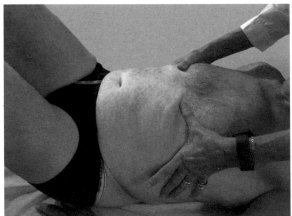

Figure 4.7

Manually repositioning of the thorax caudally helps wake up the abdominal wall and facilitate "core" mechanisms. The client then needs to learn to sustain the "new" position himself.

the abdominals in stabilizing the LPT so that the thorax and pelvis are in alignment and the reflex connections between the diaphragm and pelvic floor can be facilitated in generating IAP. The patient needs to learn to "hold" the new thorax position.

See Assessing and teaching the axial FP (p. 98).

Functional importance of the axial FP

The axial FP is an adaptable pre-movement response which helps support, align, and stabilize the spine in the neutral position before a limb movement occurs – irrespective of the direction of movement (Crommert et al 2011). In this way, the axial FP initiates preparatory control rather than movement.

In general, the spine itself does not initiate a lot of its actual movement but adaptively follows and controls movement initiated in either of the proximal limb girdles or head. Here, the center is still "contained" and remains open, although it alters

its cross-sectional shape to allow movement to freely sequence through the spine. This concept is represented in Fig. 4.8.

From control of postural alignment in and around the "neutral" zone, in movement we see that the axial pattern morphs into four subdivisions (as described earlier) based upon on the spine's movement direction away from, and returning to, the neutral posture. These are known simply as axial FP1–FP4.

- Axial FP1 contributes to: a flexible, upright neutral spine; movements into spinal extension; returning from spinal flexion (see Fig. 4.8a,b).

- Axial FP2 contributes to: a flexible, upright neutral spine; movements into spinal flexion; returning from spinal extension (see Fig. 4.8a,c).

Maintaining a flexible neutral spinal posture in the sagittal plane involves balanced coactivation of axial FP1 and FP2, as well as subtle oscillations between them to support the spine and allow it freedom to move.

This also requires good control of the first and second pelvic patterns.

- Axial FP3: controls movements into lateral weight shift, lateral flexion, and lengthening one side of the body. The sagittal alignment should also be flexibly maintained (see Fig. 4.8a,d).

- Axial FP4: links rotation between the pelvis and shoulder girdle/upper thorax – either initiated by the pelvis or the shoulder girdle and head (not shown in Fig. 4.8).

The center remains open, aligned, and "connected" in order to maintain thorax–pelvis relationship during:

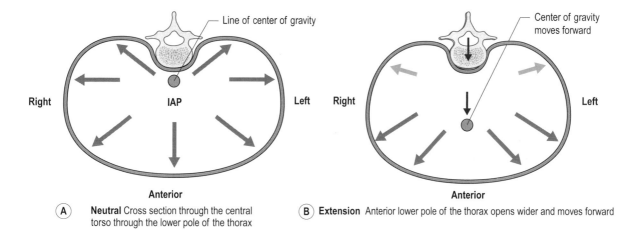

(A) **Neutral** Cross section through the central torso through the lower pole of the thorax

(B) **Extension** Anterior lower pole of the thorax opens wider and moves forward

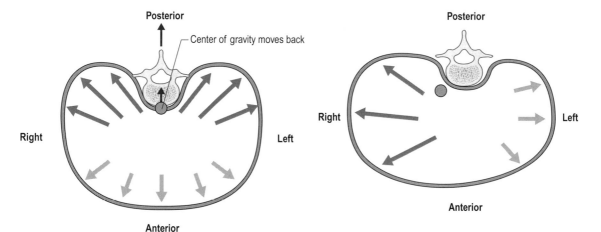

(C) **Flexion** Lower pole of the thorax moves back and widens more posterolaterally

(D) **Lengthening the right side/side-bending to the left** Right lower pole of the thorax (LPT) moves to the right and lengthens and widens more – the left side shortens and is compressed

Figure 4.8

This drawing attempts to conceptually show the spatial shifts and internal shape change in the lower pole of the thorax during axial FPs 1–3: A) neutral, B) in extension (AFP1), C) in flexion (AFP2), D) in (R) side bending (AFP3).

- forward or backward rotation of either proximal limb girdle

- opposite or contralateral proximal limb girdle rotation (as in walking)

- ipsilateral forward or backward rotation of both proximal limb girdles in the same direction (when the whole body turns – think of a golf swing or doing a spinal twist).

We can also work from the center, using the breath with through-range movement to help manipulate torso shape, thus aiding thoracic spine and rib cage mobility and smarter control (see Fig. 8.3).

I will emphasize once more that the axial FP is *the* core retraining exercise. When correctly performed, it activates the lower anterolateral abdominal wall more than the upper, primarily involving transversus and internal oblique with the diaphragm and PFM to create adaptable IAP that supports posture and movement. It also brings the thorax and pelvis into alignment.

It should not be confused with abdominal bracing, which activates all three layers of the abdominal wall (the superficial obliques with transversus) to ensure spinal stability under load (McGill 2002). The problem here is that many of your clients are already adopting such high-load strategies and rely too much on superficial trunk muscle activity, which creates excessive spinal compression, stiffness, and limited mobility. Bracing does not allow adaptable freedom of movement through the spine.

However, the abdominal wall in someone with a posterior PXS presentation needs awakening. This should occur with concurrent activation of the axial FP. Exercises 5, 6, 33 and 36 are an effective way to do this (see Ch. 7). In Ex. 36, note the legs are extended and the toes are pointing; this helps to stabilize the pelvis in a more neutral position while the client works to bring the thorax down and back.

Crunches and sit-ups are not core exercises. While they do work the abdominals, they create tension and compression stress to the lumbar spine and SIJ. They need modifying as described above.

Pulling in the stomach does not train the core either. And in the anterior PXS group, this risks further reinforcing already dominant CAC behavior and further disturbing diaphragm and PFM function. Clinical evidence has demonstrated that training transversus abdominis via the abdominal drawing-in maneuver (ADIM) or by "pulling in the lower abdomen" (Richardson et al 2004, p.186) is not nearly as effective in providing internal postural support as training the axial FP.

The axial FP underlies all other postures and movements in the therapeutic exercise sequences. For this reason it is drilled as a home routine and incorporated into all classes one way or another.

Assessing and teaching the basic axial FP

- This is initially done with gravity eliminated in supine, knees bent. Establishing and sustaining the correct action will be quite difficult for many of your clients and can require considerable patience and therapeutic skill on your part to help facilitate the correct action. Subgroup classification (see Ch. 3) will delineate the principal element to focus upon.

Most of your clients will have a stiff thorax and restricted anterior shoulder girdle myofascia, so as the lower ribs come back the shoulders will move forward. Hence it is important to support the head in the neutral position and encourage relaxing the shoulders back while working for the axial FP (Fig. 4.9).

There is a sequence of actions each of which needs to be established prior to the next being asked for:

1. The first requirement is a slow diaphragmatic breathing pattern at rest with no lift of the thorax (see Fig. 7.1). You may need to manually reposition the thorax (see Fig. 4.7) to achieve a diaphragmatic breathing pattern. This can be easier

said than done and can take a while for some to achieve.

2. The ability to actively exhale *such that the client is aware of activating the LPU* (by simultaneous palpation over the lower abdominal wall (see Fig. 4.4), with no upper chest lift on inhalation. The posterior PXS subgroup will find this difficult. They prefer to inhale - and by lifting the ribs.

3. To continue the active exhalation to the end of range so that the lower thorax moves caudad and back – and remains there on the next inhalation (see the bullet points under Formal axial FP test in supine). The pelvis slightly follows the thorax movement; it does not initiate it. Beware of the client pushing with the feet and a "butt clench."
Imagery such as "squash the beetle under your lower back ribs" can assist in maintaining the thorax position. Again the posterior PXS subgroup will find this difficult as the abdominals have to work. Watch for CAC activity in the anterior PXS subgroup. The exhalation should be driven from the lower abdomen and pelvic floor rather than by drawing in the upper abdomen.

4. To be able to sustain the "new" position of the thorax while allowing the breath to quietly come and go.

5. "Making more space for the breath": The client is instructed to gradually widen the LPT as it stays back – and sustain this opening of the center while continuing a low, slow diaphragmatic breathing pattern. The focus is to hold the thorax position/posture on both the inhale and exhale. The anterior PXS subgroup are generally "weaker" in their diaphragm – both postural and respiratory – and therefore find this action more difficult. Their upper abdominal hyperactivity makes them better at exhaling. Cues such as "think of pushing the diaphragm down to expand and widen the ribs and keep them there" can help. When correct, the infrasternal angle widens (see Figs 2.9 and 4.4). Incidentally, this is one of the few times I use the word "push" when cueing movement.
The posterior PXS group need to think more of bringing the breath down and back and to increase the exhalation – both its length of time and "oomph."

6. When the above can be mastered, the correct response is further established and challenged by maintaining stable control during various limb loading movements (see Fig. 4.9), and also by maintaining adaptive control via the appropriate axial FPs (1–4) during movement.

Recumbent training of the axial FP helps ingrain the motor pattern in the CNS. It can take some clients a while to correctly master it. Repetition and practice are necessary in order to be able to readily locate the correct action when upright.

The further challenge is its adaptable control when upright and moving – via the four axial FPs. The

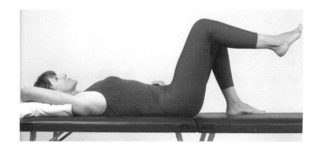

Figure 4.9

The client is palpating for lower pelvic unit activity with her (L) hand. Note that the lower pole of the thorax is in contact with the surface despite that fact that her arm is up and she has unweighted one leg. Many of your clients will need higher head support and may well struggle with bringing the ribs back in contact. Bringing the arms or legs up challenges proficiency of controlling the center and should not be attempted until the basic action is somewhat mastered.

Key Moves Core Retrainer Belt has been specifically developed to assist this (see Ch.8).

Inept axial FP control and poor proximal limb girdle control leads to a central disconnect between the upper and lower body – as a result of "central cinching" or "wringing the waist." The spine suffers.

Pelvic fundamental patterns

Free and healthy spinal movement relies on a flexible and adequately controlled pelvis. Its control in functional movement is complex and multidimensional (see Ch. 2, The pelvic fulcrum).

Some clarity can be achieved by analyzing and reinstating control of the basic pelvic actions in the three cardinal movement planes. Here, the deep system LPU not only controls the axial FP but also plays a critical role in modulating pelvic myomechanics via the pelvic FPs.

These patterns initiate movement from the pelvis and the base of the spine. They not only animate the pelvis and provide internal support and stability, they underlie its ability to change its shape and drive movement of the spine and legs.

Importantly, the pelvic FPs afford control of the pelvic rotary force couples in each plane of movement. They are actually closed-chain movements of the hips, initiated by the pelvis rather than the legs.

Note: The movements will be described as they occur in the supine crook lying position.

The primary focus in the activation of the pelvic FPs is moving from the ischial tuberosities or sit bones and tailbone. Most people will not be clear where these are; hence guided palpation helps orient them.

Palpating the ASIS will help the client more clearly sense the corresponding movements of the ischia, which occur in each of the three planes differently (Fig. 4.10). The legs remain relaxed and the feet do not push. Remember, the pelvis must initiate the movement.

The pelvic FPs are initially taught in supine or side lying without the challenge of gravity or load. When somewhat established in neutral they are appropriately drilled in various postures and movements. Here, we are aiming for their correct activation no matter what position the spine or legs are in. This is one of the aspects to consider when planning a class.

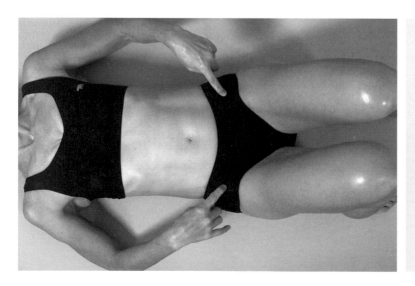

Figure 4.10

The model's fingers are palpating the bony prominences of the anterior superior iliac spines (ASIS) which correspondingly move with the sit bones mostly in an antagonistic manner; e.g., when the sit bones move back the ASIS move forward.

First pelvic fundamental pattern

Pelvic FP1 involves interior pelvic tilt/rotation and ischial outflare: the sit bones reach long, wide and back. The ASIS rotate forward and slightly approximate (Fig. 4.11). This creates:

- anterior rotation of the innominates
- nutation of the sacrum
- lordosis and extension of the low lumbar spine (and antigravity "lift" when upright)
- closing of the "superior pelvic bowl" – the ASIS approximate
- opening of the "inferior pelvic bowl" and pelvic floor as the sit bones widen and reach back, bringing the tailbone back (Fig. 4.12a,b)
- closed-chain hip flexion as the pelvis rotates anteriorly on the femoral heads. The groins deepen.

Watch for: pelvic initiation from the sit bones and movement sequencing through the spine. When the action is correct the groins deepen – and movement starts at the pelvis and ends at the head where the chin tucks (head FP1; Fig. 4.13a and see Fig. 4.11).

Compensations: Poor pelvic initiation and forward rib thrust via a CPC strategy which creates a central disconnect, resulting in movement that does not travel through the thorax. This is readily apparent in sitting (Fig. 4.13b). Simultaneously engaging the axial FP helps prevent this.

Functional importance of pelvic FP1

This pelvic pattern:

- contributes to control of the sagittal pelvic rotary force couples
- is basic in creating a neutral pelvic posture – the springboard for achieving … the neutral lumbar lordosis! Neutral lumbopelvic postures naturally activate transversus (Reeve and Dilley 2009) and other elements of the LPU, such as psoas, iliacus, and quadratus lumborum (Andersson et al 1995; Park et al 2013)
- is fundamental to all sagittal plane posturomovements which require closed-chain hip flexion; e.g., neutral sitting, forward weight shift in sitting in preparation to stand up, forward bending pattern in standing, squatting, etc. This is one of the most important patterns of movement serving daily function – hip flexion with the lumbar lordosis largely preserved
- also posturally supports "open kinetic chain" hip extension in all postures

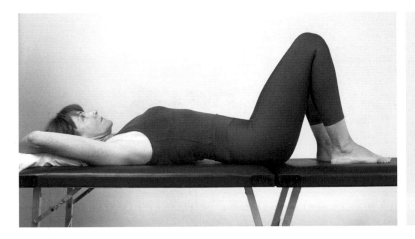

Figure 4.11

Pelvic FP1 in supine. The subject's hands are not palpating the lower pelvic unit here to make it easier to see. Note the deepening in the groins, the anterior pelvic rotation, the arch in the low back, that the ribs don't thrust forward, and that the chin tucks. The spine lengthens.

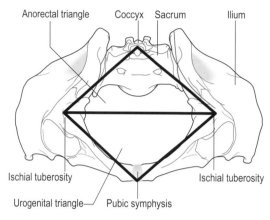

Anorectal triangle   Coccyx   Sacrum   Ilium

Ischial tuberosity   Ischial tuberosity

Urogenital triangle   Pubic symphysis

A **Neutral**

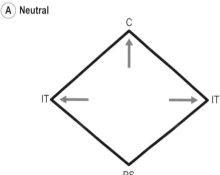

C

IT   IT

PS

B Ischial outflare 'opens' the floor = pelvic FP1

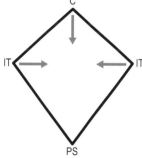

C

IT   IT

PS

C Ischial inflare 'closes' the floor = pelvic FP2

Figure 4.12

View of the inferior pelvic opening. Changes in the "diamond" shape and dimensions are modulated by the ischia and tailbone moving closer or apart: a) at rest in "neutral"; b) opening via pelvic FP1; c) closing via pelvic FP2. Reproduced from Key 2010, with permission and thanks.

- provides the stable postural set for open kinetic chain hip flexion in all postures

- pelvic FP1 is allied with the hip flexion, adduction and internal rotation lower limb movement synergy.

Also note that:

- the primary agonists in the myofascial synergy driving the pattern of movement are the lower transversus abdominis and internal oblique, iliacus and psoas, lumbar multifidus

- the antagonistic myofascia providing eccentric control of the movement are the PFM, the obturator group (the deep 6 external hip rotators), and the gluteus maximus.

Balance between agonists and antagonists is important in being able to control the pelvic rotary force couples in the sagittal plane. Control of anterior pelvic rotation, which is dependent on pelvic FP1, is predictably difficult in patient populations (so gaining a neutral pelvis is correspondingly problematic).

Pelvic FP1 is required before pelvic FP3 and FP4 can be properly achieved in sitting and standing.

Second pelvic fundamental pattern

In pelvic FP2 there is posterior pelvic tilt/rotation and ischial inflare: the sit bones move forward, closer together, and rise. The ASIS rotate back and widen slightly; this is also known as a "tail tuck" (Fig. 4.14). This creates:

- posterior rotation of the innominates

- sacral counternutation

- loss of lordosis and flexion of the lumbar spine

- opening of the superior pelvic bowl – widening of the ASIS

- closing of the inferior pelvic bowl and pelvic floor – sit bones and tailbone move closer together (see Fig. 4.12c)

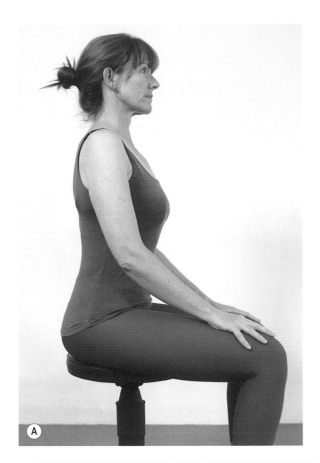

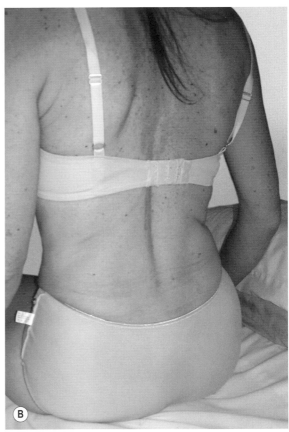

Figure 4.13

a) Pelvic FP1 in sitting ensures a neutral upright spine. The inferior pelvis is "open" to provide a wide base of inferior support (see Fig. 4.12b). b) Inadequate control of pelvic FP1 results in poor anterior pelvic rotation which is compensated for by superficial central posterior cinch or "holding patterns" higher up the spine. Note also the bilateral "Key signs."

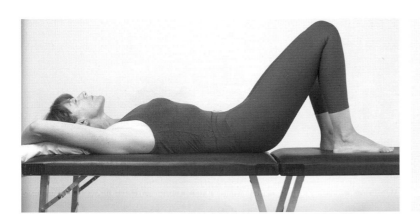

Figure 4.14

Pelvic FP2 in supine. Note that the groins become more like shallow dishes, the low back flattens, the pelvis posteriorly rotates – and the chin protrudes. The spine shortens.

- closed kinetic chain hip extension as the pelvis posteriorly rotates on the femoral heads so that the groins "open."

Watch for: pelvic initiation and movement sequencing through the spine. When the action is correct, movement starts at the pelvis and ends at the head where the chin protrudes (head FP2).

Compensations: Most patients find this pattern easy – albeit that they rely upon pushing through the feet with excessive butt clench and without much coactivation of the inner unit. In fact, they generally posture into posterior pelvic rotation and lock-in the whole posterior inferior myofascial chain of the lower limb. They are habitually stuck in pelvic FP2 and eventually the joints stiffen into this pattern. Hence mobility is reduced and they also find the eccentric control that is necessary for activating pelvic FP1 difficult, particularly during through-range hip movements.

Functional importance of pelvic FP2

This pelvic pattern:

- contributes to control of sagittal pelvic rotary force couples

- is fundamental to all sagittal plane posturomovements requiring closed-chain hip extension (e.g., sit to stand; returning to the vertical after forward bending; doing a backbend). It is particularly important in controlling the pelvic position and gaining hip extension in kneeling

- is allied with the hip extension, abduction, and external rotation lower limb synergy (Bussey et al 2009).

Also note that:

- the primary agonists in the myofascial synergy driving the pattern of movement are the PFM, the obturator group (the "deep 6" external hip rotators), and the gluteus maximus

- the antagonistic myofascial synergy is coactive – providing eccentric control of the movement pattern via the LPU (transversus abdominis and internal oblique, iliacus and psoas, lumbar multifidus).

There is commonly an imbalance controlling the sagittal pelvic rotary force couples with a bias toward excess posterior pelvic rotation or tilt – pelvic FP2. The inferior pelvic outlet is constricted (see Fig. 4.12c), "tethering" the tailbone and sit bones, and limiting free play into pelvic FP1 (and pelvic myomechanics in general). The inferior pelvis does not open well (see Fig. 4.12a,b) and the lumbar spine simply cannot assume a neutral position.

In general, I do not specifically teach the pelvic FP2 as clients can usually do it.

However, this pattern does need reinforcing when aiming to open the front of the hip and thigh, particularly if the knee is flexed – as in kneeling. The posterior PXS group find combining this with control of the axial FP really difficult. Adequate control of pelvic FP2 in kneeling is a precursor to effective control of pelvic FP3 and 4 in kneeling.

Third pelvic fundamental pattern

Pelvic FP3 involves lateral pelvic rotation in the frontal plane [the pattern is described for the left but the same actions apply to the right]: the ipsilateral (left) sit bone "sinks" in the vertical upright postures or reaches caudad in the others. In supine the ipsilateral (left) ASIS moves caudad (south); the contralateral (right) ASIS moves cephalad (north). Both ASIS remain level on the "horizon line."

This creates (Fig. 4.15):

- a lateral rotation of the pelvis on the femoral heads

- elongation of the ipsilateral (left) ischium and left side waist – and shortening of the other

- upward lateral pelvic rotation on the contralateral (right) side – and an ipsilateral downward lateral pelvic rotation (left)

- eccentric lengthening of the ipsilateral LPU myofascia (left) and concentric activity on the contralateral (right) side (see Fig. 2.13)

- ipsilateral lateral weight shift through the pelvis (to the left) in the upright postures; ipsilateral "lengthening the side" body in all postures. In supine, the weight remains centered on the sacrum, which swivels as the ischia move in opposite directions

- closed-chain hip abduction on the ipsilateral (left) side.

Watch for: Initiation from one sit bone, ipsilateral weight shift through the pelvis, and movement then sequencing through the spine. This is particularly

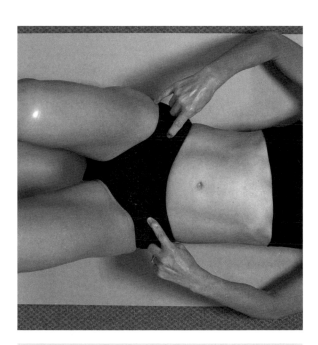

Figure 4.15

Pelvic FP3. Here, the (L) sit bone reaches south and the (L) anterior superior iliac spine also moves south; the (L) waist and side body lengthen. The weight does not shift but remains centered on the sacrum, which in fact swivels. Note how the knees remain approximately the same length.

important in the upright postures. The lower rib cage is free to follow the movement and laterally shift, which enables the side body to lengthen (axial FP3).

Pelvic FP3 and axial FP3 are thus also an effective way of breaking up CCP behavior. There will also be reciprocal 3rd pattern changes in the shoulder girdle and head (Fig. 4.16; see Fig. 7.29a,c). Try to ensure the pelvis remains in a sagittal neutral position while adding pelvic FP3.

It is important to appreciate that pelvic FP3 is not "hip hiking." While the movement may look similar, the caudal initiation by the sit bone coactivates the inner unit which is important in controlling the pelvic rotary force couple. The pelvis has to rotate in the frontal plane for the spine and center of mass of the upper body to laterally shift over the standing leg.

Try it yourself in standing: feel how effective pelvic FP3 is in activating both gluteus medius and minimus with the LPU.

Although a recent study found that standing weight shift onto one leg and hip hitch were more effective than side-lying hip abduction for activating gluteus medius and minimus (Dieterich et al 2015), clinical evidence shows that the "inner unit" is best activated by pelvic FP3 as described.

Compensations: Initiation from the center rather than the pelvis. Hip hiking is a more quadratus lumborum dominant pattern, which does not necessarily contribute to lateral weight shift through the pelvis. Hyperactivity of quadratus lumborum is part of maladaptive CCP behavior, which should not be reinforced, in the interests of spinal health (see Ch. 3). Coactivating axial FP3 helps inhibit CCP strategies (Fig. 4.16b). Another compensation is dominance of underlying pelvic FP2 where the sagittal pelvic neutral is lost.

Functional importance of pelvic FP3

This pelvic pattern:

- controls pelvic rotary force couples in the frontal plane – particularly in providing inner pelvic

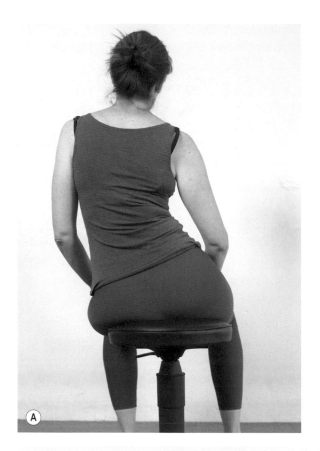

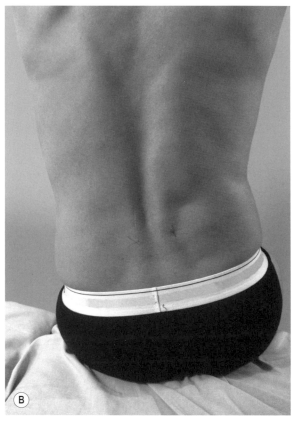

Figure 4.16

a) Pelvic FP3 in sitting. Here, the (L) sit bone sinks and the weight shifts to the (L). The spine and thorax are free to follow the movement and there are reciprocal 3rd pattern changes in the shoulder girdle and head. b) When intrapelvic control is poor and there is stiffness in the lumbo-pelvis, there is poor initiation from pelvic FP3 and the movement is attempted higher up through "cinching" and quadratus lumborum hitching on the (R) – note the divot. The weight does not laterally shift and the spine is not free to adapt in the action.

stability to balance and counter the effects of the outer myofascial activity (especially of all the glutei and tensor fasciae latae)

- is a basic requirement in lateral weight shift and load transfer through the pelvis to stand on one leg without ipsilateral pelvic shift and/or the contralateral pelvis dropping (e.g., when walking or using stairs)

- becomes the pelvic lateral weight transfer pattern in sitting, kneeling and standing. It is the pattern underlying lengthening of the side, laterality, and the ability to reach the upper limb up and laterally into space

- builds upon effective control of pelvic FP1 in sitting and standing and on pelvic FP2 in kneeling.

Also note that:

- the primary agonists in the myofascial synergy driving the pattern of movement are the ipsilateral gluteus medius and minimus; and the LPU synergy – specifically iliacus and psoas, which act to both move and stabilize the pelvis and spine in concert with transversus, multifidus, and quadratus lumborum (see Fig. 2.13)

- the eccentric antagonists contributing to the pattern of movement are likely to be the ipsilateral multifidus, iliacus, psoas, with transversus, quadratus lumborum, PFM, and the adductors.

The Key pelvic lateral weight shift test examines the ability for pelvic FP3 in sitting and standing (Fig. 4.17). Note the pelvic initiation and inclination, and adaptive movement in the spine and upper limb girdle. Further testing challenges the ability to sustain the frontal plane pelvic rotation while tapping the foot or unweighting the leg in various ways.

Patient populations commonly posture more onto one leg by hanging on the iliotibial band, dropping the contralateral pelvis, and flexing that knee – and then have difficulty maintaining a level pelvis in the frontal plane when standing on one leg. The one leg standing test, also known as the stork, Gillet or kinetic test, gives a positive result when control of pelvic FP3 is inadequate (Fig. 4.18a,b).

Training single muscles (e.g., gluteus medius) as a remedy for contralateral lateral pelvic drop overlooks the importance of inner pelvic control and does little to improve control of the pelvic rotary force couples needed to function effectively. It is my clinical impression that overtraining the glutes in isolation, without considering the other contributors in triplanar rotary force couple control, may contribute to the increasingly high incidence of gluteal, hamstring, and other tendinopathies.

The "pelvic drop" exercise (standing on a step and maintaining both knees extended while lowering

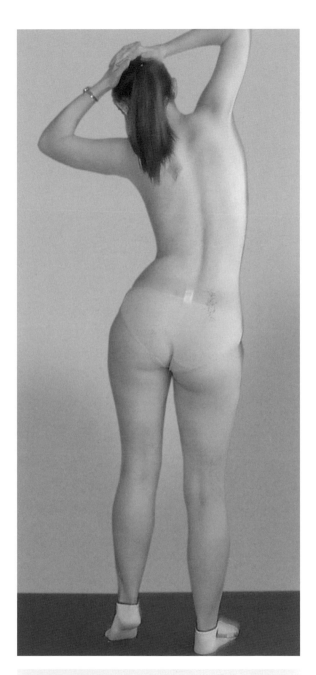

Figure 4.17

The Key lateral pelvic weight shift test – assesses the ability for lateral pelvic rotation and adaptive lateral bending movement through the spine. Here the (R) heel "grounds" to help the (R) sit bone drop while the (L) lifts.

107

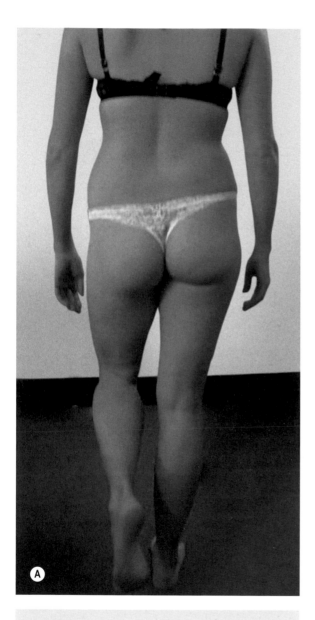

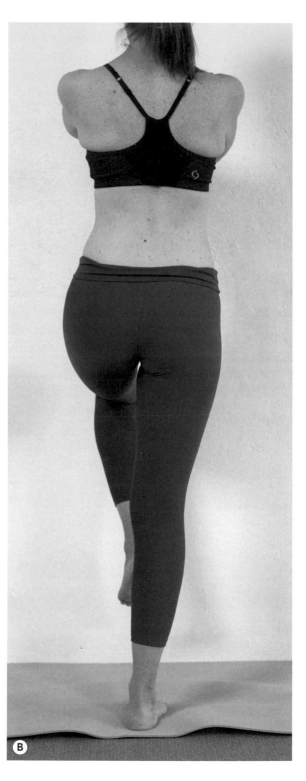

Figure 4.18

a) When control of pelvic FP3 is inadequate, standing on one leg results in the pelvis dropping on the non-weight-bearing side. Note the subject leans slightly over the weight bearing leg and tries to stabilize her spine via central cinch pattern activity. b) When load transfer through the pelvis is effective, the pelvis remains level and the body is balanced above it when standing on one leg.

one foot to the floor and returning it to the step) is a good exercise which activates the inner glutei (O'Sullivan et al 2010) and addresses the frontal plane force couple control through pelvic FP3. However, the exercise as described only returns the pelvis to the horizontal.

The Key pelvic frontal plane test (pelvic FP3) asks for pelvic rotation from the horizontal to upward tilt on the non-weight-bearing side in order to initiate the weight shift through the pelvis and spine.

In standing, pelvic FP3 can be further progressed to a really strong workout by carrying the pelvic drop exercise into pelvic FP3 in order to work the frontal plane pelvic force couple through its full range (Fig. 4.19a,b).

Fourth pelvic fundamental pattern

Pelvic FP4 is concerned with "distorsion" (intrapelvic rotation and sacral torsion): the ipsilateral (right) sit bone reaches long, back, and wide (drops down from the horizon line) while the contralateral sit bone (left) rises and moves slightly medially. (Again, the pattern is described for the right, but the same actions apply to the left.)

The ipsilateral (right) ASIS rotates forward and rises above the horizon line; the contralateral ASIS (left) rotates back and drops below the horizon line. Here, unlike in pelvic FP3, the weight will shift slightly across the pelvis to the medial left buttock and SIJ. The weight will also shift slightly more to the left scapula and the head will rotate to the right (the obverse occurs in rotation to the left).

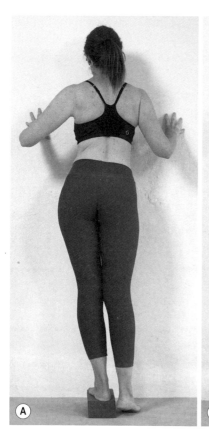
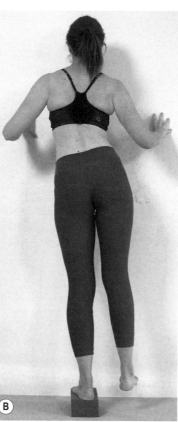

Figure 4.19

a) The pelvic drop test lowers one foot to the floor and returns it level with the step. b) Carrying the movement into end-range pelvic FP3 creates a really strong through-range workout for control of lateral pelvic rotation.

This is a combination of pelvic FP1 on the ipsilateral (right) side and pelvic FP2 on the contralateral (left) side – hence some familiarity and ability in these patterns is advisable before asking for this pattern.

This creates (Fig. 4.20):

- antagonistic innominate rotations in the sagittal plane which distort the pelvic ring

- pulling of the sacrum into torsion

- resultant intrapelvic rotation (which I have called distorsion). This brings about:

- rotation of the whole pelvis and rotation through the spine from the bottom up – in the example here, rotation to the right

- in particular in the joints over the lumbosacral junction, move into "closing" on the right

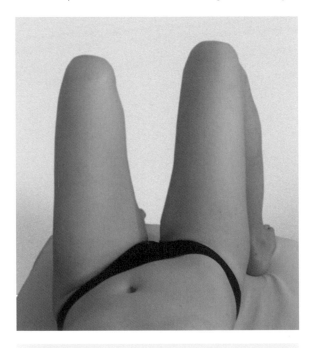

Figure 4.20

Pelvic FP4 initiating with the (R) sit bone. Note the weight shift to the (L).

(extension, right rotation) and a corresponding opening on the left

- antagonistic rotations in the hip joints – in the example here, internal rotation on the right and external on the left.

Watch for: Movement starts from the sit bones and sequences through the spine into rotation up to the head, which also slightly rotates. Watch the thorax because the movement wave should sequence through it and the client should feel the ipsilateral (right) scapula unweight slightly while the point of the right shoulder falls back. Simultaneously engaging the axial FP4 helps control thoracopelvic alignment (Fig. 4.21a).

This can be a difficult pattern for some to achieve. To help facilitate a better response, imagine both innominates as wheels (Franklin 2002) – the ipsilateral (right) wheel rotates forward while the contralateral (left) wheel rotates back. Similarly "growing the knee away" on the ipsilateral (right) side and growing the contralateral (left) knee shorter can also help. Thinking or imagining the movement helps create a more refined perceptuomotor response.

Compensations: The client will want to butt clench and push with the feet, bringing the hip into endrange external rotation and extension to crudely rotate the pelvis as a whole rather than find the intrapelvic action. This is usually associated with CCP strategies which "pop the ribs forward" or wring the waist, which creates a central disconnect, thus disturbing segmental health and blocking the movement wave traveling up through the thorax (Fig. 4.21b). Asking the client to only weight bear through the toes can help to inhibit the mass pushing response in the legs.

When upright, the increased antigravity demands require adequate control of the sagittal plane patterns and pelvic FP3 for effective support and lateral weight shift to facilitate good activation of pelvic FP4 (see Fig. 7.29d). Without this there is increased central cinch activity (Fig. 4.22).

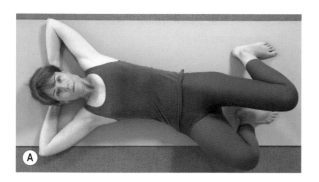

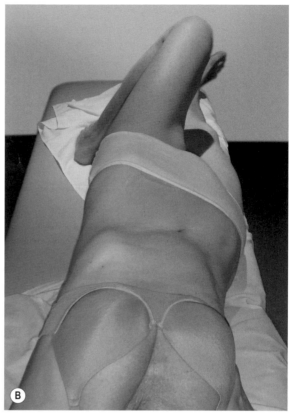

Figure 4.21

a) Pelvic FP4 initiated by the (L) sit bone. Note how the (L) knee has lengthened and the weight has shifted slightly to the (R) and the movement carries through the thorax. b) Incorrect action: shown with one leg extended. While the weight has shifted through the pelvis the subject is using the common dysfunctional pattern of heel push and butt clench with a central posterior cinch. This creates a "central disconnect" – the pelvis goes one way and the thorax the other, and the movement does not sequence through the spine.

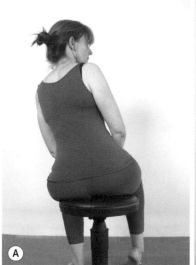

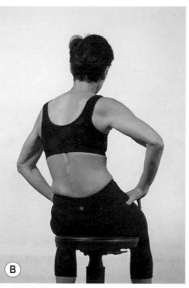

Figure 4.22

Pelvic FP4 in sitting. Note the weight has shifted to the (L) to unweight the (R) sit bone so that it can initiate (R) backward pelvic rotation. b) Incorrect action – the pelvis does not initiate the movement, so there is little weight shift and the spine collapses. Central cinch activity is unusually minimal in this subject – there is more action in the shoulder girdle.

Chapter 4

Functional importance of pelvic FP4

This pelvic pattern:

- controls pelvic rotary force couples in the horizontal plane (forward/backward pelvic rotation)

- controls intrapelvic rotation, and rotation of the pelvis as a whole, which drives rotation in both the spine and hip joints and underlies all axial rotation necessary (e.g., for walking)

- is important in the transitioning from one posture to another, which involves weight shifts and pelvic/axial rotation, particularly those involving level changes (e.g., getting up from the floor)

- underpins the physiological patterns of rotation within the body axis that underlie all sporting prowess

- enables flexibility into distorsion, which is also required in order to gain full range open-chain movements of the hip in opposite directions (e.g., the dancer's high kick – where anterior rotation of one innominate supports full hip extension, and posterior rotation of the other supports full hip flexion).

Pelvic FP overview

The pelvic FPs are functional patterns of movement which "wake up" the pelvis and hips, integrating function between them and the lower spine. Some clients will initially find it difficult to disengage their habitual, dominant superficial muscle strategies in the legs which just lock-in the pelvis. The task is to be able to achieve movement initiation from the pelvis regardless of what position the hip/thigh is in.

Gently guiding the pelvic FPs in side lying is a very nice way of settling low back pain in someone with a very acute presentation because it decompresses and frees the spine. Pelvic FP4 is particularly useful for this. Remember: they are small, discrete movements.[1]

[1] If you search on YouTube for "Side Lying Pelvic Patterns" you can find an accomplished performance by Maria Kirsten, yoga teacher, at: https://www.youtube.com/watch?v=DiHWrPgohx4&t=21s [Accessed 20 March 2018].

Note: The pelvic FPs have been described above in supine, based upon the direction of movement of the sit bones. Taking the example of pelvic FP1: the sit bones "reach long, wide and back," then they drop. In prone their action is still long, wide and back – but they lift. This is also important to consider in all the other postures.

The pelvic patterns, in combination with the axial and other patterns, are practiced repeatedly in various postures and through the various planes of movement. By this means it is possible to create a diverse array of physiological functional movement sequences.

The pelvic patterns are key points of control. The focus is always on initiating the movement from them in lower quadrant movements. This is particularly important when "stretching" tight lower limb myofascia and joints.

Anyone with low back and pelvic pain – and many lower limb disorders – will have poor control of the pelvic FPs. Reinstating them will bring your client on a journey to improved function and less pain.

Shoulder fundamental patterns

The shoulder fundamental patterns give life to the upper spine, thorax, and shoulders (see Ch. 2, The upper quadrant). Grasping these relies on appreciating the key role the claviscapular unit plays as a decoupler between the spine and upper limb in posture and movement.

The shoulder FPs are three-dimensional closed-chain movements of the shoulders that are initiated by the claviscapular unit, not the arm. They underlie all open-chain and closed-chain arm movements.

They are fundamental to our being able to alter and control posture, and initiate movement and shape change, in the upper torso. In addition, they help reestablish control of the shoulder girdle rotary force couples in each movement plane.

The shoulder FPs improve muscle performance problems as well as flexibility. Through them we can access bound/tight myofascia and stiff joints in the torso upper quadrant and arm. Functionally, they are allied with the head fundamental patterns.

The primary focus in their activation is a gentle lift and protraction of the manubrium and movement initiated from the anterosuperior point of the shoulder at the acromion. I often place a paper dot on the upper manubrium and front points of the shoulders to aid the client's awareness of these initiation points (Fig. 4.23). Also focusing upon the associated movements of the nipples can help the patient get the right feel of the spino/claviscapular movements.

The shoulder FPs are initially taught in sitting with the hands placed on the iliac crests, as shown in Fig. 4.23. If the client has insufficient shoulder mobility they can be performed with the arm hanging by the side. Whichever position, the client needs to consciously relax the arms to gain claviscapular initiation.

Ensuring that your client has as near a neutral pelvis and lower spine as is possible helps to facilitate these movements in the upper quadrant (Caneiro et al 2010).

The movements can also be taught unilaterally in side lying, which is a more comfortable position for the acute patient.

We are eventually wanting the client to be able to activate the shoulder FPs no matter what position the arm is in (e.g., hands on head). This is an important aspect to consider when planning a class.

First shoulder fundamental pattern

Shoulder FP1 involves posterior rotation or tilt of the shoulder girdle in the sagittal plane: the manubrium slightly lifts and protracts while the front points of the shoulder initially lift, widen, and draw back before gently dropping. This creates (Fig. 4.23a,b):

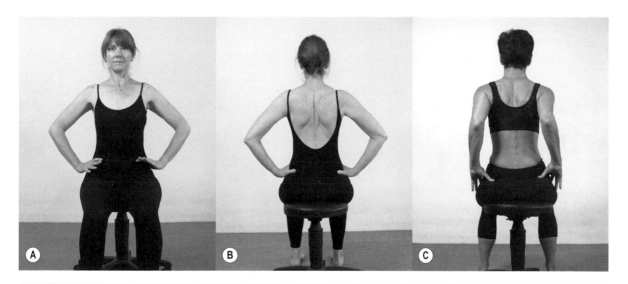

Figure 4.23

Shoulder FP1. a) Correct anterior view: the manubrium moves forward and slightly up and the points of the shoulders move back. The top chest opens. b) Correct posterior view: Note the elbows remain wide and there is good tone in the posterior lower scapular stabilizers – and no central posterior cinch activity. c) Incorrect: The elbows pull back and there is excess activity over the posterior rotator cuff. This subject shows better activity in the posterior lower scapular stabilizers than is usual – and less activity over the lower pole of the thorax than is clinically common.

- posterior tilt of the scapulae, with an associated retraction and inferior translation

- associated upward rotation of the clavicles

- lifting of the anterior upper rib rings via the manubrium while the posterior ribs "drop"

- movement of the spine over the cervicothoracic junction and upper thorax into neutral – and extension

- "lift" in the cervical spine and head above such that they can find their neutral position – the posterior neck lengthens

- lifting and widening of the nipples

- assumption by the shoulder girdle of a neutral position for organizing adaptable stability to optimally support upper limb function

- coactivation of the rotator cuff – the humeral head moving back with slight closed-chain flexion of the glenohumeral joint.

Watch for:

- The manubrium and point of shoulder initiate the movement – they move up, wide, and back before sliding slightly down.

- The elbows are wide and do not pull back, which helps to facilitate the posterior lower scapular stabilizers and anterior rotator cuff to center the humeral head in the glenoid fossa.

- The arms are relaxed with the hands on the iliac crests if possible. This helps to free the clavicle, slightly lifting it off the upper ribs. This is helpful in those with an over-depressed girdle.

- There is simultaneous movement in the manubrium and over the cervicothoracic/upper thoracic spine. The cervical spine is relaxed and able to adaptively lengthen.

Compensations: Where there is poor manubrial contribution, the client will attempt the action by leading back with the elbows rather than the acromion. In so doing, they will tense the arms and overactivate the pectoralis minor and posterior rotator cuff and teres, which will "pop" the anterior shoulders forward and down and protract the scapulae instead. There is no associated movement in the spine (Fig. 4.23c; and see Fig. 3.24). The neck invariably tenses and shortens

When the lower scapular stabilizers are "forgotten" and axial FP control is poor, the client may also compensate by overengaging the thoracolumbar extensors and popping the lower ribs forward (see Ch.3 on CCPs). The manubrium should present forward and the lower ribs "go back" through IAP.

Functional importance of shoulder FP1

This shoulder pattern:

- provides the posterior contribution to balancing the shoulder sagittal rotary force couples

- corrects poor posture by achieving and controlling a neutral spine in the upper quadrant

- assists in mobilizing the lower cervical and upper thoracic spinal region into extension. This is particularly important over the joints of the cervicothoracic junction, which is commonly stiff and flexed with an apparent gibbous or "dowager's hump"

- provides the appropriate postural set to support bringing the head and neck back (e.g., when looking up overhead)

- is an important starting point for effective shoulder rehabilitation, the goal of which is the ability to gain static and dynamic control of the scapula in posterior tilt (and external rotation) – a major component of scapular retraction (Kibler et al 2008). Here the serratus anterior and middle and lower trapezius work together to stabilize the scapula

- supports upper limb movements pulling in toward the body

- is allied with elevation and abduction, external rotation, and extension movements of the upper limb.

Second shoulder fundamental pattern

Shoulder FP2 is responsible for anterior rotation or tilt of the shoulder girdle in the sagittal plane: the points of the shoulder move forward, approximate, and drop as the manubrium drops and retracts.

This creates (Fig. 4.24a,b):

- movement of the scapulae into anterior tilt, with an associated protraction and superior translation

- associated downward rotation of the clavicles

- dropping of the anterior upper rib rings via the manubrium, and lifting posteriorly

- movement of the cervicothoracic junction and upper thoracic spine into flexion

- approximation and dropping of the nipples

- forward movement of the head and shortening of the posterior neck

- forward movement of the humeral head with closed-chain extension of the glenohumeral joint

Watch for: There is little to worry about here as most of your clients will find this pattern easy. However, look for point of shoulder initiation with elbows remaining wide and arms relaxed. Check that there is not excess tension in the cervical spine.

Functional importance of shoulder FP2

This shoulder pattern:

- provides the anterior contribution to balancing shoulder rotary force couples in the sagittal plane

- brings the head and arms down and forward

- supports upper limb movements of reaching forward and pushing away from the body

- is allied with depression, adduction, and internal rotation movements of the upper limb.

When posturally sustained the shoulder girdle is in a non-ideal position for organizing adaptable stability to support the changing demands of upper limb function in elevation.

Imbalance between the first and second shoulder patterns is common, with control of FP1 predictably difficult in patient populations. Most of us work with our head and arms forward and down most of the day

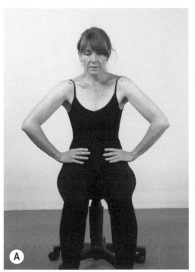 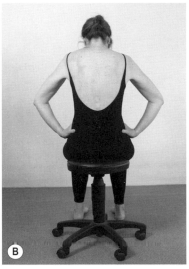

Figure 4.24

Shoulder FP2. a) Anterior view; b) posterior view.

and so we risk becoming stuck in shoulder FP2, which then becomes the default postural set supporting upper quadrant function.

Resulting adaptive myofascial restrictions and ensuing joint stiffness make it even more difficult to move into shoulder FP1. For this reason I rarely prescribe shoulder FP2 except to exaggerate its postural position as one extreme of the available movement between it and shoulder FP1. Oscillating between the two patterns with an emphasis on shoulder FP1 mobilizes the regional spinal segments.

The significance of shoulder FP1 is usually missed in spinal and shoulder rehabilitation. Balance between the first and second shoulder patterns allows a neutral sagittal alignment of the shoulder girdle and upper spine, which is the prelude to gaining good execution of shoulder FP3 and FP4 – and optimal neck function.

Third shoulder fundamental pattern

Shoulder FP3 involves lateral rotation of the shoulder girdle in the frontal plane. From the sagittal neutral shoulder girdle position (the client usually needs to be cued into shoulder FP1 to achieve this): the ipsilateral (right) point of the shoulder lifts and moves to the right as the manubrium shifts to the right and the contralateral (left) point of shoulder drops. There is minimal forward movement of both points of the shoulder. [The pattern is described for the right scapula leading, but the same actions apply to the left.]

This creates (Fig. 4.25a,b):

- backward rotation and elevation of the lateral end of the right clavicle and upward scapula rotation with superior translation

- a corresponding downward scapula rotation, with inferior translation on the left and associated clavicular depression

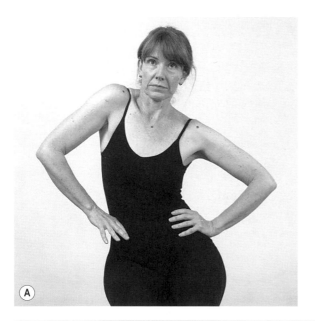 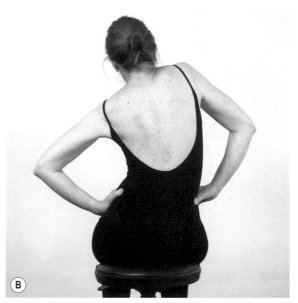

Figure 4.25

Shoulder FP3. a) Correct anterior view. The (R) point of the shoulder initiates the movement. b) Correct posterior view. Note the lateral opening through the (R) thorax and armpit chest.

- lateral shift of the manubrium and upper rib rings to the right, with lateral rib "fanning" and elongation of the lateral "armpit chest"

- lifting, and movement to the right of the right nipple

- left side bending of the cervicothoracic spinal segments together with (left) rib approximation and shortening of the left lateral armpit chest

- slight side bending of the head and neck

- closed-chain glenohumeral adduction on the upward rotating scapula (with hands on hips)

- closed-chain glenohumeral abduction on the downward rotating scapula.

Watch for: Ensure the point of the shoulder leads the movement and the elbows remain wide with arms relaxed. Keeping the point of the shoulder back helps ensure a sustained sagittal neutral posture and that the scapulae ideally remain in some retraction. Expect to see lateral movement in the upper thoracic spine.

Encourage the claviscapula lifting with upper thoracic lateral shifting action rather than the dropping of the other scapula.

Compensations: The lower pole of the thorax initiates the movement via CCPs. There may be loss of sagittal neutral spine and dominance of shoulder FP2. Most patients will also attempt to overemphasize the scapula depression and jam the scapula down as they punch the point of the shoulder forward. In other words, ensure that scapula depression is "soft" – and scapula is retracted not protracted (see Fig. 4.25).

Functional importance of shoulder FP3

This shoulder pattern:

- controls lateral scapular rotation, particularly upward rotation of the claviscapular unit to support arm elevation

- Initiates lateral weight shift through the upper quadrant

- mobilizes the upper thoracic spine and thorax.

Oscillating the action between sides helps to mobilize the lower cervical and upper thoracic spinal region by encouraging lateral shift of the upper thorax and contralateral side bending. This helps mobilize the cervicothoracic junction and upper thorax, which is commonly stiff into extension, lateral flexion, and rotation.

The upward-rotation shrug of the shoulder with the glenohumeral joint in 30° abduction (shoulder FP3 with hands on hips) has been shown to be more effective in activating the upper and lower trapezius force couple and facilitating upward scapular rotation than the standard shrug with the arms by the side (Pizzari et al 2014).

Shrug exercises with the arm in 90°, and particularly 150° of abduction, elicit greater activity of the lower trapezius and serratus anterior relative to the levator scapulae and can be effective in reducing a depressed and downwardly rotated claviscapular unit posture (Choi et al 2015) (see Fig. 7.27a).

It has also been found that retracting the scapula (a combination of shoulder FPs 1, 3 and 4) with the arm overhead is a most effective way to activate the medial lower scapular stabilizers (Castelein et al 2016) – and has the added advantage of also creating eccentric myofascial lengthening of the commonly tight posterior rotator cuff and teres myofascia (see Fig. 7.27b).

Fourth shoulder fundamental pattern

Shoulder FP4 is responsible for backward and forward shoulder rotation in the horizontal plane. From the sagittal neutral shoulder girdle position (the client usually needs to be cued into shoulder FP1 to achieve this): the manubrium moves forward and the ipsilateral (right) point of the shoulder widens and draws back and the manubrium rotates to the right. The opposite point of the shoulder (left) moves forward. [Backward shoulder rotation on the right is described.]

This creates (Fig. 4.26a,b):

- right scapular external rotation, posterior rotation or tilt, and retraction – and an associated upward rotation and retraction of the right clavicle

- a corresponding left forward shoulder rotation involving left scapular internal rotation, anterior rotation or tilt, and protraction – and an associated downward rotation and protraction of the left clavicle

- drawing of the manubrium, upper ribs, and cervicothoracic spine into right rotation

- the right nipple leads the left into right rotation

- the head will usually follow into right rotation – however, this is not obligatory.

Watch for: A sustained sagittal neutral posture and that the point of the shoulder leads the movement back - not the elbow. Expect to see scapula retraction with backward shoulder rotation and rotation in the upper spine and head.

Similar to the fourth pattern in the pelvis, shoulder FP4 is a combination of the first and second shoulder patterns.

Compensations: The posterior rotator cuff overengages – in concert with pectoralis minor which blocks the movement; emphasis on forward shoulder rotation rather than backward rotation; the movement is initiated via CCP activity around the lower pole of the thorax; there is little movement in the spine and increased neck and arm tension (Fig. 4.26c).

Functional importance of shoulder FP4

This shoulder pattern:

- supports rotary movements initiated in the upper limb girdle (e.g., cocking the arm up and back for a tennis serve)

- provides appropriate postural sets to support head and neck movements

- contributes to rotary mobility of the cervicothoracic spine

- initiates rotation in the upper body (e.g., forehand and backhand in tennis)

- contributes to energy efficiency in functional movement (e.g., contralateral arm swing in walking).

Shoulder FP overview

These functional patterns of movement mobilise the upper thorax and wake up the neuromuscular control of the posterior upper thoracic and claviscapular myofascia, integrating function between the shoulder girdle and spine. They help to mobilize the lower cervical and upper thoracic spinal region and thorax – particularly into extension, lateral shift, and contralateral side bending. They are basic to shoulder function as they reinstate important patterns of movement commonly lost in people with upper quadrant pains.

The shoulder FPs have been described in sitting. The same actions apply in all other postures, where they are repeatedly drilled in various arm positions through all planes of movement. The focus is always that the shoulder FPs initiate upper quadrant movements. This is particularly important when stretching tight myofascia and joints.

Scapular stabilization exercises have been a common focus in rehabilitation. The "scapula setting" or "scapular orientation exercise" is frequently prescribed but acknowledged as difficult for patients to learn accurately (Mottram et al 2007). This is not surprising given the commonly found deficits in the medial lower scapular stabilizers (middle and lower trapezius and serratus anterior) and related poor control of the three-dimensional scapular rotary force couples. McQuade and colleagues (2016) challenged the scapular stability paradigm, pointing out that the scapula can only function as a robust energy transfer system when it is capable of movement variability

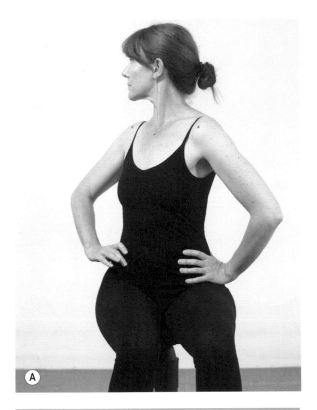

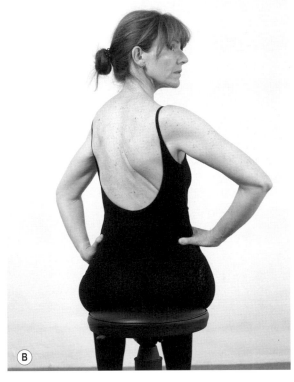

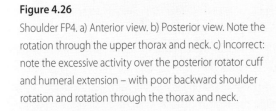

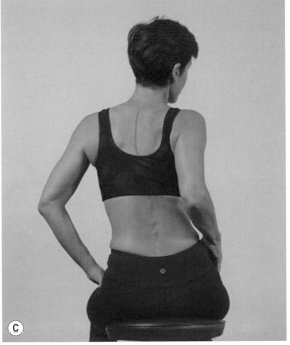

Figure 4.26
Shoulder FP4. a) Anterior view. b) Posterior view. Note the rotation through the upper thorax and neck. c) Incorrect: note the excessive activity over the posterior rotator cuff and humeral extension – with poor backward shoulder rotation and rotation through the thorax and neck.

(which gives it a resilience that is more desirable than static stability).

In the rehabilitation of shoulder function, restoring three-dimensional control of the scapula into posterior rotation or tilt, external rotation, and upward rotation are important (Kibler et al 2013). The lower scapular stabilizers are best activated in specific functional patterns (as opposed to isolated muscle activity) where the serratus anterior and lower scapular stabilizers are coactivated as stabilizers in retraction. The first, third and fourth shoulder patterns are the foundations that enable this movement.

Performing the FPs in different arm positions improves adaptive control. Shrugging with the arm overhead (see Fig. 7.27a) favors the trapezius upward rotation force couple (desirable) over rhomboids and levator scapulae (undesirable). Retraction performed here engages the medial scapular muscles (Castelein et al 2016) and is more likely to facilitate increased lower trapezius activity and less upper trapezius activity (De Mey et al 2013) (see Fig. 7.27b).

As a prelude to more advanced scapular retraction exercises with resistance and/or involving the whole trunk and lower extremity functional kinetic chain, it is important that the client can properly execute and sustain shoulder FP1, FP3 and FP4 to avoid "lock-in" compensations in the shoulder and upper trunk.

A common mistake is to add inappropriate load, resistance and/or an unstable surface without adequate control of the shoulder FPs; for example, performing a push-up (press-up) can overactivate the superficial upper trapezius and glenohumeral muscles (pectoralis major) while scapular muscle activity is actually decreased (De Mey et al 2014). Loading the shoulder without control of the fundamental patterns reinforces aberrant patterns and loading – the likely cause of the initial problem.

Often underappreciated is the degree to which shoulder girdle movement dysfunction adversely affects the spine. Similarly, segmental dysfunction in the upper thoracic and cervical spines significantly contributes to most shoulder and upper limb pain disorders (see Ch. 1, On injuries).

While improving scapular control early in shoulder rehabilitation is a common goal, the coupled movements of the clavicle and spine via the sternum are usually not well appreciated.

Gaining correct control of the shoulder FPs will improve upper quadrant function and lead to improved treatment outcomes in the management of all upper quadrant pain disorders (i.e., of the spine, shoulder, and upper limb) irrespective of the varying pathological diagnoses.

Head fundamental patterns

These are discrete, well-localized movements, with the axis of movement at the top of the neck – "think it" at about the base of the ear! Correctly performed, they restore mobility to the upper spine. (See also Chapter 2, The upper quadrant.)

Like the other FPs, they are in fact rotations with associated translations in the three movement planes. Unlike the other FPs, however, the points of initiation are different in each plane of movement.

Head FP1 is best initially taught in supine. Later, when well controlled, it and head FP3 and FP4 can be taught in sitting while actively controlling head FP1 to maintain a sagittal neutral head position. Visual feedback from a mirror is useful to encourage the client to move their head but not their neck.

First head fundamental pattern (in lying)

Head FP1 is responsible for anterior sagittal rotation of the occiput on the upper neck. Ensure the head is appropriately supported in supine crook lying with a neutral pelvis: the chin fully drops and retracts; the back of the head slides north.

This creates (Fig. 4.27a):

- flexion of the head on the upper neck; nodding as in saying "yes"

- (when performed in sitting) an associated posterior shift or retraction of the head in space. This is ideally co-associated with shoulder FP1. The neck lengthens (see Fig. 3.31b).

Watch for: The movement is localized to the upper spine. Cue it with: "Feel that you have four double chins," and "Feel the muscles working under your jaw." Looking downward also assists the movement. Increasingly sustain the action while breathing naturally. Head FP1 aims to preferentially activate the deep cervical flexor muscles, hence the sternomastoids should be minimally active. Head FP1 in lying has also been described as the craniocervical flexion test (Jull et al 2008).

Progression: The exercise can be carefully progressed by maintaining the position while attempting to just unweight the head from the support (O'Leary et al 2007). The forehead leads the movement (see Fig. 4.27b) rather than the chin (Fig. 4.27c).

Compensations: Poor upper cervical movement and excessive mid- and lower cervical flexion; overactivity of the sternomastoids in both head support and particularly when attempting to unweight the head (whereby the chin lifts and protracts and the occiput posteriorly rotates instead). It is important that the pelvis is not in habitual posterior tilt, which, because of the head/tailbone functional connection, makes head FP1 more difficult to achieve. Try it yourself (and then note that it is easier when the pelvis is in FP1).

Functional importance of head FP1

This head pattern:

- provides anterior force couple control to balance the head on the top of the spine and allows appropriate adaptive postural support

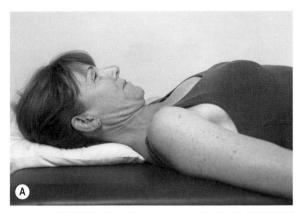

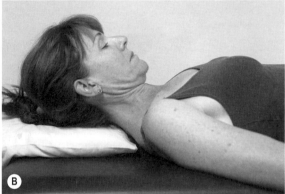

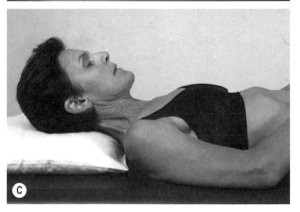

Figure 4.27

Head FP1. Correct craniocervical flexion (a) is maintained during unweighting the head (b); and note how the forehead leads the movement. Incorrect unweight (c): note the craniocervical flexion is not maintained and the increased tension in the superficial neck muscles.

- initiates flexion in the upper spine and torso in supine

- contributes to patterns of movement supporting looking down, facial expression, swallowing, phonation, etc.

- contributes to forward weight shift patterns.

In patient populations head FP1 is also commonly non-automatic and difficult to "find" when upright and moving. This is especially the case when attempting to sit up straight. Lengthening the spine relies upon coactivation of head FP1 with pelvis FP1 (see Fig. 4.2). Falla et al (2007) showed that postural reeducation in sitting, in order to create a neutral pelvis and spine, greatly improved craniocervical deep flexor activity automatically.

Performing neck retraction or "posterior gliding" exercises in the absence of some ability in head FP1 and shoulder FP1 risks shearing and overworking the mid-cervical segments. However, with attention to detail in coactivating head FP1 with shoulder FP1 (see Figs 3.31b and 7.26a), it is a great way to train both the lazy deep neck flexors and lower scapular stabilizers in healthier patterns of spinal postural control.

Second head fundamental pattern

Head FP2 controls posterior sagittal rotation of the head on the neck. The chin protracts and lifts. The back of the skull slides south.

This creates:

- extension of the head on the neck

- associated protraction and anterior shift of the head in space when upright (Fig. 4.28).

Watch for: Movement is well localized to the upper cervical spine – looking up can assist this.

Compensations: Most patients are "strong" in this pattern, albeit it poorly localized to the upper segments.

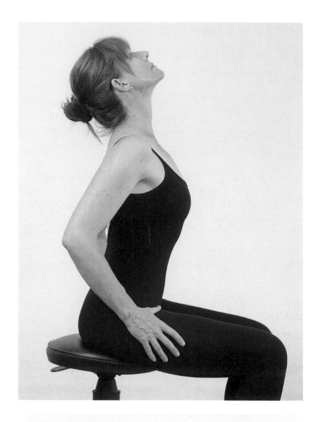

Figure 4.28
Head FP2 sitting. The occiput posteriorly rotates on the upper neck.

Functional importance of head FP2

This head pattern:

- makes the posterior contribution to sagittal force couple control – although this is usually dominant

- contributes to patterns of movement supporting looking up/overhead, facial expression, jaw opening, etc.

Third head fundamental pattern (in sitting or standing)

Head FP3 is responsible for lateral occipital rotation in the frontal plane. From the sagittal neutral head position (clients usually need prior cueing into the first patterns in the pelvis and shoulder girdle): "Think of moving your left ear slightly to the left and lifting it and point the right ear to your shoulder."

This creates (see Fig. 7.26b):

- right lateral tilt of the head and upper cervical spine.

Watch for: Lateral rotation of the head on the neck.

Compensations: Loss of sagittal neutral head position and movement poorly localized, with lateral flexion of the mid-cervical spine instead (Fig. 4.29).

Functional importance of head FP3

This head pattern:

- helps orient the head for auditory acuity and facial expression

- allows appropriate adaptive head movements in response to lateral weight shift through the spine and proximal limb girdles

- is involved in postural righting reactions.

Fourth head fundamental pattern

Head FP4 controls head rotation in the transverse plane. From the sagittal neutral head position (the client usually also needs prior cueing to obtain this): the eyes lead the head turning – to about 45°.

This creates (see Fig. 7.26c):

- head rotation on the upper neck.

Watch for: The ability to isolate head/upper cervical rotation and maintenance of alignment via head FP1 during the movement.

Compensations: Most commonly, movement occurs mainly in the mid-cervical spine; the sagittal alignment is lost, and the rotation is accompanied by lateral flexion (Fig. 4.30).

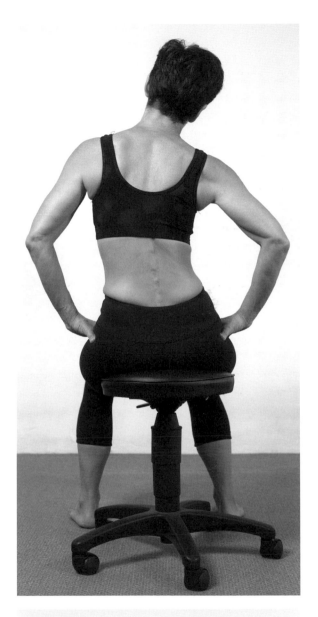

Figure 4.29
Head FP3. The lateral movement of the head on the neck is poorly localized – the mid-cervical levels overwork.

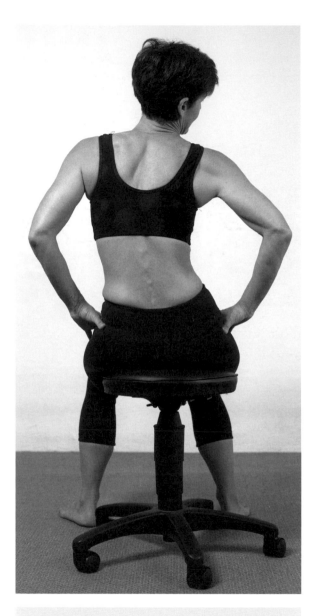

Figure 4.30
Head FP4. Rotation of the head on the neck, particularly at C1–2, is poorly localized – the movement mostly occurs over the mid-cervical levels – and this also involves side bending.

Functional importance of head FP4

This head pattern:

- initiates rotation in the upper spine
- initiates weight shift in the upper body
- orients head positioning for sensory acuity.

Eye movements: There is a close coupling between eye movements and head FP1, FP2, and FP4. The eyes, however, are themselves also capable of independently rotating in the transverse and sagittal planes, and combinations thereof, while the head remains still. Asking for synchronous or asynchronous eye movements while the head is both stable or moving is a nice way to break up tension in the posterior suboccipital muscles and facilitate deep cervical flexor activity.

Jaw movements: There is a close functional relationship between the temporomandibular joint (TMJ) and the joints of the cervicocranial junction. TMJ problems are invariably related to defective upper cervical joint function and head FP control – particularly of head FP1.

Head FP overview

The role of the head in movement is often overlooked. It being our primary communication center and information gatherer means that balancing it well on the top of the spine is one of the neuromuscular system's major tasks. Receptors as the base of the skull influence muscle tone throughout the body. The head initiates a lot of upper spinal movement – particularly in the sagittal and transverse planes. Yet our modern lifestyle finds the head hanging forward as we stare at a screen for much of the day, and our arms are similarly used down and forward. The spine follows – and in time gradually loses its sagittal control and ability for easily sustained upright support. The office-bound human literally "leads with his chin" in movement generally, compensations set in, and sensory acuity is dulled. Spinal movement suffers and so do we.

The eight basic postures and their variations: the platforms for initiating movement

The fundamental patterns are initially taught as described above and become a basic template for incorporating into all movement patterns in which the FPs initiate and guide the movements.

They are drilled in many and varied ways in various postures in the three planes of movement so as to aid their integration into the person's movement behavior. Varying the limb positions in each of the postures effectively targets myofascial restrictions in both the limbs and torso in different ways.

The basic postures are as follows:

- Supine

- Side lying – and also arm supported side lying

- Prone

- All fours – and variations with this

- Sitting variations:

    ○ upright in a chair with hips and knees at a right angle

    ○ long (legs extended)

    ○ sitting kneel

    ○ side

    ○ cross-legged

- Kneeling: upright and half kneeling

- Standing

- Inverted postures: head, shoulder and hand standing (for the advanced!).

Note: In all sitting variations except for the first, it is highly likely that you will need to provide appropriate support under the pelvis to accommodate stiffness in the hips and/or restrictions in posterior

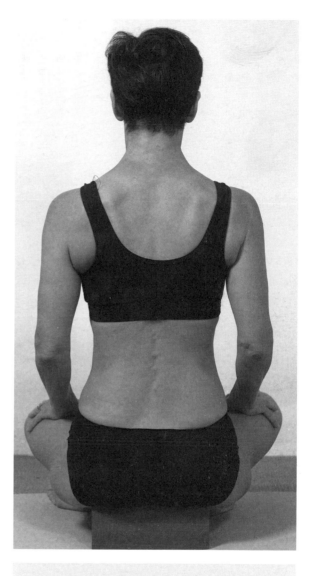

Figure 4.31
Support under pelvis helps the subject achieve a neutral pelvis and spine in cross leg sitting.

myofascial chain. In so doing you are helping the client to achieve a sagittal neutral pelvis and spine (Fig. 4.31).

Equipment is useful to accommodate restricted range of movement, open stiff areas, and provide different types of support from which to work the FPs

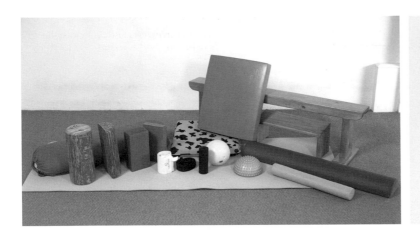

Figure 4.32
Some of the common props which we variably incorporate in classes (L) to (R): Bolster; Rolla; small D roll; large foam block; small foam block; Key Moves Core Retrainer Belt; flat cushion; rigid strap; small Blackroll; 3" firm foam cushion; small ball; spiky pod; long D roll; small noodle – and behind: kneeling stool and bench.

(Fig. 4.32). For example, a supine posture can be lying flat on the floor; lying back over a bolster, D roll or spiky pod in various configurations; lying along a bench; or lying back over a ball.

In postures which open the proximal limb girdles (e.g., Ch. 7, Exercises 2, 4, 39, 41, 56, and 57), supporting the limb may be necessary in order for the client to relax into the stretch.

Recommended reading

Franklin E (2002) Pelvic power for men and women – Mind/body exercise for strength, flexibility posture and balance. Hightstown, NJ: Elysian Editions, Princeton Book Company.

Key J (2010) Back pain: A movement problem. A clinical approach incorporating relevant research and practice. Edinburgh: Churchill Livingstone Elsevier.

Kolar P, Kobesova A, Valouchova P, Bitnar P (2014) Dynamic neuromuscular stabilisation: Developmental kinesiology: breathing stereotypes and postural locomotor function. In: Chaitow L, Bradley D, and Gilbert C (eds) Recognising and treating breathing pattern disorders. Edinburgh: Churchill Livingstone Elsevier.

Kyndall l, Boyle PT, Lewis C (2010) The value of blowing up a balloon. Am J Sports Phys Ther 5(3):179–188.

Myers T (2014) Anatomy Trains: Myofascial meridians for manual and movement therapists, 3rd edn. Edinburgh: Churchill Livingstone/Elsevier.

References

Andersson E, Oddsson L, Grundström, Thorstensson A (1995) The role of psoas and iliacus muscles for stability and movement of the lumbar, pelvis and hip. Scand J Med Sci Sports 5:10–16.

Brumagne S, Dolan P, Pickar JG (2013) What is the relation between proprioception and low back pain? In: Hodges PW, Cholewicki J, Van Dieën JH (eds) Spinal control: The rehabilitation of back pain. State of the art and science, Edinburgh: Churchill Livingstone Elsevier.

Bussey MD, Bell ML Milosavljevic S (2009) The influence of hip abduction and external rotation on sacroiliac motion. Man Ther 14(5):520–525.

Caneiro JP, O'Sullivan P, Burnett A et al (2010) The influence of different sitting postures on head/neck posture and muscle activity. Man Therapy 15:54–60.

Castelein B, Cools A, Parlevliet T, Cagnie B (2016) Modifying the shoulder joint position during shrugging and retraction exercises alters the activation of the medial scapular muscles. Man Ther 21:250–255.

Choi W-J, Cynn HS, Lee CH et al (2015) Shrug exercises combined with shoulder abduction improve scapular upward rotator activity and scapular alignment in subjects with scapular downward rotation impairment. J Electromyogr Kinesiol 25(2):363–370.

Crommert ME, Ekblom MM, Thorstensson A (2011) Activation of transversus abdominis varies with postural demand in standing. Gait Posture 33(3):473–477.

De Mey K, Danneels L, Cagnie B et al (2013) Kinetic chain influences on upper and lower trapezius muscle activation during eight variations of a scapular retraction exercise in overhead athletes. J Sci Med Sport 16:65–70.

De Mey K, Danneels L, Cagnie B et al (2014) Shoulder muscle activation levels during four closed kinetic chain exercises with and without Redcord slings. J Strength Cond Res 28(6):1626–1635.

Dieterich A, Petzke F, Pickard C et al (2015) Differentiation of gluteus medius and minimus activity in weight bearing and non-weight bearing exercises by M-mode ultrasound imaging. Man Ther 20(5):715–722.

Falla D, O'Leary S, Fagan A, Jull G (2007) Recruitment of the deep cervical flexor muscles during a postural correction exercise performed in sitting. Man Ther 12:139–143.

Franklin E (2002) Pelvic Power for men and women – Mind/body exercise for strength, flexibility posture and balance. Hightstown, NJ: Elysian Editions, Princeton Book Company.

Hodges PW, Gandevia SC (2000) Changes in intra-abdominal pressure during postural and respiratory activation of the human diaphragm. J Appl Physiol 89:967–976.

Hodges PW, Sapsford R, Pengel LHM (2007) Postural and respiratory functions of the pelvic floor muscles. Neurourol and Urodyn 26:362–371.

Hodges PW, Tsao H, Sims K (2015) Gain of postural responses increases in response to real and anticipated pain. Exp Brain Res 233:2745–2752.

Ishida H, Watanabe S (2013) Changes in lateral abdominal muscles' thickness immediately after the abdominal drawing-in maneuver and maximum expiration. J Bodyw Mov Ther 17(2):254–258.

Jull GA, O'Leary SP, Falla DL (2008) Clinical assessment of the deep cervical flexor muscles: The craniocervical flexion test. J Manipulative Physiol Therap 31(7):525–533.

Kibler WB, Sciascia AD, Uhl TL et al (2008) Electromyographic analysis of specific exercises for scapular control in early phases of shoulder rehabilitation. Am J Sports Med 36(9):1789–1798.

Kibler WB, Ludewig PM, McClure PW et al (2013) Clinical implications of scapular dyskinesis in shoulder injury: The 2013 consensus statement from the "scapular summit". Br J Sports Med 10.1136/bjsports-2013-092425.

Kolar P, Neuwirth J Sanda J et al (2009) Analysis of diaphragm movement during tidal breathing and during its activation while breath holding using MRI synchronized with spirometry. Physiol Res 58:383–392.

McGill S (2002) Low back disorders: Evidence based prevention and rehabilitation. Champaign, IL: Human Kinetics, p.210.

McQuade KJ, Borstad J, de Oliveira AS (2016) Critical and theoretical perspective on scapular stabilisation: What does it really mean, and are we on the right track? Phys Ther 96(8)1162–1169.

Mottram SL, Woledge RC, Morrissey D (2007) Motion analysis study of a scapular orientation exercise and subjects' ability to learn the exercise. Man Ther 2009 14(1):13–18. Epub 2007 Oct 1.

O'Leary S, Jull G, Kim M, Vicenzino B (2007) Specificity in retraining craniocervical flexor muscle performance. J Orthop Sports Phys Ther 37(1):3–9.

O'Sullivan K, Smith SM, Sainsbury D (2010) Electromyographic analysis of three subdivisions of gluteus medius during weight bearing exercises. Sports Med Arthrosc Rehabil Ther Technol 2:17.

Park RJ, Tsao H, Claus A et al (2013) Changes in the regional activity of psoas major and quadratus lumborum with voluntary trunk and hip tasks and different spinal curvatures in sitting. J Orthop Sports Phys Ther 43(2):74–82.

Pizzari T, Wickham J, Balster S et al (2014) Modifying a shrug exercise can facilitate the upward rotator muscles of the scapula. Clin Biomech 29:201–205.

Reeve A, Dilley A (2009) Effects of posture on the thickness of transversus abdominis in pain-free subjects. Man Ther 14(6):679–684.

Richardson C, Hodges P, Hides J (2004) Therapeutic exercise for lumbopelvic stabilization. A motor control approach for the treatment and prevention of low back pain, 2nd edn. Edinburgh: Churchill Livingstone.

Tsao H, Galea M, Hodges PW (2010) Driving plasticity in the motor cortex in recurrent low back pain. Eur J Pain 14(8):832–839.

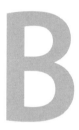

B

Getting to work rebuilding enhanced spinal movement control

Body posture is a key aspect of spinal health. The astute movement therapist is able to read the body for the clues it offers about altered function in the postural/movement system. Seeing "the wood for the trees" is a practiced art.

In both sitting and standing, the body gives clues about the likely quality of movement control. Essentially we are interested in the "line of the body" (how the major units of mass are organized in postural alignment) and its kinematics (the shape it carves in movement). We are also keen to read the muscle contours and shape of the body axis, which give clues about the quality of inner support and control mechanisms.

The quality of movement, however, is of prime interest. We need to know: *how* it happens; where it starts; how it sequences through the body, and its ease and integration with breathing.

This is a whole body approach. Understanding the continuous body-wide nature of the fascial system helps see the interconnectedness of dys/function and symptoms.

However, in the clinic you will usually be dealing with a regional problem, such as neck pain, where you would look for possible features of the shoulder crossed syndrome, and examine the head and shoulder FPs, control of the center, and breathing before deciding on a relevant, appropriately staged, specific exercise program. Needless to say, you would also be advising on pelvic position for sitting well.

In a class situation you will be working with the whole body and the functional movement relationships between regions and their interaction with the center. This is further developed in Chapters 7 and 8.

The following is a clinical assessment battery: a guide to what to look for and possibly test. Treat it as a reference rather than thinking that you need to do all the tests with each client.

Noticing signs of the clinical syndromes, inferior tethers, and other features of altered movement behavior described in Chapter 3 gives clues as to the likely movement strategy the client will adopt in the tests below, and also helps hone your observational and cueing skills in a class situation.

The "failed movement test" becomes the exercise therapy. But there are likely to be many!

When observing movement in both the formal tests and during a class, it is important that you can begin to identify the "key" missing patterns: those which, when reinstated, will improve the quality of the movement.

With practice you will be able to prioritize which of the fundamental patterns need to be reestablished first. In addition, you will want to ascertain which functional movements are required most, so that the relevant patterns can be drilled for improved function.

Assessment algorithm

Initial assessment

Observation

Your first contact with a client is usually with them sitting, fully dressed, as you get their story. This is an important observation time where they will not realize what you are doing, so it can yield valuable information.

Note:

- their habitual sitting postures, readiness to move, level of arousal, etc.

- their breathing pattern – when dysfunctional, the shoulders and/or upper chest lift on inhalation and a notable gasping may be apparent when they speak

- any breath holding in some of the specific tests.

Standing assessment

Observation

For formal observation to be informative, the patient needs to be in their underwear. Diagnosis is based upon simple observation of postural alignment, body shape, muscle contours, and the quality of spinal stabilization and movement in simple movement tests.

If a test movement does not reproduce pain, that does not mean it is normal. Aberrant movement will more than likely cause pain sooner or later. If pain is reproduced, it shows the system is indeed struggling. To repeat: it is the *quality* of control that is important.

Patients in each pelvic crossed syndrome subgroup exhibit distinct features of kinesiopathological movement creating predictable stresses on the spine.

The following assessment guide includes the most common tests and possibilities you may observe and find

Side view: informs the quality of sagittal alignment (see Ch.3):

- Evidence of pelvic crossed syndromes? Subgrouping will provide further clues as to what to expect in movement and will guide exercise choice.

- Evidence of the shoulder crossed syndrome?

From behind: observe the body shape, muscle contours and limb positions. Active muscles are bulky with well-defined contours.

- Balanced spinal curves and even myofascial tone? Is there a lordosis? If so, where is it? CPC activity can lead to a high lumbar pseudo lordosis instead of a normal low lordosis (see Fig. 3.19).

- Symmetry in the spine and pelvis? Alternatively, is there a pelvic lateral shift and/or rotation with scoliosis? (This can either be structural or due to an acute psoas spasm.)

- Layer syndrome? Bands of torso myofascial hyperactivity and hypoactivity give clues as to the quality of habitual spinal movement (Fig. 5.1; see Fig. 3.2a).

- Evidence of the "Key sign"? Presence indicates poor core support and control (see Figs 5.1; 3.12 and 3.13).

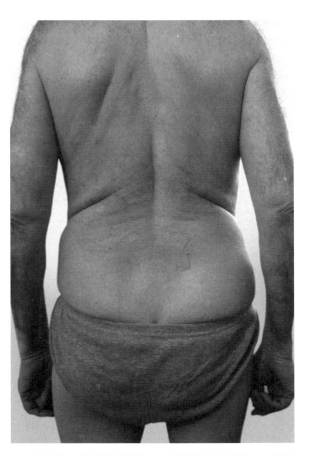

Figure 5.1

Layer syndrome. Note the banding of myofascial activity – particularly the central posterior cinch and associated Key signs – and the poor myofascial tone over the interscapular and lumbosacral areas.

In the **lower quadrant**, check for evidence of pelvic inferior tethers.

- Stance position – equal weight through both legs? "Propping" (see Fig. 3.16) with hyperextended knees? Hanging on one leg and the iliotibial band?

- Foot position – centrated, pronated, or externally rotated? Increased external rotation is common on the symptomatic side in lower quadrant pain disorders and can indicate an SIJ problem and/or asymmetrical pelvic inferior tethers (see Fig. 3.35a).

- Tail tuck? If so, is there also either "butt clench" or passive reliance on the iliofemoral ligaments together with poor gluteal activity? (Fig. 5.2a,b).

In the **upper quadrant**, check for evidence of shoulder crossed syndrome (Fig. 5.3):

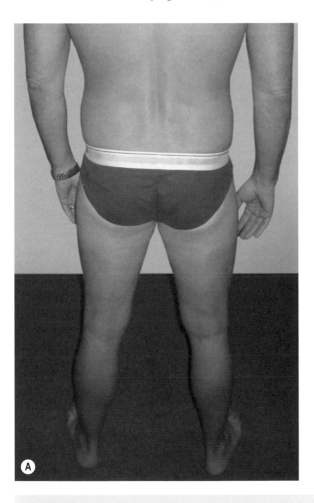

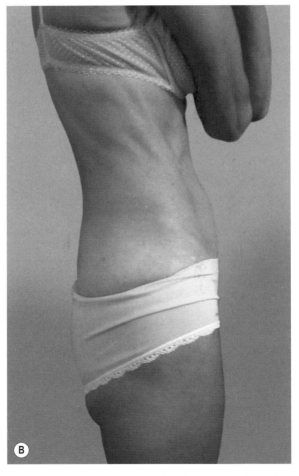

Figure 5.2

a) Creases in the pants can indicate active butt clenching, which is usually part of a more dominant lower limb synergy of external rotation/abduction/extension. The inferior pelvis is "drawn in." It usually occurs in a posterior PXS or mixed syndrome. b) Hanging end range on the iliofemoral ligaments with poor gluteal tone usually indicates an anterior PXS. Both strategies feed into the development of pelvic "inferior tethers."

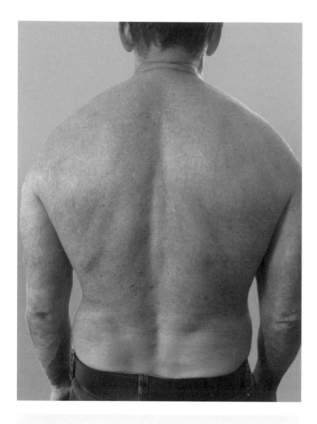

Figure 5.3

Shoulder XS from behind. Note the increased kyphosis and shoulder girdle protraction and downward rotation – and that the arms are postured in flexion/internal rotation. The client presented with shoulder pain.

- Increased internal rotation of one or both arms?

- Scapula in abduction/protraction, anterior tilt, internal rotation?

- Increased thoracic kyphosis/dome and cervico-thoracic gibbus?

- "Upper Key Sign"? (See Fig. 3.23). This usually indicates dominant shoulder inferior tether activity and related thoracic joint and rib involvement – common in shoulder and upper limb pain disorders (e.g., rotator cuff or tennis elbow).

Anterior view: again observe the body shape, muscle contours and limb positions:

- Is there evidence of layer syndrome? (see Ch. 3) – observe the abdominal wall in particular as this greatly helps with subclassification (Fig. 5.4; also see Figs 3.2b, 3.6).

In the **lower quadrant**, check for the following:

- Alignment of the legs, inner thigh, and quadriceps contours – position of the feet and/or patellae (turnout/turn in) may indicate a hip rotation bias.

- What position are the feet in? Any sign of hallux valgus? These can indicate persistent medial loading; prominent long toe flexor tendons indicate poor intrinsic activity.

In the **upper quadrant**, check for apparent shoulder inferior tethers:

- Observe the anterior neck muscle contours – is there prominence of the sternomastoids and/or scaleni? (usually apparent in a shoulder XS) (see Fig. 3.25).

- Bulk and symmetry in the pectorals?

- Claviscapular spatial position? Point of shoulders drawing down/in?

- Arm is postured in some flexion and internal rotation? This will be the case when the upper limb flexor myofascial chain is dominant.

Simple movement testing in standing

In the **lower quadrant**, check the following:

- Habitual forward bending pattern – look for hip/pelvis initiation vs spinal initiation. Note evenness of segmental movement, willingness to move and whether this produces pain (Fig. 5.5a,b; see Fig. 3.17).

- Ability to modify the forward bending pattern with cueing to "let the knees move forward

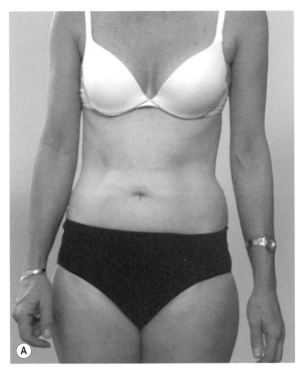

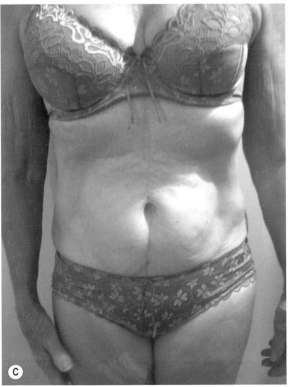

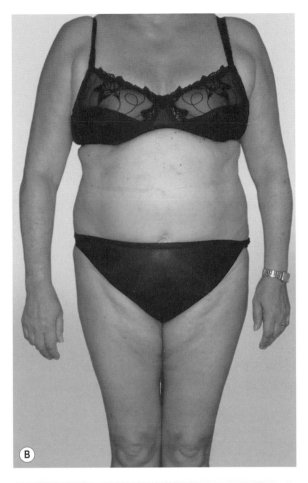

Figure 5.4

Anterolateral abdominal wall (ALAW) dysfunction. a) Anterior PXS with hyperactivity of the upper ALAW. b) Posterior PXS with underactivity of the whole ALAW. c) Mixed syndrome on a primary posterior PXS picture: this presentation usually occurs when the subject has been diligently pulling in the stomach – resulting in abdominal "suck in" and lift of the thorax.

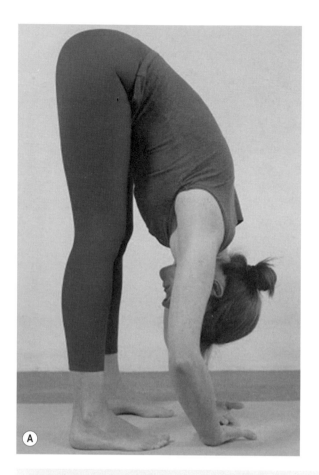

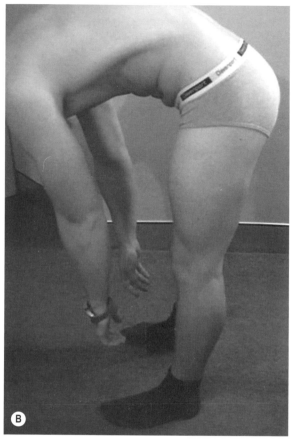

Figure 5.5

Forward bend pattern. a) This is perfect forward bending in a yogi! You can see the length in the posterior inferior myofascial chain and the full anterior pelvic rotation which allows the spine to drape forward. In particular, note the high point of the ischial tuberosities. b) Dysfunctional forward bend. Note the posterior inferior myofascial chain tethering which prevents both the pelvis from rotating anteriorly and ischia from lifting; the spine compensates by over-flexing. The subject was a personal trainer who presented because of low back pain.

while the sit bones move up back and wide." If pain was present in the habitual pattern, does it change with modifying the kinematics? What is the quality of pelvic control in this? Does CPC activity increase here? (Fig. 5.6)

- Any fixed distorsion in the pelvic ring on forward bending. Distorsion is a natural movement but problems arise when it becomes fixed on

one side (see Ch. 2, Pelvic fulcrum and Fig. 2.14; Ch. 4, Pelvic FP4).

The distorsion test is indicated if there are unilateral symptoms in the spine, pelvis, hip or lower limb. Stand behind your client and place your thumbs on the posterior inferior iliac spine (PIIS) – coming onto this from below (Fig. 5.7a). Note whether they are level or if one is lower. Follow the movement of the PIIS during the

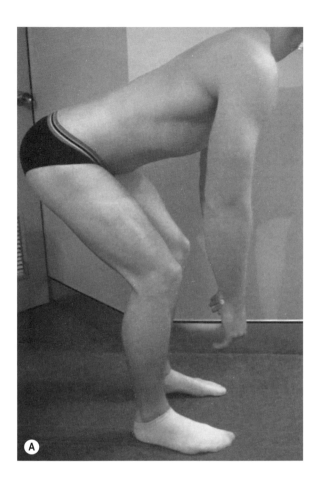

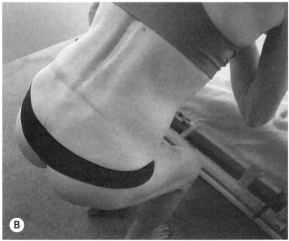

Figure 5.6

Ability to modify the forward bending pattern.
a) The same subject shown in Fig. 5.5b had an adaptable neuromyofascial/articular system and was able to change his pattern in one visit. b) Entrenched dysfunction. Intrapelvic/hip/spinal joint and myofascial restrictions and reliance on central cinch patterns because of poor core support make changing the pattern difficult. This is why we need to work for pelvic and core control at the same time. The subject was a "gym junkie" and had undergone decompression surgery for a (R) sciatica and footdrop.

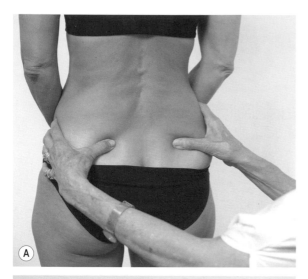

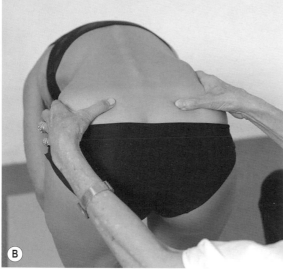

Figure 5.7

Testing for pelvic "distorsion" in forward bending. a) Start position. b) Asymmetrical response – the (R) posterior inferior iliac spine moves south, which indicates a problem on the (R).

forward bend, noting whether they remain level (if they were) – or not. Commonly, the PIIS on the symptomatic side will "stop" or "tug south" on the symptomatic side (Fig. 5.7b). This occurs because of more joint and/ or myofascial restrictions in the ipsilateral posterior inferior myofascial chain (over the hip/pelvis or in the hamstrings or calf) or all through. These limit anterior rotation of the innominate (and pull the sacrum into a torsion such that it and L5 on the decreased anterior iliac rotation side are "stuck open" – as is that SIJ. This will likely lead to joint and neural bother, and further tightness of the relevant myofascia. A vicious cycle sets in that can explain chronic SIJ pain, sciatica, hip bursitis, gluteal tendinopathies, femoroacetabular impingement, and many other lower limb pain disorders.

A positive test is likely to be paired with decreased ipsilateral "closing" of the lumbosacral junction on the pelvic lateral weight shift test to the contralateral side (see below).

- *Extension/back bending.* Does the pelvis anteriorly translate? Is there even segmental movement into extension in each region, or does the CPC activity "lock" the spine over the thoracolumbar region with little movement in the thorax and pelvis (i.e., posterior PXS; Fig. 5.8a)? Alternatively, does the pelvis shift anteriorly without much intersegmental movement into extension (i.e., anterior PXS; Fig. 5.8b)?

- *Pelvic spatial shift in the three planes.* Note any asymmetry, pain, and spinal segmental movement, and the ability of the pelvis rather than CCPs to initiate the movement (Fig. 5.9a,b). Decreased closing and/or pain may be apparent over the lumbosacral junction, particularly in lateral shifting.

- *The Key pelvic lateral weight shift test* (see Ch. 4, Pelvic FP3). This provides a lot of information about the spine, regarding not only the ability for pelvic initiation and adaptive spinal control

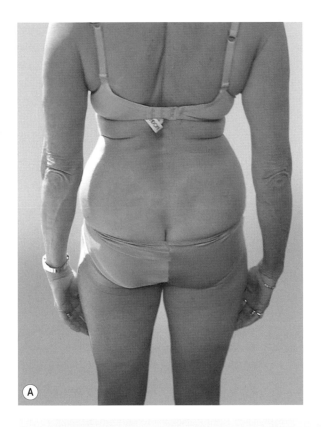

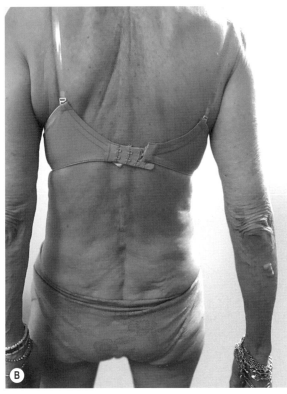

Figure 5.8

Spinal extension. In a posterior PXS or mixed syndrome there is little anterior pelvic shift and usually an increase in central posterior cinch "locking" without much segmental movement – particularly over the lumbosacral levels. b) In an anterior PXS the pelvis shifts more anteriorly with very little intersegmental movement through the spine.

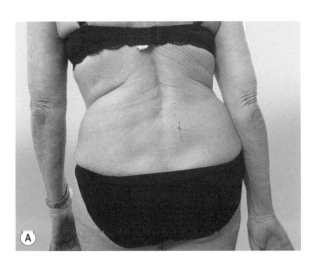

Figure 5.9

Asymmetry in spatial lateral pelvic shift. Note the lack of movement within the pelvis and over the low lumbar levels – particularly extension and the "closing" movements (notably over the (R) lumbosacral region). Also note the marked central posterior cinching and Key signs. The X marks the site of the client's local back pain. She also had a (R) gluteal bursitis.

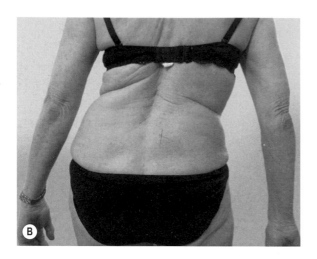

Figure 5.9 *continued*

but also the evenness and quality of intersegmental movement (Fig. 5.10a,b). When pain is produced it can give insights into its source. For example, if right leg pain is produced with weight shift onto the right leg, the source could be either the spine, SIJ, hip or knee. If right leg pain is produced with a left lateral weight shift, the source is likely to be in the spine.

- *Standing on one leg.* Look for the ability to maintain a neutral triplanar pelvic position and the quality of spinal stabilization by checking whether the inferior tethers are being utilized for control (Fig. 5.11a,b; see Fig. 4.18b).

- *Squat pattern.* Observe free-form kinematics and ability to control pelvic FP1 without central posterior cinching. Watch for pelvic inferior tether dominance and the pelvis rolling into posterior tilt. Is there flexibility in the leg kinetic chain? (See Fig. 3.15)

- *Limb load tests.* If hunting down a problem, look for quality of pelvic/spinal alignment and control with triplanar open-chain hip movements. Does hip extension lead to central posterior cinching or hip flexion lead to lumbar flexion? Both of these are caused by poor pelvic control in anterior rotation (Fig. 5.12a,b).

- *Walking pattern.* I find it easier to look from behind: does the pelvis drop on the "swing" leg side and/or does the person laterally lean over the stance leg to bring the center of gravity over the leg (Trendelenburg effect)? These both indicate weakness of pelvic FP3. Is there contralateral rotation between the pelvis and shoulder girdle? Is there rotation within the thorax? Rotation should be maximal through the dorsal hinge around T7. A dome and stiff thorax will prevent this. Look for creases in their clothing when they walk, because most of the movement will be occurring here. With CCP behavior the excessive creases are over the high waist. Do the arms swing, or are they held in flexion which blocks rotation via shoulder FP4?

- If your client is a runner, check their running style, keeping the above points in mind.

Sitting assessment

Observation

- Habitual posture (this will usually be adopted all day long; see Fig. 3.32). Look for pelvic position, as it dictates the quality of spinal support. Are all the sagittal curves present?

- Evident shoulder crossed syndrome? Look from the side, front, back, and obliquely (see Figs 3.9 and 5.3). If the client complains of shoulder or upper limb pain, observe for any fullness of the infraclavicular and supraclavicular region and "tenting" of the scaleni (Fig. 5.13).

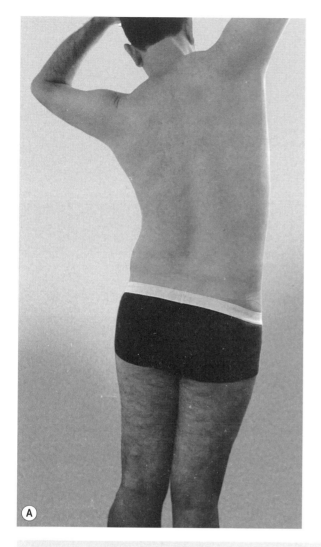
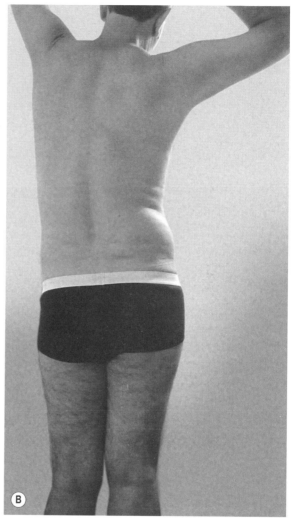

Figure 5.10

Key pelvic lateral weight shift test (KPLWST) shows up differing patterns of pelvic and related spinal movement. a) In the (R) KPLWS the client somewhat laterally rotates his pelvis and comes onto the (R) leg with reasonable adaptive spinal movement. b) In the (L) KPLWST he shows poor lateral pelvic rotation and (R) lumbosacral closing, plus weight shift over the (L) leg. Note the poor closing/tissue bunching over the (R) lumbosacral region and how he then compensates over his (R) thoracolumbar junction. Also note the (R) lateral waist bulge indicative of a weak transversus. He also shows features of a layer syndrome, has generally poor lumbosacral movement and had (R) sciatica.

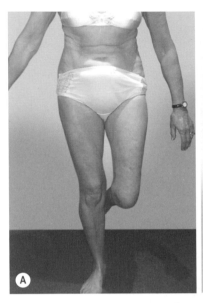

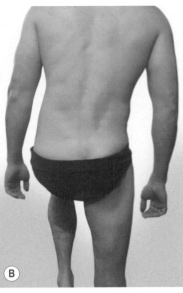

Figure 5.11

Standing on one leg. One should not only look at the quality of triplanar pelvic control but also weight shift and the pattern of spinal stabilization. a) Poor pelvic control is compensated for by marked central anterior cinching in an anterior PXS subject. b) Inferior tethers limit pelvic control, which is associated with poor weight shift through the pelvis and compensations in the spine (skin redness is a post-treatment effect).

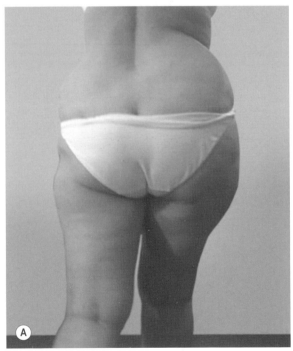

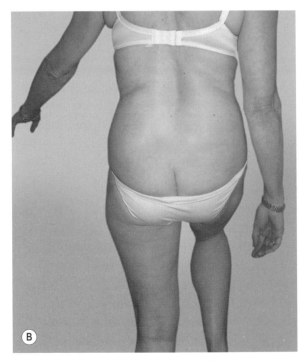

Figure 5.12

a) Hip extension without the pelvis moving into anterior rotation results in increased central posterior cinch activity and also inclining the trunk forward. b) Hip flexion becomes lumbosacral flexion There is no life in the pelvis, occasioning central cinching in an attempt to stabilize the spine – and there is little weight shift, hence balance is poor.

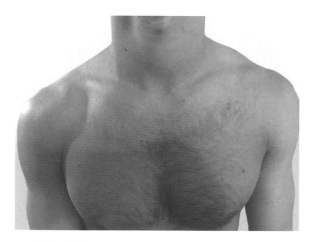

Figure 5.13

Shoulder XS signs. There is increased sternomastoid activity and scaleni "tenting" (R) > (L). Note the divot and (R) clavicular depression because of increased pectoral activity. Also note the fullness of the (R) 2/3 costosternal junction. The subject had (R) shoulder pain.

- Note the breathing pattern. If the spine is collapsed, lifting the upper shoulders and chest is likely – but unhealthy. Are the accessory breathing muscles (the scaleni, sternomastoids, pectorals) prominent? (See Fig. 5.13.)

Simple movement testing

In the **lower quadrant**:

- Can the client sit up and align the pelvis and spine in "neutral" (without CCPs, upper body tension and breath holding)? (See Figs 3.33, 4.2, and 4.13.)

- What is the quality of axial alignment and stabilization in response to active limb load? Ideally the spine remains in neutral (Fig. 5.14a) and there is no central cinch activity as shown in Fig. 5.14b and c.

- After cueing a neutral pelvis and spine, what is the quality of pelvic alignment and stabilization when

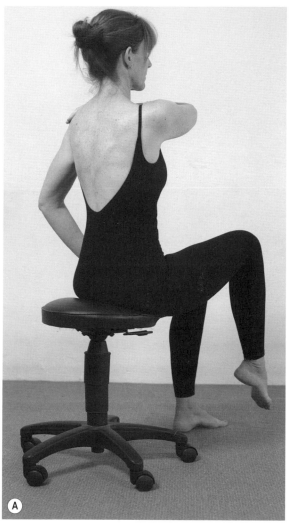

Ⓐ

Figure 5.14

Hip flexion core challenge in sitting. a) Pelvic and spinal alignment is maintained.

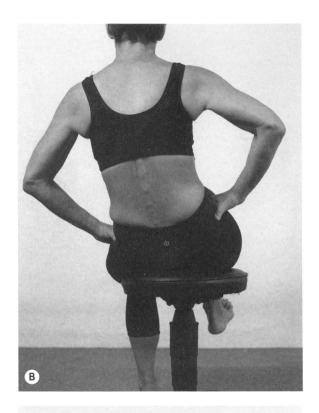

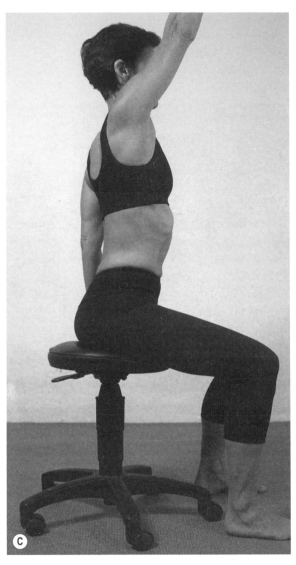

Figure 5.14 *continued*
b) Unhealthy control with loss of sagittal neutral plus lateral "Leaning Tower of Pisa." c) The model attempts to demonstrate increased central posterior cinch activity and loss of sagittal alignment upon arm elevation, which is barely discernible as her function is so good!

knee extension is asked for in sitting? Pelvic inferior tethers will make an upright neutral difficult due to tightness in the posteroinferior myofascial chain, limiting both hip flexion and knee extension. Poor LPU activity results in loss of pelvic stability on knee extension (Fig. 5.15a). It is advisable to palpate the PIIS here – I do not like there to be any movement at all. If the pelvis can remain neutral, is there active posterior (or anterior) cinch activity (Fig. 5.15b)? Ideally, there should be none.

- Test the breathing pattern. From behind, gently wrap your hands around the lower rib cage and feel for posterolateral basal expansion (Fig. 5.16). The thorax should not lift, neither should the scapulae lift and/or anteriorly tilt (which would indicate an upper chest breathing pattern).

- Test the client's ability in performing the axial FP and "opening the center" (see Ch. 4, Controlling the center, Figs 4.4 and 4.5). Slightly lower your

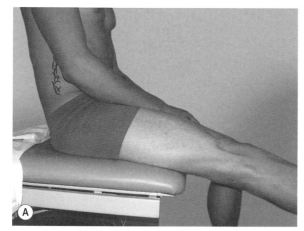

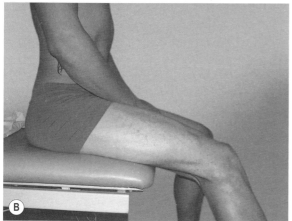

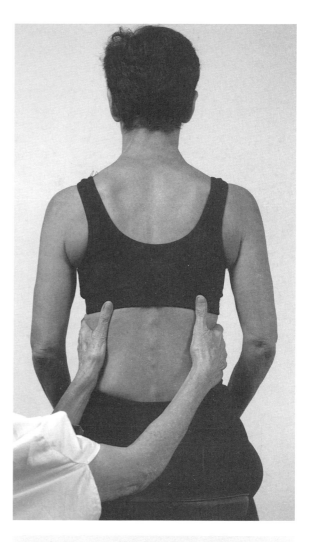

Figure 5.15

a) Poor intrapelvic control leads to posterior tilt and spinal collapse on knee extension. b) Here the client manages to control the pelvis but central cinch activity is evident. He also needs to keep working at integrating better axial FP control as he controls the pelvis well.

Figure 5.16

Practitioner hand-hold position for testing posterior basal breathing and lateral expansion.

hands from the breathing test position so they encircle the lower rib cage and your thumb tips are over the end of the 12th rib and ask, "Can you expand back and wide into my thumb and hands?" Look for sustained activation and a regular breathing pattern.

There should be a firming over the lower abdominal wall and under your thumbs. If competent, you may decide to challenge this further by adding limb load.

- Test performance of the pelvic fundamental patterns (see Ch. 4): Look for the pelvis initiating and the ability of the spine adaptably following the pelvis:

  o Pelvic FP1 – see Fig. 4.13

○ Pelvic FP2 – I do not test this as a rule. I may ask clients to do it for clarity of the opposite movement to pelvic FP1

○ Pelvic FP3 – see Fig. 4.16. This is the Key pelvic lateral weight shift test in sitting. It requires some underlying control from pelvic FP1

○ Pelvic FP4 – see Fig. 4.22 and Fig. 7.29d. This requires some ability in control of pelvic FP1 and pelvic FP3.

• Test weight shift initiated in the pelvis:

○ Pelvic FP1 is carried into forward weight shift – look for pelvis initiation (see Fig. 7.30a) – not the head and shoulders (Fig. 5.17)

○ Test backward weight shift through pelvic FP2. Does the thorax posteriorly translate into axial FP2 (Fig. 5.18a)? Or is "jacking" apparent because of weak abdominals, central posterior cinching and psoas fixing, which are common in posterior PXS (Fig. 5.18b)?

○ Pelvic FP1 + FP3 is carried into lateral weight shift of the whole torso (see Fig. 4.16). Placing the hands on the head helps inform about the ease of myofascial flexibility and joint mobility in the upper quadrant (see Fig. 7.49a) – as well as the ability to control the center through axial FP1 and axial FP3 (Fig. 5.19).

• Moving from sitting to standing – and from standing to sitting:

○ This involves further forward weight shift initiated through pelvic FP1 to unweight the pelvis before moving into pelvic FP2 to stand up. On return to sitting pelvic FP1 still initiates. Does the pelvis initiate the movement in both directions, or do the head and shoulders initiate through head FP2 and shoulder FP2 in a more primitive pattern of "total flexion" of the axis – and probably pushing up through the upper limbs (Fig. 5.20).

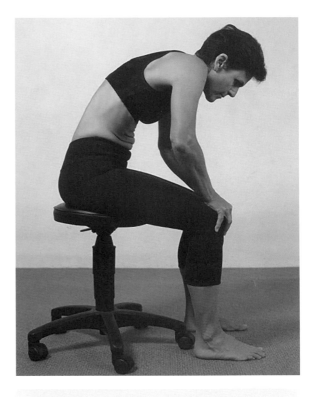

Figure 5.17

Poor control of pelvic FP1 leads to poor forward weight shift initiated in the pelvis. Instead, the head and shoulders lead the movement and the pelvis is left behind.

In the upper quadrant, perform the following:

• Test diaphragmatic breathing pattern and ability in the axial FP (see Figs 4.5 and 5.16).

• Test active neck and head movements: flexion/extension; rotation; side bending:

○ What is the quality of upper quadrant spinal alignment prior to testing?

○ What is the contribution of adaptive postural support in the thorax/shoulder girdle to support neck movements? (Fig. 5.21) Is there segmental movement between C6 and T6?

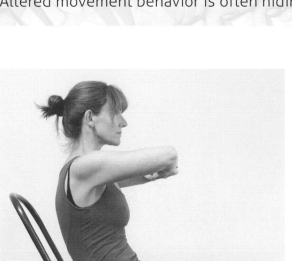

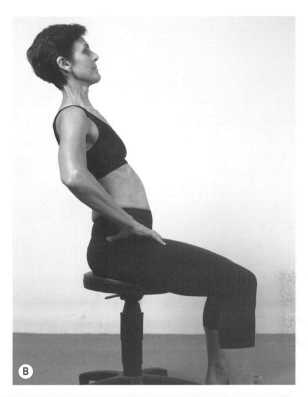

Figure 5.18

a) Integrated control between pelvic FP2 and the axial FP2 in backward weight shift – the spine adapts to the movement and the posterior thoracolumbar region "opens." b) Poor control of the axial FP in movement leads to poor backward weight shift and adaptive control of the center, which is replaced by "jacking" with central posterior cinch activity and associated holding with psoas.

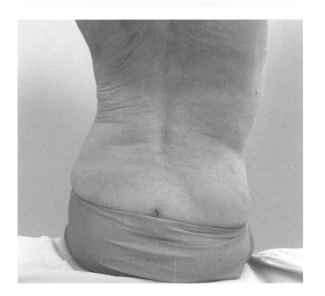

Figure 5.19

Poor initiation and control of the pelvis in both the sagittal and, particularly, the frontal plane. There is little adaptive weight shift and movement through the spine and thorax. Note: because of a reliance upon central cinch patterns, the (R) thoracolumbar region does not open and there is poor control of the center.

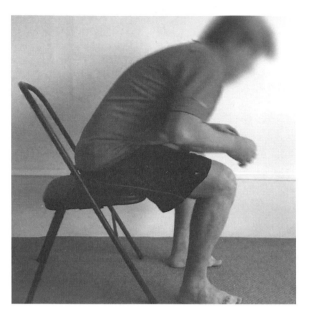

Figure 5.20
Unhealthy sit/stand in total spinal flexion and arm push –
the head and arms lead.

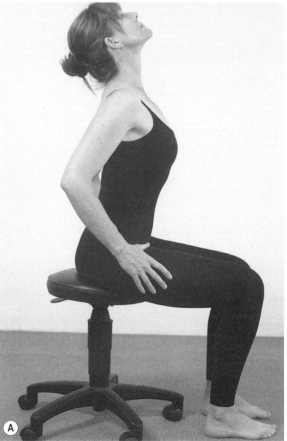

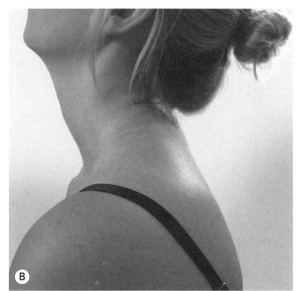

B

A

Figure 5.21
a) Cervical extension is supported by good posturo-
movement in the upper pole of the thorax into extension.
b) Poor/no thoracic intersegmental postural setting into
extension to support neck extension. Despite her youth,
note the gibbous over the cervicothoracic junction and
relative "hinge" in the movement around C5–6.

○ What is the pattern of segmental movement in the cervical spine? In particular, is there a sense of movement in the cervicocranial and cervicothoracic junctions, or "hinging" in the mid cervical spine? (Fig. 5.22.)

• Test active open-chain shoulder movements: elevation in flexion and abduction; extension; horizontal flexion and extension; hand behind back and head (see Ch.4, Fundamental shoulder patterns).

Look for appropriate positioning and stability of the shoulder girdle and ability to maintain axial alignment.

Hand behind back is interesting: shoulder inferior tethers and associated glenohumeral internal rotation deficit (GIRD) limit this activity. As a result, the client compensates by over-engaging shoulder FP2 and

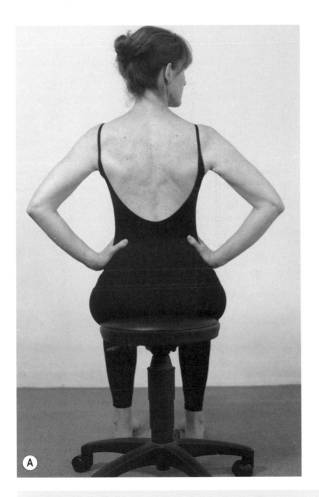

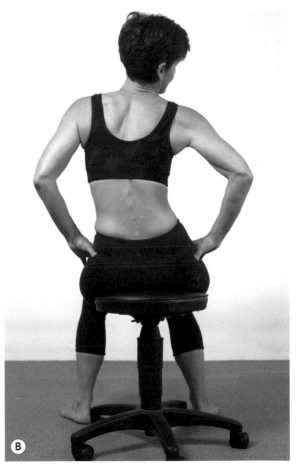

Figure 5.22

a) Good rotation in the cervical spine relies upon good control of the head on the neck, with adaptive postural support through the cervicothoracic junction and upper thorax; the head remains poised and well-balanced on top of the spine. b) When movement and control through the cervicocranial and cervicothoracic junctions and upper thorax is defective, rotation mainly occurs in the mid-cervical spine and is often associated with lateral flexion.

further depressing and anteriorly tilting the clavis-capular unit, thus losing alignment. Pain is common (Fig. 5.23). See also Figs 3.24, 3.26, 3.28, 3.29, 3.30.

- Test performance of the shoulder FPs (see Ch. 4, Shoulder fundamental patterns). Look for ability to initiate from the claviscapular unit and movement sequencing through to the spine; arms remaining soft and no central cinching and/or neck tension. If the client is unable to place their hands on their hips, test the shoulder FPs with arms by their side

  - Shoulder FP1 – see Figs 3.24 and 4.23

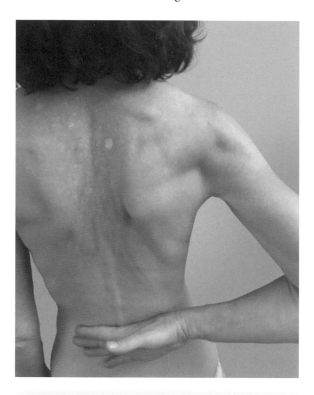

Figure 5.23
GIRD is well seen in placing the arm behind the back. The lack of flexibility in the posterior rotator cuff is compensated for by increased anterior inferior tether activity which anteriorly and downwardly rotates the claviscapula (shoulder FP2). Note also the increased activity of levator scapulae, upper trapezius, and rhomboids.

- Shoulder FP2 – as in pelvic FP2, I usually do not test this

- Shoulder FP3 – see Fig. 4.25. This is responsible for lateral weight shift through the upper quadrant. It requires some underlying control from shoulder FP1

- Shoulder FP4 – see Fig. 4.26. This requires some ability in control of shoulder FP1 and shoulder FP3.

- Test performance of the head FPs and the quality of neck movements (see Ch. 4, Fundamental head patterns). Ability in the head patterns is closely allied to ability in the shoulder patterns – especially shoulder FP1 – in gaining a neutral upper quadrant alignment. The head patterns also functionally relate to the pelvic patterns in movement

  - Head FP1 – see Fig. 7.26a

  - Head FP2 – see Fig. 4.28. I usually do not test this, because it is commonly the habitual posture

  - Head FP3 – see Fig. 7.26b

  - Head FP4 – see Fig. 7.26c.

Supine lying assessment

Observation

- What posture does the body assume? To which subgroup does the person belong? Posterior PXS people will have a lifted thorax (see Fig. 4.6); anterior PXS subjects assume a more fetal posture. Postures are a reflection of the dominant patterns of myofascial activity, so particularly note both the pelvic position (is it tucked in posterior tilt; Fig. 5.24a?) and the lower limb position (Fig. 5.24b).

- Identify the breathing pattern.

Specific movement testing

- Ability to change the breathing pattern if indicated?

- Ability to perform the axial FP (see Ch.4, Assessing and teaching the basic axial FP).

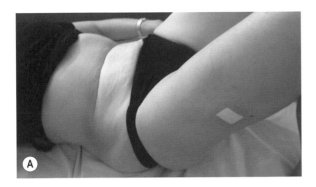

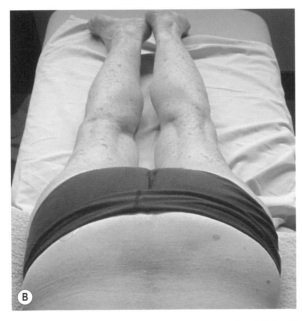

- Pelvic crossed syndrome subgrouping helps delineate likely performance difficulties.

- Passive range of movement testing in the pelvic/hip and thorax/shoulder girdle – for any myofascial and joint restrictions as a result of pelvic and shoulder girdle inferior tethers.

- Discrete ability in performance of the pelvic patterns (see Ch. 4, Fundamental pelvic patterns, and Figs 4.11, 4.15 and 4.20).

- Limb load tests such as the ASLR test. Note that this is quite a high load test which should not be attempted if your client has a lot of pain. Also note the quality of axial stabilization: is the axial FP active (see Ch. 4: Controlling the center), or is there central anterior cinching? (See Figs 3.6; 3.11) Conversely, in a posterior PXS client, underactivity of the abdominal wall and poor stability of the lower thorax is common – and this may also involve a diastasis recti abdominis (Fig. 5.25). Proper control of the axial FP usually eliminates the latter.

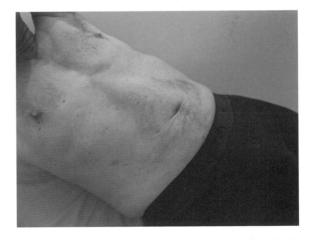

Figure 5.24

In supine crook lying an anterior PXS subject invariably postures the pelvis into posterior tilt, indicative of pelvic "inferior tether" hyperactivity. The supraumbilical fold is indicative of hyperactivity in the upper abdominal wall. Noticing this helps predict what you might find when testing the axial FP. The subject suffered from incontinence and had been rigorously "pulling in her tummy" and tightening her pelvic floor. Continence dramatically improved with ceasing these activities plus manual treatment and more appropriate exercise prescription. b) Excess external hip rotation and asymmetry is usually (but not always) predictive of the major symptoms being on the more externally rotated side.

Figure 5.25

A diastasis recti abdominis can be common in the posterior PXS subgroup. It will often disappear when the axial FP becomes properly reestablished.

Chapter 5

Prone lying assessment

Observation

- General myofascial tone of the back. With the patient relaxed there should be no activity at rest. CPC activity at rest is evidence of the layer syndrome (Fig. 5.26).

Movement testing

- Ability to perform the axial FP prone. In a healthy pattern there is evident posterolateral expansion of the lower pole of the thorax. Is there ability to sustain this opening with regular slow diaphragmatic breathing?

- Sphinx position: this demonstrates spinal mobility into extension – or otherwise (Fig. 5.27a). Note the natural extension in the young baby (Fig. 5.27b).

- Ability in performing the pelvic patterns – notably pelvic FP1 – without coexisting CPC activity. Backward pelvic rotation (see Ch.7, Exercise 16) involves pelvic FP4. Poor pelvic

FP4 initiation results in cinching and "winding" at the waist together with lack of movement sequencing through the thorax (Fig. 5.28).

- Pattern of axial stabilization on limb load or lifting the head. Is there healthy axial FP control in hip extension (Fig. 5.29a) – or unhealthy CPC on lifting the leg or head (Fig. 5.29b)?

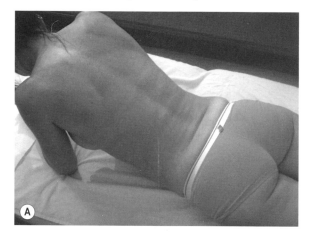

A

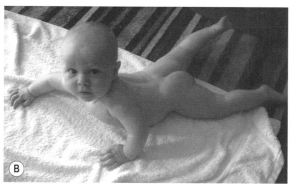

B

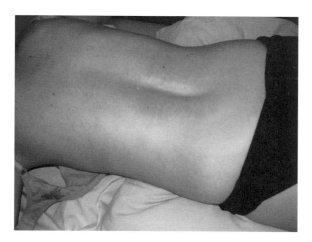

Figure 5.26
Active central posterior cinch activity at rest usually indicates underlying irritable local/regional spinal joints; this is in addition to CNS "hard wiring" of "cinch patterns" for postural control.

Figure 5.27
Sphinx is often very informative. Look for: lack of extension (the spine should be able to accommodate the position); evenness of segmental movement; regional skin pleating like overstretched elastic (which can indicate how much of the time that part of the spine is postured and moved in flexion); and segmental spasm, which can indicate symptomatic levels. Stiffness and discomfort is common. b) Note the flexible extension in the 6-month-old baby.

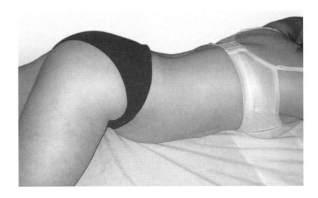

Figure 5.28

Prone backward pelvic rotation should involve lower pelvic unit activity (LPU) and deepening in the groins. Note here the poor LPU contribution, which is compensated for by excess central posterior cinch activity (thus fixing the lower pole of the thorax and blocking the weight shift and rotation) and movement sequencing up through the thorax to the head and neck.

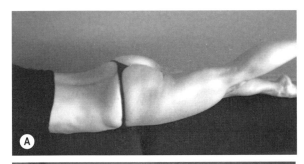

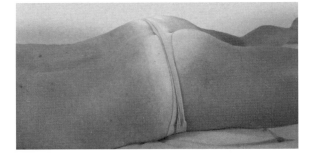

Figure 5.30

Poor core support mechanisms result in inadequate posturing of the pelvis in some anterior rotation to support the hip extension (see Fig. 5.29a), so once again there is excessive central cinch pattern activity. Also note the increased hamstrings tone. This is the same subject seen in Fig. 5.29b (and Fig. 5.6b).

Figure 5.29

a) Healthy axial FP control on hip extension. Note also how the pelvis has gone into anterior rotation to support the hip extension. b) Unhealthy central posterior cinch activity on lifting the head. Note the poor intersegmental movement through the upper thorax which should occur to support lifting the head. The subject has undergone lumbar surgery.

- Adaptive pelvic support for hip extension. Is pelvic FP1 adequate in providing appropriate anterior pelvic rotation to support hip extension (Fig. 5.29a)? Alternatively, do the hamstrings and glutei pull the pelvis into posterior rotation because of poor control of pelvic FP1 in providing adequate stabilization (Fig. 5.30)? (This is usually associated with CPC activity.)

- Ability in performing the shoulder patterns (particularly shoulder FP1; see Fig. 7.42 and 7.43) without simultaneous CPC activity (Fig. 5. 31).

Chapter 5

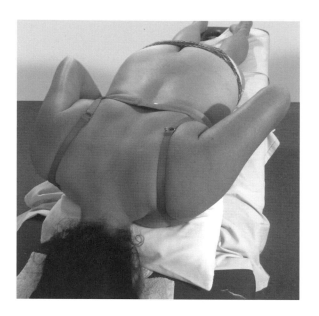

Figure 5.31
Attempting to activate the posterior lower scapular stabilizer myofascia in shoulder FP1 also involves central posterior cinch activity; "Key signs" are also just visible. The client is also over-activating the upper trapezii and the posterior rotator cuff. Neck tension and breath holding occur. Note the correct isolated lower scapular stabilizer activity in Fig. 4.23b.

Thoughtful review

Recognizing the "deep" myofascial system movement deficits and compensatory strategies of spinal control usually helps explain the development and perpetuation of symptoms.

Has your assessment built a picture of dysfunction in your client to explain their pain?

- Which regions of the myofascial envelope are overactive and tight?

- What is the effect of this on joint function?

- Which part of the myofascial system do we want to enliven more so that the spine and proximal limb girdles have more balanced control and improved function?

- Which FPs are likely to best do this?

- Which planes of movement might it be best to work in? For example, commonly, clients lose spinal extension.

Working for this is a priority to enable better function in the other movement planes – so you may prescribe passive extension over a bolster, or Sphinx (Ch. 7, Exs 2 and 3, respectively) and work for some fairly fail-safe active control as in Ex. 20: Half Sphinx to amphibian – or more challenging control in prone as in Ex. 45: Slow heel kick.

In a class situation you may construct a class around sagittal plane control and improving extension, which would include the transitional postures and movement phrases involved moving to and from it, by incorporating the relevant FPs. You may choose various postures in which to do this (e.g., prone lying on the floor; all fours; prone over a chair or ball; even supine).

In the early stages of using this approach, formal testing will help you pick up and understand individual components of aberrant control. With practice, you will find that you can easily notice deficits – even with a brief glance in a class situation.

CASE STUDIES

Case study

David – aged 23 – elite runner with chronic low back pain and left-sided leg pains

David suffered recurring left hamstring problems and an achilles tendinopathy. He also had a history of left knee pain. He had a regular gym program which included "core work" and a heavy weights program – both machine based and squats with 100 kg weights, which he had undertaken for 3 years, 3 times a week.

David had consulted a range of health practitioners to address his injuries, never gaining more than temporary relief. Physiotherapy for his leg injuries had only involved local treatment. Scans of his back were unremarkable. There were no features in the pain behavior to indicate concerns re insidious pathology.

Assessment

Standing:

- David presented as a mixed pelvic crossed syndrome – probably on an underlying anterior PXS picture. He had an evident layer syndrome, associated axial and pelvic inferior tethers – and a Key sign (see Figs 3.2a, 3.12, 3.13, and 5.1). I later concluded that his training regimen had had a significant effect on his appearance.

- Predictably, in forward bending, he hyperflexed his spine with reduced pelvic/hip control, inflexibility of the hips, and posterior inferior myofascial chain (see Fig. 3.17). Here, he also had asymmetry: his left PIIS remained "further south" on the left, his symptomatic side (see Fig. 5.7).

- Spinal extension was uneven, reduced, and slightly painful in the low back.

- Standing hip flexion produced lumbar flexion, whereas hip extension created increased CPC activity and showed poor anterior pelvic rotation for postural support of hip extension.

- The Key pelvic lateral weight shift test showed uneven intersegmental movement, with reduced closing over the left > (more than) the right lumbosacral junction and ipsilateral (L) LBP. There was associated reduced contralateral lateral shift of the thorax and "opening" over the thoracolumbar spine (see Fig. 5.10, and also Fig. 3.14b).

- In squatting his pelvis rolled into posterior tilt early in range with increased CPC activity (Fig. 5.32, and see Fig. 3.15).

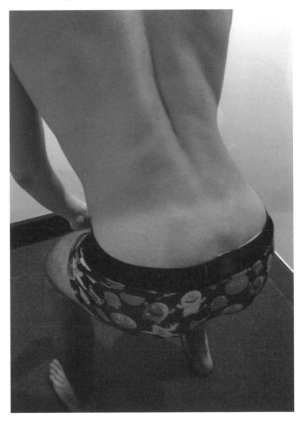

Figure 5.32

Poor squat pattern with inadequate pelvic and core support. The pelvis and lumbosacral levels are pulled into posterior rotation and end-range flexion early in range. Note the reactive L4–5 joints on the (L) just below his suntan demarcation, hyperactive central posterior cinch patterns (L) > (R), and also the thoracolumbar tissue reactivity (L)> (R).

- Distortion test (see Ch. 7, Ex. 56) revealed marked tightness of his hip flexors (L) > (R).

Sitting:

- David habitually sat in pelvic and spinal collapse. He was unable to assume a neutral pelvis and spine, compensating with increased CPC and some CAC activity (see Figs 3.33, 4.2 and 4.13b).

- He could not activate the axial FP (see Ch. 4, Controlling the center).

- Hip flexion in sitting resulted in increased CPC activity and he leaned to one side because of poor axial FP control, hence spinal stabilization suffered (see Fig. 5.14).

- Knee extension created lumbopelvic flexion (see Fig. 5.15a).

Supine:

- When testing the axial FP in supine, the upper abdominal wall dominated and the pelvis tipped into posterior tilt. David could not achieve the second stage test of widening the lower ribs postero-laterally.

Prone:

- In the prone Sphinx position David had pain, guarding, and stiffness.

- Palpation revealed marked stiffness and irritability when testing for sacral nutation, which was worse on the left. Likewise, L5 was stiff, irritable and "back" on the left > right.

- The L4–5 segment was flexed, accompanied by intersegmental spasm and "bogginess" left >right. Palpation from T10–L3 revealed loss of joint play, markedly reactive myofascial tissues and local allodynia, particularly from T11–L2 left > right.

In summary, the L4/5 segment appeared to be the significant "weak link" with all the other levels variously contributing to his symptom picture.

Exercise history

David's gym exercise program had consisted of:

1. Rowing machine, bike and cross-trainer

2. Sitting resisted knee extension

3. "Core strengthening": crunches, sit-ups, and planks

4. Squats: free form with Kettlebell weights and against a wall with a gym ball behind his back

5. A series of stretches:

   a. Supine: pulling knees to chest (Fig. 5.33)

   b. Supine buttock stretch (Fig. 5.34)

   c. Prone sit back on heels stretch for the low back (Fig. 5.35)

   d. Sitting adductor stretch (Fig. 5.36)

   e. Sitting hamstrings stretch (Fig. 5.37)

   f. Standing hamstrings stretch (Fig. 5.38)

   g. Standing quadriceps stretches (Fig. 5.39).

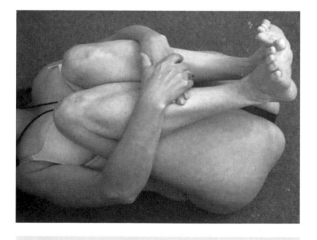

Figure 5.33

Supine: pulling knees to chest. The low back gets more stretch than anything else.

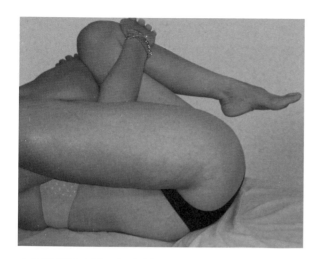

Figure 5.34

Supine buttock stretch. Note that the pelvis is in end-range posterior tilt and the most stretch is to the low back, not the buttocks. When the low back is further bothered, the buttocks will continue to be tight.

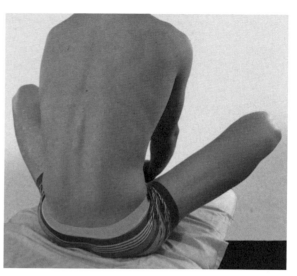

Figure 5.36

Sitting adductor stretch. There is no control here in either the pelvis or spine – just collapse of the spine into end-range flexion loading, and perpetuating problems.

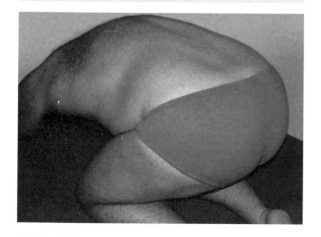

Figure 5.35

Prone sit back on heels stretch for the low back. The tightness over the client's posterior hips does not allow him to flex them – and so most of the stretch is to the lower back. He had undergone repeat injections at L4–5 in an attempt to settle discogenic symptoms and sciatica. Symptoms quickly settled when his exercise program was properly addressed.

Assessment review

David's exercise program was not appropriate. He was typical of someone "working for strength" without adequate patterns of underlying deep system control. He relied on, and was reinforcing and strengthening, his inferior tethers, which was why he was symptomatic. His exercise program did not address his functional needs but simply entrenched his problems in the following ways:

- He lacked spinal extension – both passive and active control. Yet just about all his exercises pulled or worked his lumbopelvic spine into end-range flexion. This repetitive end-range joint loading created segmental stress and in time "neural bother" (see Ch. 1, On injuries). The myofascial tissues within the L4–S2 postcode: the gluteals, hamstrings, and calf muscles became "fired-up," tight, and lost free slide. Hamstring problems and achilles tendinopathies should not be a surprise. David's lumbopelvic control became further compromised. A vicious

157

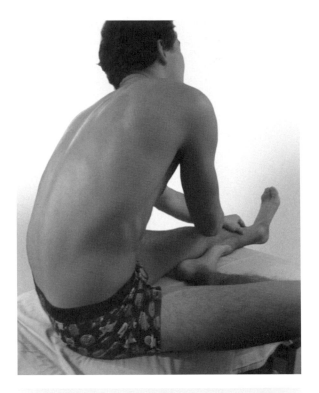

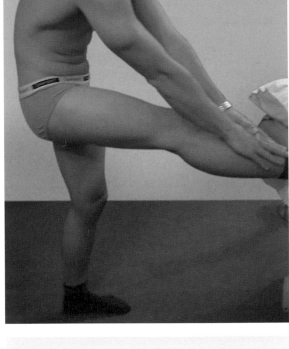

Figure 5.37
Sitting hamstrings stretch. You can easily see how this is bothering the spine, which itself seems to be squirming. This is the actual case study subject. If he continues to impose such extreme end-range flexion loading to his spine, the cycle of neural bother will continue – and predictably so will his hamstrings and Achilles symptoms.

Figure 5.38
Standing hamstrings stretch. Again there is no pelvic control. You can see how the tight posterior inferior myofascial chain including the hamstrings pulls the pelvis into posterior tilt and lumbosacral flexion. The more bothered the back, the tighter will the hamstrings become. A vicious cycle ensues unless checked with more suitable exercises. Incidentally, notice that he is reinforcing his shoulder inferior tethers and thoracic "dome."

cycle ensued – and he suffered chronic low back pain.

- Poor control of the axial FP and pelvic FP1 meant he could not assume a neutral sitting position – hence using the rowing machine and doing resisted knee extension resulted in the spine and pelvis being postured and moved into end-range flexion/posterior tilt. The same applied with the bike.

- His Key sign and inability to activate the axial FP indicated a weak core. His crunches, sit-ups, and planks did nothing to reestablish effective deep

system core support and control. Instead, they worked the spine into flexion – a pattern in which he was already strong – and he took to overly "bracing" with his superficial abdominals creating a compressive load to the spine.

- In a squat, his poor control of the axial FP and pelvic FP1 meant he relied upon axial and pelvic inferior tethers, further reinforcing their dominance, and compromising the spine. I do not

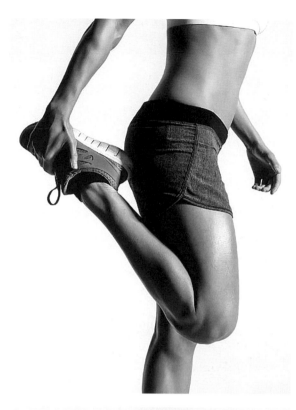

Figure 5.39

Standing quadriceps stretches. If the quadriceps are tight it is usually related to high lumbar problems and tight hip flexors. For the stretches to be effective and safe for the spine (i.e., maintain alignment), good control of the axial FP and pelvic FP2 are required.

consider wall squats with a ball behind the back to be functionally sound. In healthy kinematics, the pelvis needs to posteriorly shift in space and anteriorly rotate in order that the spine is not compromised. Wall squats also impart a high loading stress to the knees.

- The lack of control was also apparent in all his stretches. These are commonly prescribed exercises, but done in this manner they all (with the exception of the calf stretch, and perhaps the quadriceps stretch) would variably impart a lot

of stress to the spine. Note how in stretches a–f (see Figs 5.33–5.38) the pelvis is in posterior tilt and the spine in end-range flexion!

It is the chronic stress imparted to the spine that further drives these distal myofascial and joint restrictions.

Alternative approach

David needs to aim to gain control of natural upright sitting and be able to sustain this when studying, doing knee extensions and using the rowing machine (see Ch. 7, Exs 23 and 50).

With adequate control here, the above stretches should be modified by placing the ischial tuberosities on blocks to accommodate the posterior myofascial chain restrictions while requiring pre-activation of both the pelvic FP1 and the axial FP to help him to assume a neutral pelvis and spine. By driving further anterior pelvic rotation via pelvic FP1, he will more effectively access the tight myofascia in his legs (Fig. 5.40a,b). Also see Fig. 8.9 and Ch.7, Exs 53, 56 and 57).

The following is an appropriate initial prescription for exercise at home (see Ch. 7):

- *Ex. 2: Constructive rest position*. This affords passive extension in supine while using a bolster to gain improved pelvic and spinal mobility.

- *Ex. 3: Sphinx*. This is another avenue for improving passive spinal extension.

- *Ex. 4: Rotation in side lying*. This helps to lessen the expected stiffness in coming out of the passive extension poses; helps break up the "holding patterns" and opens the posterolateral hip/pelvis and improves rotation through the thorax.

- *Ex. 5: Pinning the beetle*. To establish axial FP control in supine – and when adequately controlled with diaphragmatic breathing, add appropriate limb load challenge.

- *Ex. 7: First pelvic pattern*. Establishing pelvic FP1 with the axial FP in supine, and sitting – and mindfulness about adopting this always when sitting. This is

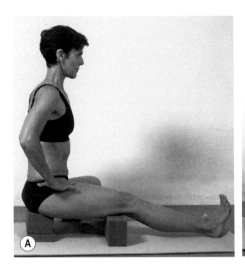

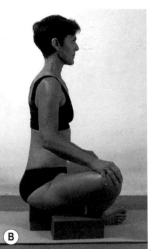

Figure 5.40
Modifying stretches help the client achieve active control. a) Hamstrings and b) adductors. The client needs sufficient height under the pelvis and support for the legs to enable her to engage and control the pelvic FP1 to lead the stretch (together with the axial FP to maintain spinal alignment and control and the effectiveness in the stretch). While she does not look as though she is achieving much range of movement, she is controlling her pelvis well – and is at the limit of her available hamstrings length.

prerequisite before expecting adequate control for hip and leg stretches as shown in Fig. 5.40.

- *Ex. 32: Forward bend pattern.* This is drilled to reestablish pelvic control for bending, sit to stand and squat.

Case study

Susie – aged 38 – working mother with SIJ pain and stress incontinence

Susie worked in a demanding desk job in the fashion industry. She had a longstanding history of right SIJ pain and intermittent stress incontinence. She recalled a bruised coccyx in a snowboarding accident sometime before the pain onset.

She had seen a physiotherapist who told her that her SIJ was unstable and prescribed drawing in the lower abdomen to activate her core (see Ch. 4: Functional importance of the axial FP, ADIM); "glute strengthening" exercises (i.e., clams; bridging and squats using Theraband resistance); and isolated pelvic floor exercises. Susie also believed that clenching her buttocks was helpful.

These exercises had not brought about any real improvement in Susie's symptoms, and being concerned about her shape and "big tummy," she had decided to try Pilates for toning and strength. She had been attending twice weekly for the previous 3 months – a floor class (25 participants) and a reformer class (9 participants).

She had recently developed headaches and neck tension, and marked right lateral hip pain – diagnosed as bursitis by one doctor and gluteal tendinopathy by another.

During the subjective examination I noted that she was an upper chest breather and gasped when she spoke. She appeared anxious.

Assessment

Standing:

- Susie had a pure anterior pelvic crossed syndrome presentation – with generalized low muscle tone, poor buttock development and tail tuck. She either hung on her iliofemoral ligaments in end-range hip extension and posterior pelvic tilt or dropped one side of her pelvis and hung on her iliotibial band.

- She had hyperactivity of the upper abdomen (CAC) and hypoactivity of the lower (see Fig. 3.6), some evidence of CPC activity, and a Key sign (see Fig. 5.1).

- She had evident pelvic inferior tethers – stood in "turnout" right more than left, and (predictably) when she bent over she hung off her hamstrings in posterior pelvic tilt and end-range lumbar flexion.

- She had a fixed pelvic ring distorsion on the right in neutral, which increased on forward bending (see Fig. 5.7).

- In squat, Susie had limited posterior pelvic shift and anterior rotation. Because of her poor control of pelvic FP1 she lost control of her lumbosacral lordosis early in range.

- Spinal extension was reduced and she compensated by shifting her pelvis further forward (see Fig. 5.8b).

- Lateral pelvic shift to the left produced pain over her right low back and SIJ.

- The Key pelvic lateral weight shift test onto the left leg also reproduced right lumbosacral pain as well as her right hip pain. The same test onto the right leg produced a mild pulling over her right lateral pelvis and general lumbosacral discomfort (see Fig. 5.10) together with uneven segmental movement.

- When standing on one leg (R more than (>) L) the pelvis rolled into posterior tilt and dropped slightly on the contralateral side with evident central conical cinch pattern activity in attempting stability (see Fig. 5.11a,b and Fig. 4.18).

Sitting:

- Susie habitually slumped when she sat down.

- She could not achieve a natural neutral spine. When attempting this she initiated with a central conical cinch because of poor control of pelvic FP1 and the axial FP.

161

- She was unable to widen the lower rib cage on testing the axial FP.

- When attempting the lateral weight shift test her pelvis slightly rolled into posterior rotation, and she could not initiate the movement from pelvic FP3 – initiating it instead via hip hiking and CCPs (see Figs 4.17 and 5.19).

- Rotation showed poor initiation from pelvic FP3 and FP4 and "wringing the waist" (see Fig. 4.22).

- She had poor control of the shoulder fundamental patterns.

Supine:

- Susie had a poor diaphragmatic breathing pattern and found it difficult to inhibit lifting her chest and shoulders on inhalation.

- Requesting her to pull in her lower abdomen or pull up her pelvic floor, as she had been prescribed, resulted in increased CAC activity, poor lower abdominal activity, and breath holding. Predictably, this same pattern was evident during the supine ASLR test.

- She was unable to activate the axial FP and widen the lower pole of her thorax.

- When attempting the pelvic FP1 she found it difficult to inhibit pushing with her legs and throwing her lower ribs forward; consequently there was poor deepening in the groins.

- Predictably, she was unable to unweight her pelvis in pelvic FP1 – her bridging and roll ups were entirely in pelvic FP2 with the lumbar spine in end-range flexion.

- Joint palpation in prone. Her L4/5 segment was very bothered and reproduced the lateral hip pain. In addition, she was stiff and irritable over L5 and sacrum, and the joints of her thoracolumbar junction R>L – all of which will contribute to and drive her lower quadrants symptom picture.

Assessment review

Despite doing specific exercises and going to Pilates twice weekly, not only were Susie's SIJ pain and incontinence unchanged, she now had hip pain, headaches, and neck tension. What caused this?

- Pilates is an excellent fitness workout if you are young and supple. However, in those with stiffness and poor deep system control it needs careful modification and fine-tuning.

- Pulling in her stomach and pulling up her pelvic floor inhibits good diaphragm activity and disturbs the balance and timing of the IAP core support mechanism. She compensates with central cinch activity, particularly anteriorly. The diaphragm and pelvic floor suffer further. In Pilates, the sequencing usually asks for abdominal/pelvic floor activation before breathing. The diaphragm should engage first.

- Increased pelvic floor and oblique abdominal activity is common in people with incontinence. Pelvic floor activity is also often delayed (see Ch. 3, Other common features of altered movement). The pelvic floor also needs to have elasticity and extensibility; ability in pelvic FP1 helps this.

- Training the gluteus muscles in isolation without coactivating the inner unit and working for dynamic control of the three-dimensional pelvic force couples can reinforce the pelvic inferior tethers. These hold the sacrum in counternutation and result in loss of intrapelvic mobility. Rather than being unstable, the pelvis/hip is in fact stiff R>L.

Susie finds it hard to activate her pelvic patterns – particularly pelvic FP1 – and when cued in class to find a neutral spine, she cannot get there. She needs specific cueing to pre-set her axial and proximal limb girdle FPs so that they can initiate and control movement.

Control of pelvic FP1 is important for gaining a neutral spine, sitting, forward bending and squatting, where the glutes are required to eccentrically lengthen to allow the hips to flex. This is particularly important when working for strength; otherwise, the challenge invariably results in the pelvic inferior tethers "locking in" to the second pelvic pattern. Both the spine and pelvis suffer.

The poor initiation of movement from the pelvis also leads to problems when stretching. For example, attempting to stretch the hamstrings in long sitting is often initiated from the head and shoulders rather than from the pelvis (see Figs 5.37, 5.38, 5.40 and 8.9).

- The poor pelvic control is associated with both disturbed control of the "center" and over-reliance on the upper limbs to compensate. Further, poor control of the shoulder FPs means that when attempting, say, bicep curls or a "plank," Susie will lock-in with shoulder and axial inferior tethers – leading to increased tension, neck stiffness, and headaches.

Alternative approach

The following is an appropriate initial prescription for exercise at home (see Ch. 7):

- *Ex. 1: Diaphragmatic breathing.* First and foremost Susie needs to master a diaphragmatic breathing pattern and the foundations of control provided by the axial FP and the limb girdle first fundamental patterns.

- *Ex. 2: Constructive rest position.* Susie's neuromyofascial system imbalance has led to spinal stiffness. Passive extension should be introduced: in the short-term, supine bolster is preferable to the Sphinx exercise in order to avoid exacerbating her headaches and neck tension.

- Susie then needs to incorporate the FPs into movement drills – in all planes of movement – and maintain correct patterns of control with increased loading. She needs help to establish effective sagittal plane control as a basis for gaining control in the frontal and transverse planes.

- Movement therapy that promotes flexibility and gains control of important underlying basic patterns, in a variety of multiplanar movements, will allow Susie to experience movement freedom without pain.

One of the potential shortfalls of Pilates-based exercises is the dominance of sagittal plane movements.

In addition, "working for strength" without adequate underlying patterns of support and control from the deep system leads to reinforcement of the inferior tethers. This becomes a lot more likely with large classes and inadequate supervision.

When the fundamental patterns can initiate and control movement, Susie will master all her failed movement tests – particularly those into rotation. Drilling these becomes part of her exercise therapy.

Case study

3. Gloria – aged 51 – executive with acute left shoulder pain

Gloria was a chief executive who had been diagnosed with a frozen shoulder (adhesive capsulitis) by one doctor and tendonitis by another. Three injections into the shoulder had provided short-term relief.

Physiotherapy was initially helpful, but progress plateaued. While the shoulder pain was paramount she had also experienced some intermittent forearm and hand symptoms. She was feeling rather desperate because the pain kept her awake at night. Despite the irritability of her pain, there was nothing in her history to indicate "red flags."

Gloria also suffered chronic "low grade" LBP and knee pain (L>R) and neck stiffness. Previous X-rays and MRI of her back and knees showed generalized degenerative changes. An ultrasound of her shoulder showed full-thickness tear and tendonitis of the supraspinatus tendon and bursitis with bursal impingement.

She liked to walk and had been doing yoga twice a week for about a year, but had ceased due to the shoulder pain.

Assessment:

Standing:

- Gloria displayed a posterior PXS with an active butt clench. She had an evident shoulder crossed syndrome (see Fig. 3.9) and an upper Key sign (see Fig. 3.23). The layer syndrome, and both axial and pelvic inferior tethers were also apparent.

- She had a thoracic "dome" and her left arm postured in more internal rotation (see Figs 3.22, 5.3).

Sitting:

- Shoulder inferior tethers were apparent L>R with concomitant fullness of the supraclavicular fossa (see Figs 3.25 and 5.13).

- Left arm elevation in abduction and flexion was painful early in range and very restricted by both pain and stiffness (see Fig. 3.26). She could neither place her left hand on her hips nor reach behind her back (Fig. 5.41).

- Cervical movements were pain free, but reduced, particularly left rotation – she said her neck felt a bit stiff. There was little or no adaptive spinal movement below about C5 in extension and rotation (see Figs 5.21b and 5.22b).

Lying:

- Cervical joint palpation revealed marked reactive changes and local pain C456. There was stiffness with local pain over C1–2 and between C6 and T2.

- Thoracic joint palpation revealed marked allodynia and restriction at T1–6 and the

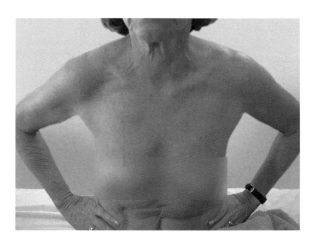

Figure 5.41

While this subject is able to place her hands on her hips, it is instructive as we see the effects of the (R) shoulder inferior tethers – pectoralis minor in particular. Placing one's hands on hips requires claviscapular unit elevation and sufficient glenohumeral internal rotation. Clinically, shoulder anterior inferior tethers and GIRD go together. The humeral head pops forward. The subject had (R) shoulder and neck pain and breathing pattern dysfunction.

adjacent ribs L>R. T2–4 and adjacent ribs referred pain to her left shoulder.

- Gloria had marked restriction with acute shoulder pain on passive testing of claviscapular elevation in side lying (Fig. 5.42).

- Passive glenohumeral testing produced painful restriction at about 80° elevation, with no internal rotation at available abduction – attempting this smartly increased her pain.

- Modified brachial plexus tension testing was positive on the left and slightly so on the right.

Assessment review:

In the short term Gloria required extensive manual therapy to settle her pain, and restore joint and myofascial flexibility and function, in her left upper quadrant. Her initial home exercise program consisted of:

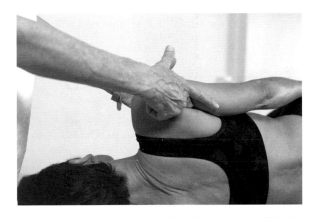

Figure 5.42
Passive testing of claviscapular mobility on the chest wall. The relaxed middle fingers of the practitioner's hand hook under the anterior and posterior axillary fold and draw the scapula cranially, exploring mobility in the available movement vectors. It is also informative to feel the quality of the myofascial tone under the operator's hands.

- *Ex. 2: Constructive rest position.* This provides modified passive extension over a bolster, with head and arm support as necessary to open the top chest and anterior shoulder girdle, and the arm myofascia.

- *Ex. 13: "Temperature check" rotation.* This can be used both to open the upper pole of the thorax and shoulder and to connect shoulder FP4 with head FP4.

- *Ex. 12: Rag doll.* This helps mobilize the joints and myofascia of the upper thorax.

- *Ex. 25: Shoulder fundamental patterns.* FPs 1, 3 and 4 with, at first, arms by her sides (as she could not place her hands on her pelvis), progressing to hands on pelvis when range and pain allowed.

She would need pain relief and a lot more specific mobility before she could join a class.

Gloria is typical of many who "break down" with injuries while trying to exercise. Seeing and appreciating the ramifications of her clinical syndromes helps us understand why she has likely developed her problems.

A stiff sedentary office worker, she needs help in reestablishing and fine-tuning the FPs (the "foundations of control") so that she can both access her stiff restricted regions – particularly her thorax and shoulder girdle – and find the inner patterns of control to support the yoga poses.

> Practiced well, yoga is an excellent discipline which balances inner and outer control, as it largely asks for maintaining sagittal alignment and breath control in the three-dimensional manipulation of shape in the various poses.
>
> However, teachers need to be aware that when control from the FPs is inadequate, clients will rely upon all of the inferior tethers for control, especially when over-challenged. These compromise the spine and drive symptom development.

It proffers a reliable and practical approach for spinal rehabilitation and reawakening the spine.

The general aims of the "Key Moves" approach

1. To redress the described postural movement faults seen in people with spinal dysfunction, and in so doing also reduce their concomitant effects on the joint, myofascial, breathing, and continence systems (see Ch. 3). People with spinal pain disorders are heterogeneous in that no two people will have the same biopsychosocial construct. However, in terms of the "bio" element, common movement dysfunctions are variably apparent.

   Arguably, the strength of this approach is that it maps and describes the features of altered control and also directly addresses these in prescribing therapeutic exercise specific to the problem.

2. In particular, interventions aim to:

   - improve joint and myofascial mobility, and regain a more flexible spine capable of being moved into neutral and beyond in three-dimensions. We want to achieve better intersegmental movement generally, and particularly into lost directions of movement (e.g., extension). This will include regaining a lumbar lordosis, and obtaining more flexibility in the thorax and proximal limb girdles. The process also involves rebalancing neuromuscular activity

   - reestablish good foundations of spinal movement control (i.e., the FPs). We aim to improve discreet control and coordination and to fine-tune movement. Problems arise in people working for strength if underlying patterns of deep system control are inadequate

   - restore functional spinal movement and enhanced freedom to move by integrating the FPs into a more varied movement repertoire. Appreciating the features of healthy movement

(see the beginning of Ch. 4) helps guide your approach and choice of movement tasks such that the quality and diversity of the client's sensorimotor skills of the torso are enhanced.

Guiding principles of the Key Moves approach

The overarching principle is reactivating and moving principally from the deep myofascial system

Rather than focus on outer muscle shape "burn" and strength in exercise, the focus is inward – upon the body's internal spaces and postural support, and the intrinsic movements of the torso.

Breath control

Ensuring a three-dimensional diaphragmatic breathing pattern at rest, which can be maintained during all postures and movement. Breathing entrained to movement is infrequently adopted and, when used, it is usually on exhalation to wake up the LPU and abdominals.

However, the breath is a valuable assist tool when "working the center" to improve opening in the lower rib cage and ability in all four parts of the axial fundamental pattern.

Reestablishing ability in the fundamental patterns

These components of movement are a blueprint for corrective exercise for the spine. Consider the FPs as a template that can be used in all postures and in all planes of movement.

The (most important) axial FP, the pelvic FPs, and head FP1 are initially taught in supine before expecting competent upright control. We then connect the FPs in movement and explore the functional relationship between them; for example, pelvic or shoulder FP3 initiates axial FP3. The head patterns functionally relate to the limb girdle patterns.

Competency in underlying FP control is a prerequisite before being able to safely "work for strength." We are rebuilding control through mastering these basic building blocks of movement.

Lengthening the spine and its neutral alignment in all postures and related movements

In particular, we focus upon the head–tailbone connection, which is deeply embedded in our evolutionary movement patterns. Mastery of the FPs helps to reestablish healthy patterns of spinal antigravity control. In the early/acute stages the appropriate FPs are initially practiced with gravity eliminated to help reprogram the habitual responses of the postural system to gravity. We work for postural endurance (the ability for sustained postures with adjustment in them); for example, gaining and sustaining an upright neutral spine involves adaptable integrated control between the first patterns in the pelvis, shoulder, and head with the axial FP (see Fig. 4.2).

"Opening the center" and controlling it in all postures and movement

Effective core control (the axial FP) supports the spine internally, contributes to a neutral thorax/pelvis alignment and creates space for the breath. It is always defective in variable measure in your clients. Competent core control inhibits CCP activity. We also need to actively work the center to inhibit likely CCP behavior while activating the pelvic, shoulder, and head patterns – and when adding limb load. This also applies when actively elongating tissue – otherwise known as stretching.

Point of initiation in movement

All movement involves weight shifts over the base of support – ideally initiated by the FPs – particularly those of the head and proximal limb girdles. The FPs initiate spinal movement, which sequences *from* the point of initiation. We need to set up our clients for a correct movement – to specifically cue the FPs to preengage the deep system preparatory control usually missing in their movement. This is important in building capacity in core control – it has to be "on" and capably sustained, such as during a back extension, otherwise the patient will utilize their habitual practice – inevitably "superficial muscle grab" and excess tension. The FPs initiate proximal control, thereby providing axial stability for distal limb movement.

Redressing myofascial imbalance and joint stiffness

We aim to both facilitate patterns of deep system control and inhibit or "bank down" dominant superficial myofascial activity. Muscle tightness and reduced fascial slide distorts the myofascial envelope's tensegrity, contributing to axial joint stiffness in one or more planes. With practice, overused and tense muscles begin to release and gain flexibility; underused and flaccid muscles begin to develop tone and robustness.

Rebalancing myofascial tension and improving joint mobility, particularly of the hip and shoulder joints, is achieved through both passive poses and active control initiated in the FPs. This includes gaining control of the three-dimensional rotary force couples in the pelvic and shoulder girdles. As distinct from usual stretches, working in this way actively involves the nervous system in active elongation of tight myofascia, aiding neuroplasticity through focused attention.

Deficient proximal control in your clients is compensated for by increased activity in the limbs. Hence excess myofascial tension and reduced flexibility in the limbs is also addressed.

Yielding to the base of support

Sensing our weight, and "giving it" to the ground through whatever the base of support, is a valuable tool in letting go excess tension and the tendency to "hold oneself up" away from the earth. In the passive supported poses, the more one can yield to the base of support on the underside body, the more the myofascia on the top body opens (as in Ch. 7, Ex. 2: Constructive rest position, or as in Ex 4: Rotation in side lying). Letting go superficial tension helps liberate the breath. Yielding to the base of support is also particularly important in gaining elongation and release of bound limb myofascia through active FP control (e.g., Ex. 53: V to Z hip stretch).

Grounding the base of support

Movement is a combination of "sinking" and connecting down to the earth to "ground" us so that we can engage the ground reaction force to push us "up." This is how we learned to exploit gravity (see Ch. 2). Grounding is particularly important when the hands or feet are the base of support. When they are well grounded, we can better find the reflex connections between them and the proximal limb girdles. The heel–sit bone connection, for example, helps facilitate the pelvic FPs. But no less important are the sit bones, ASIS, symphysis pubis, knees, elbow, etc., as grounded bases of support facilitating reflex postural control. Good grounding also ensures that the base of support is well centrated rather than being off-center.

Moving slowly with minimal effort and no tension

The FPs are discreet micro-movements which initiate and control natural movements. Fine-tuning these movements relies upon mindful focus, sensory perception and time to organize adjustments. Moving slowly requires more accomplished control – hence your clients usually want to move quickly. Accessing restrictions in the myofascial system requires slow and sustained movements in order to switch off habitual/reflex neuromuscular overactivity and then engage fascial creep and hysteresis, helping the tissues to begin to give.

Effort and speed disrupt the ability to "feel" the movement. Owing to fascial tensegrity, deep system neuromuscular activation only needs to be about 10–15% of a maximum voluntary contraction to be effective. Less effort allows increased perceptuo-sensori-motor ability in finely tuned control. This is important because spinal movement consists of lots of small segmental movements. Effort also increases the likelihood of dominant superficial muscle activity and tension, which limits movement and creates stiffness.

Staying in it – and being in it

Research shows that dysfunction in the postural control system underlies spinal pain problems (see Ch. 1, p. 6; Ch. 2, p. 21; Ch. 3). The postural system is built for endurance against gravity. Sustaining a pose challenges the system. Here, attention to yielding and grounding the base of support while activating the relevant FPs both releases the tissues and improves postural control. "Being in it," one can notice any tension and protective holding against any likely discomfort, which enables a refocus on grounding, opening the center, specific activation, the breath pattern, and letting go. Redirecting a busy and overwhelmed mind into relaxing and focusing on the quiet spaces inside helps connect into deep system awareness and control.

This is allied to other mindfulness movement approaches, such as Yin yoga and tai chi.

Breaking up the holding patterns

Clients "hold" reflexly and habitually, usually via inferior tether strategies. These are usually a bilateral response (particularly around the center) which distort sagittal alignment and control and hold the spine and proximal limb girdles centrally in the frontal plane. Weight shift and rotation becomes limited. The Bobath method employs what are termed reflex-inhibiting postures – often in rotation – to relax spasticity. Similarly, adopting asymmetrical postures such as side sitting (see Fig. 7.52) or side lying rotation (see Fig. 7.4) helps inhibit CCP activity, thereby allowing for improved axial FP and proximal limb girdle FP control.

Locking the elbows when weight bearing through the arms (common when on all fours), indicates reliance on shoulder inferior tethers and poor shoulder FP control. Working in side sitting or side lying helps break the pattern (see Fig. 8.5).

Similarly, we work to unlock the legs out of "propping" by either using kneeling and half-kneeling as postures for movement or working the pelvic patterns in standing with flexed legs (e.g., Ex. 32: Forward bend pattern) or standing with one foot on a bench or chair and employing the pelvic patterns to open the anterior and posterior myofascial chains in the leg.

Sensorimotor enrichment – and learning

A client's habitual posturo-movement control feels normal even when it is dysfunctional. This is because of altered interoception and proprioception, where clients often have a poor sense of their inner selves – of muscular effort, weight, and spatial relationships – particularly behind – and movements "going back". An effective sensory system and effective deep system control go together. Sensory awareness helps refine movement. As the deep myofascia is abundantly innervated with sensory receptors, its activation provides a rich source of sensory information to the CNS, which will further help organize more refined movement responses.

For this reason, in class we initially work a lot in recumbent poses where the body is more supported. This reduces demand in the postural system enabling "new" patterns of control to be more easily introduced. In addition, owing to the large area of body surface contact, it is likely that sensory receptors in the skin are stimulated which contribute to interoception or perception of our internal state. We are helping the client focus more clearly on inner awareness and reactivating their "lost" patterns of deep system movement control.

Similarly we always work in bare feet to exploit the foot's natural input into the system.

In this and other ways, we help clients to focus upon and appreciate the "felt sense" of posturo-movements. We demonstrate, describe or prompt them to work out the required task, which encourages the felt sense of the movement. In some cases, if clients are finding it difficult, we may passively do the movement for them so they can experience what is required.

We use various cues – verbal, tactile, imagery, etc. – to help clients sense their weight, effort, and movement flow. For example "sinking" the sit bones via pelvic FP1 in sitting activates the postural system, thus creating natural lift in the spine without effort or tension. Exploring other movement options, such as reaching out into space, then becomes easier.

Learning occurs through attention, perception, experience, and repetition. The more mindful we are about how we choose to organize ourselves against gravity, and the more we practice long forgotten movement behaviors, these new patterns start to become better represented in our CNS – and in due course become part of automatic postural movement behavior. This is neurological reprogramming.

Adopting the Key Moves in practice

- Gauging your client's abilities, and staging and tailoring exercise accordingly, is important. A common error is to prescribe a regimen that is beyond their capacity, which results in compensations being further reinforced. The purpose of this book is to help you fine-tune therapeutic exercise and reestablish important foundations of control to improve the quality and variety in movement. As I have said before: as a house needs sound foundations, so does the movement system.

- Distilling the essence of what is important in rebuilding healthy patterns of control can seem daunting at first. In the clinic you will have to prioritize which exercises are going to give you the best mileage. Keep it simple and go back to basics, such as sitting advice; restoring flexibility into extension to help establish control of the axis; staged control of the axial FP, and those limb girdle FPs and related movements most appropriate to the primary pain problem.

A home program should consist of appropriate, relatively failsafe exercises (e.g., Ch. 7, Exs 2, 4, and 13), whereas classes allow a lot more scope to explore and refine movement (see Ch. 9).

- Assessment delineates what is needed. To facilitate a better contribution from the deep sensorimyofascial system, your cues are important. These are usually auditory but can be any (or a combination) of visual demonstrations, gentle touch and facilitating the movement by placing your hand on the part which should be initiating the movement.

Here are some of the words that I might use to invite and encourage deep system activation. Less is literally more:

imagine or think of … ; reach long/wide; go slowly; soften; lengthen; float; sink; melt; sense … ; feel … ; be aware of … ; notice … ; open … ; let go … ; we only want micro-movements; yield … ; widen … ; grow the movement slowly – don't throw the movement; make it sensuous or … languorous or … lazy; be interested rather than ambitious; don't harden; enjoy … ; play with it; explore … ; bring your brain to (e.g.) your sit bones an … ; stay in it and … ; don't try so hard; move smarter rather than harder; where does the movement start? could you go to sleep doing …?

Further guiding principles for adopting this approach in practice

The following additional aspects of movement function should also be appreciated and incorporated into a tailored spinal rehabilitation program which aims to restore "lost" features of movement ability in people with musculoskeletal pain (described in Ch. 3).

- *Breath awareness*: Breathing is a sensitive indicator of the state of the nervous system (see p. 20 and Ch. 3). Hyperarousal is particularly manifested in altered breathing patterns – and interoceptive dysfunction leads to poor awareness and control of this. Many clients over-breathe and/or hold their breath hence we remind them to be mindful of their breathing pattern (how and where), and of whether they hold their breath, particularly when doing unfamiliar, difficult or "releasing" movements. Be aware that commonly, when you draw a client's attention to their breathing, they will tend to further overdo it. As an alternative, I ask them to relax the shoulders and open the center to make space for the breath (the axial FP) and simply just allow it to come and go – redirecting the breath rather than "making it."

- *Control of the center (axial FP)* in lying is basic and needs to be achieved before expecting ability when upright, where there is more demand on the postural system (The Axial FP: Ch. 4 – p. 93). Proper mastery of the axial FP involves "functional core control" – the ability to coordinate the postural response of IAP with breathing, both at rest and when moving. Unless your clients are familiar and somewhat competent with the axial FP in lying, they cannot find it when up and moving. This is important.

- A *"neutral spine"*: Competence in the axial FP provides mastery of uprightness in the sagittal plane – the ability to adopt a "neutral spine" in a healthy manner. Axial sagittal plane control underlies effective frontal and transverse plane control – the ability for weight shift and rotation through the axis. Nevertheless, do not expect to get perfect sagittal control before asking for movement in the other planes – but know its importance and that it underlies effective control in these other planes of movement.

- *Ensuring that the FPs are a point of initiation which lead the spinal movement* – "all good leaders have followers." Your cues should set up the correct pattern, which in healthy control automatically comes on before a movement. We are honing their ability to activate, sense, and adjust these functionally important small adjustments and "micro-movements."

- *Neural re-patterning and neuroplastic change.* Activating single muscles is not functional – and can lead to further dysfunction, e.g., pulling in the stomach.

- The brain organizes movement patterns. It likes tasks, and the clearer the intention of a movement, the better organized the response. If your cues are correct, the brain will sort out which muscles to use in achieving the correct pattern of movement. The quality of the client's response will lead you to further cues if necessary in order to improve the movement pattern being asked for.

- *Visualization* is another avenue for tapping into the senses to improve movement. Visualizing a movement primes the sensorimotor pathways and "lights up the brain" – akin to the approaches of various body/mind somatic awareness methods, such as ideokinesis (Todd, Sweigard, Dowd, Bernard, and Franklin, etc.), Rolfing, Alexander, Somatics and Feldenkrais.

- *Psychological aspects of movement*: How you move affects how you feel – and, naturally, how you feel influences how you move. Clients are often tense, "try too hard" and have "performance anxiety" – all of which tends to engender even more superficial muscle activity and tension. Hence, although the response may not be as good as you might wish, encouragement is important for the person's sense of self-worth, and aiding "letting go" and improving mastery.

Clinically, moving from the deep system seems to be connected to the limbic system in the CNS – it has a calming, pleasurable quality. The client's eyes will go glassy and breathing becomes relaxed. This is particularly evident when using rotation in recumbent movements; Feldenkrais knew about this.

- *Working with different aspects of control* helps improve the client's movement versatility: growing the movement slowly; eccentric control and the reversibility of a movement; and ability in playing a movement back and forth, particularly in sustained postural loading. We are aiming to improve the client's ability to sense and adjust intrinsic micro-movements as opposed to his habitual large, more extrinsic gross/coarse movements.

We are also working for fine-tuning the ability to differentiate and discriminate movement – to dissociate one part from another (e.g., hip from lumbar spine).

- *Exploring spatial reach – particularly reexperiencing "going back" in space.* Control of weight shifts over the base of support enables movements directed into the space around us. Particularly important are those behind us – into that part of the kinesphere to which we become unaccustomed. An example is Ex. 32: Forward bend pattern, where pelvic FP1 is drilled in standing – the sit bones and tailbone *need to go back* when we bend forward. Other examples include backward shoulder rotation – Exs 25c and 46a; backward pelvic rotation – Exs 16, 46b; hip extension in Exs 45 and 54; head retraction in Exs 17, 26a – and so on.

- *Diagonal and rotary movement patterns* are utilized both to engage the various oblique vectors in the myofascial envelope (e.g., Exs 13, 20, 39a) and to encourage freer weight shifts over the base of support. Single limb movements facilitate this, e.g., Exs 27, 44.

Chapter 6

We also work for flexible weight bearing through the limbs with weight shift initiated in the limb girdle FPs, e.g., Ex. 21.

- *Pain should not be exacerbated by movement.* This needs clarifying: warn your clients that when addressing joint and myofascial restrictions, discomfort is to be expected – but not pain.

  If pain is provoked, check the movement quality – invariably you will find they are using habitual superficial muscle dominant strategies – likely the inferior tethers. Pain is a messenger.

  In fact, deep system movements usually improve pain. For someone with acute pain (usually in the clinic), quietly focusing on the breath, letting go, and doing gentle FP movements in a recumbent, unloaded position is a great way to obtain relief.

  After a class, I love it when people spontaneously say "that was challenging [tasking the brain so] – but I feel so relaxed, tall and free."

- *Working for more capacity and endurance in the postural system.* As control of the fundamental patterns improves, we ask for the sustaining of more demanding postures and organizing of more complex movements – even working for strength. *The Golden Rule, however, is that "maintaining the line" and quality control in the pose is paramount.* If performance deteriorates, we go back and bed down the basic patterns to a greater degree before more sensitively adding load (longer levers, longer holds, and such like).

Recommended reading

Franklin E (1996) Dynamic alignment through imagery. Champaign, IL: Human Kinetics.

Franklin E (2006) Inner focus - outer strength. Using imagery and exercise for health, strength and beauty. Hightstown, NJ: Elysian Editions, Princeton Book Company.

Hackney P (2002) Making connections. Total body integration through Bartenieff Fundamentals. New York: Routledge.

Hartley L (1995) Wisdom of the body moving. An introduction to body-mind centering. Berkeley, CA: North Atlantic Books.

Myers T (2014) Anatomy Trains: Myofascial meridians for manual and movement therapists, 3rd edn. Edinburgh: Churchill Livingstone/Elsevier.

References

Adkins DL, Boychuk J, Remple MS, Kleim JA (2007) Motor training induces experience-specific patterns of plasticity across motor cortex and spinal cord. J Appl Physiol 101(6):1776–1782.

Remple MS, Bruneian RM, VandenBerg PM, Goertzen C, Kleim JA (2001) Sensitivity of cortical movement representations to motor experience: Evidence that skill learning but not strength training induces cortical reorganisation. Behav Brain Res 123(2):133–141.

Tsao H, Galea MP, Hodges PW (2010) Driving plasticity in the motor cortex in recurrent low back pain. Eur J Pain 14(8):832–839.

Van Dieën J, Kingma I (2013) Spine function and low back pain: interactions of active and passive structures. In: Hodges PW, Cholewicki J, Van Dieën JH (eds) Spinal control: The rehabilitation of back pain. State of the art and science. Edinburgh: Churchill Livingstone Elsevier, p.52.

Key Moves 2:
Kinesthetic therapeutic movement exercises for spinal health
and well-being

7

The exercises presented here, which involve mindfulness, the breath, discrete control, and ease of movement without pain, are best considered as "movement explorations."

Dysfunctional patterns of motor control lead to distinct patterns of joint and myofascial dysfunction. Assessment should delineate a picture of dysfunction which helps explain the symptoms and joint findings. Understanding why the problem has occurred points the way to appropriately redressing it with movement therapy.

Explaining the usual relationship between altered movement and pain is important in reassuring your client that pathological structures (if found) are not necessarily the cause of their symptoms.

Where to start?

Settle the acute pain first. In my experience the spinal joints are the primary source of pain – which in turn leads to changes in the neuromyofascial system – which further compromises joint function.

If spinal joints are "angry," it is unrealistic to think that you can dramatically improve their motor control. Appropriately mobilizing the joint(s) and related myofascia, however, switches off the pain and much of the associated disordered neuromuscular activity and related myofascial symptoms, both locally and referred. We can then work to restore patterns of movement which protect and support the spine while giving it more freedom to move.

However, not all your clients will require manual therapy prior to exercise therapy. When pain, joint, and myofascial dysfunction is less entrenched, appropriate movement therapy can restore flexibility,

functional patterns of control, and ease what pain there is.

In my practice, clients usually receive specific spinal manual therapy to settle their pain and restore joint and neuromyofascial function.

From the start, they are expected to be mindful about changing provocative postural habits and perform a basic home exercise program which aims to specifically restore lost or deficient aspects of function. The prescribed home exercises complement the manual therapy – both arms of therapy working toward the same goal; for example, improving spinopelvic mobility and control into lumbosacral extension or nutation.

If the problem is complex or acute, I will not necessarily prescribe a home exercise on day 1. Getting to the source of the spinal problem and delivering effective manual treatments can be complicated. Here, I may only offer simple postural advice and prescribe a basic exercise, such as Ex. 4 (Rotation in side lying), to encourage "letting go" and diaphragmatic breathing. As the pain settles the client is expected to do more.

When symptoms have settled sufficiently, we encourage clients to attend our Key Moves therapeutic exercise and movement classes. Ideally, their treatment and home program paves the way to restoring enough basic mobility to do so.

Improving posturo-movement function involves a considerable sensorimotor relearning curve. There are numerous aspects of function we need to restore. We have to improve joint mobility plus myofascial balance and flexibility as well as neuromotor control. An important aspect of this will be reestablishing the foundations of control – the fundamental patterns (FPs).

Supporting your client "where they are at"

People with spinal pain are stiff! We need to support them in ways that accommodate their current regions of stiffness, but which also encourage opening and discourage unwanted compensations. The creative use of various props (see Fig. 4.32) can help the client achieve more mobility and better control. Importantly, they can also be used to help modify a certain base of support (see Fig. 4.31) so that the client can better "center" and "ground" this. In turn, this helps facilitate better spinal "lift" and more ideal alignment, and initiation from the FPs.

Inventory of Key Moves clinic exercise handouts

The following exercises are designed to improve flexibility and skilled performance of the FPs – the important basic building blocks of healthy spinal movement. They are suitable as supervised clinic or studio handouts and for incorporating into classes.

The Key Moves require focused attention in following the prompts to achieve the specific desirable actions. Even so, bear in mind that motor control problems can be difficult to address without considerable supervised learning; so do not give out too many exercises, and check them frequently. Getting them right is not easy.

Your choice of exercise will obviously depend both upon the acuteness and irritability of the client's problem and on the goal of the exercise in relation to that person's principal defects. Attend to the basics first! We are rebuilding control.

I like to give exercises that deliver "3 for the price of 1" (e.g., addressing control, release, and alignment). The exercises address missing aspects of regional function and contribute to overall spinal flexibility and control.

Some exercises in this chapter are described for one side; obviously they are repeated on the other. In classes these exercises are also incorporated with other movement sequences. **Note:** The focus in all the exercises is on the point of initiation: controlling the center and initiating movement from either the pelvic or shoulder or the head patterns.

IMPORTANT: These exercises are designed to help the client move without pain, and that should be possible provided that all the prompts are carried out. If your client experiences undue pain, check their performance carefully; or, if you are the client, consult your therapist.

Table 7.1
Recommended exercises

Basic beginners
A. Correct breathing This is basic to activation of the "core." While you won't necessarily do this on day 1 in the clinic – especially if you are dealing with a complex pain problem – I have placed it first as it is the first competency. We find that clients with dysfunctional breathing patterns often need considerable one-on-one attention. Our Key Moves Preliminary Program focuses a great deal on establishing correct diaphragmatic breathing patterns and control of the axial FP (which, incidentally, is often easier said than done!)
1. Diaphragmatic breathing
B. Restoring joint mobility, myofascial length, slide, and opening in the tissues These are basic, more passive, and somewhat fail-safe exercises, although the client still has to be mindful and work at achieving alignment, letting go, and "opening the center":
2. Constructive rest position 3. Sphinx 4. Rotation in side lying

Table 7.1 *continued*

C. Basic motor control competencies	
a) Supine	5. Pinning the beetle
	6. Baby pose: building further core control
	7. First and second pelvic fundamental patterns
	8. Third pelvic fundamental pattern
	9. Fourth pelvic fundamental pattern
	10. Isolating hip flexion
	11. Head fundamental pattern 1 and eye patterns
	12. Rag doll
b) Side lying	13. "Temperature check" rotation
c) Prone	14. Prayer stretch: connecting breath, core and pelvic patterns
	15. Windscreen wipers
	16. Backward pelvic rotation
	17. Happy neck exercise
	18. Praying mantis
	19. Wide wings
	20. Half Sphinx to Amphibian
d) All fours	21. Cat/Camel
	22. Supplicant pose
D. Being mindful of practicing these "deep system movement drills" through the day	
a) Sitting	23. Healthy sitting
	24. "Opening the center"
	25. The shoulder fundamental patterns
	26. The head fundamental patterns
	27. Shoulder shrug and slide
	28. Windmills
	29. Pelvic dancing in sitting
	30. Sit to stand
b) Standing	31. Healthy standing
	32. Forward bend pattern

MORE ADVANCED EXERCISES

E. Increasing the challenge of deep system control	
a) Supine	33. Basic abdominal exercises for a healthy spine
	34. Pelvic reach and roll
	35. Pelvic hovercraft
	36. Advanced abdominal exercise for a healthy spine
	37. Smart hamstring stretch
	38. Brainy buttock release
	39. Windswept poses
	40. Half baby to Cross-over
b) Side lying	41. Twister
c) Prone	42. Shoulder pattern combo
	43. Double arm triangles
	44. Spreadeagle
	45. Slow heel kicks
	46. Shoulder and pelvic backward rotation in lying
	47. Mini press to Seal

Table 7.1 *continued*

d) Sitting	48. "Core" challenge sitting
	49. Lateral weight shift pattern
	50. Hamstring releases in sitting
	51. Shoulder and chest opener
e) Side sitting	52. Pelvic rock and roll in side sitting
	53. V to Z hip stretch
f) Kneeling and all fours	54. Butt booster on all fours
	55. Rebooting your iliopsoas and core
	56. "Distorsion" progressing to Crescent stretch
	57. Prone piriformis stretch
g) Standing	58. Foot exercises
	59. Calf stretches in standing
	60. Table-top stretches

These exercises have also been differently regrouped at the end of this chapter to further assist your exercise prescription skills,

At the back of this chapter you will also find a patient assessment summary and exercise prescription sheet to help you keep track of which exercises you have prescribed for each client. This will also provide insights as to your functional goals in prescribing an exercise – and help staging. For example

Ex #2: Constructive rest position is a fairly safe way of improving mobility of the joints and soft tissues as a prelude to working for active control of the axial and first fundamental patterns

I have also included a copy of the Patient-specific functional scale, which can be a useful tool in managing some of your clients with more troublesome musculoskeletal problems.

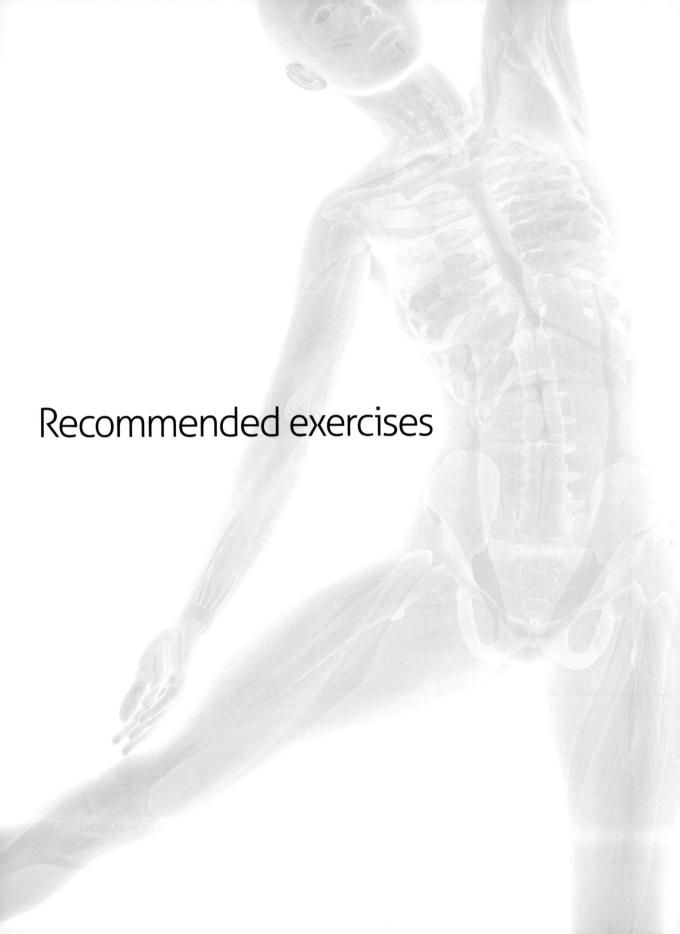

Recommended exercises

Chapter 7

1 — Diaphragmatic breathing

This is basic to achieving control of your "core."

Purpose: Reestablish a correct diaphragmatic breathing pattern.

Benefits: Helps everything! Poor posture, stress and tension can lead to habitual upper chest breathing patterns that put us in "fight and flight" mode and anxious frames of mind. This is associated with many musculoskeletal pain complaints. Healthy breathing patterns aid relaxation, contribute to better posture, and improve the body's chemistry and general well-being.

Position: Lie on your back with comfortable support under your head. Bend your knees. First, discover your habitual breathing pattern: place one hand on your chest, the other on your stomach and simply notice your breath, without making any deliberate attempt to change it (Fig. 7.1). Which hand moves first?

- Do you breathe through the mouth or your *nose*?

- Do you breathe into and lift the upper chest or *down low into your belly and back/side ribs*?

- Are your breaths short and sharp or *long and slow*?

- Is your *out breath longer* or shorter? Is there a *pause* between breaths?

  Note: The responses in italics are the desirable ones. If your top hand moved first, you are an upper chest breather. You need to change this.

Key moves in this exercise: Relax! Particularly your shoulders and neck. Drawing attention to one's breathing invariably leads to trying too hard and over-breathing.

1. Instead, think of widening the lower ribs to create more space for the breath – and simply let it come and go. You are not "making" the breath but simply redirecting it. As you breathe through your nose you should not hear any sound or "sniffing." There should be no movement in the upper chest. Can you sense the breath down into your pelvis and, equally, into the front, back, and sides of your lower ribs and waist? Can you keep the lower ribs wider and breathe regularly? Your lower stomach will gently firm. Do not pull your stomach in as this stops you breathing properly.

2. Gradually slow your rate of breathing – and lengthen both the exhalation and the pause between breaths.

   A good breathing pattern approximates the following ratio:

   ○ Inhale for 2

   ○ Exhale for 3 and

   ○ Pause before the next inhalation for 1 (or longer)

   ○ You can further lengthen the breath length but try to keep the same ratio between them.

Deep breathing is not the same as big breathing! Most people misunderstand this. Healthy breathing is not about trying to take a big breath but rather a deep breath down into the body. You are not attempting to increase the volume of air inhaled, but rather to bring the air low into your "core."

When consciously lengthening the exhalation, "let go" of the areas where you are holding tension; pause as long as you comfortably can before the next inhalation, which will come when it is ready. *Allow* the inhalation rather than "trying" and rushing it. Can you sense the diaphragm descending down through your body like the plunger in a coffee pot or a parachute opening out?

Just be aware and simply sense the breath coming through your body.

Compensations: Lifting the upper chest and shoulders on inhalation; inability to fully exhale; holding excess tension in the abdominals (which inhibits the diaphragm); breathing too hard and fast; inability to achieve posterolateral basal expansion; mouth breathing.

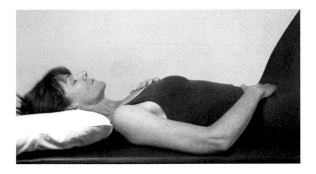

Figure 7.1
Diaphragmatic breathing.

Chapter 7

2	**Constructive rest position**

Purpose: Improve spinal flexibility into extension; open up the anterior myofascial chains, hips and shoulders – and the diaphragm – and direct the focus to the inner body.

Benefits: Helps all spinal pain disorders. Most of our day involves us bending forward in one way or another and we become stiff. Lying back over a bolster unravels the day's impact on the body and allows a time for recharging the batteries – to relax and let go and have the time to focus on slow diaphragmatic breathing.

Position A: Lie back along a bolster as it is the ideal support. If you are really stiff, start with a pillow(s) behind your head and no pillows behind your back then progress to placing two (or more) pillows lengthwise under your spine. As you become more flexible you can use a bolster rather than pillows.

Key moves in this exercise: Gently work your sit bones away so that they drop down off the end of the bolster. Think of your sacrum as being like Niagara Falls – your sit bones drop down, back and wide (first pelvic pattern). When on a bolster they will probably not quite touch the floor. The tailbone drops down and back.

Place a pillow under your head if your neck is uncomfortable or your chin pokes forward.

1. Place the legs and arms in any of the variations shown, let them go heavy, and give your full weight to the bolster (Fig. 7.2a–c; *note:* 7.2c is an "advanced" leg position).

2. Gently draw the points of the shoulders and sit bones back and wide: feel the increased opening over the top of the chest/shoulder and upper arm, and in the hips/pelvis and thighs.

3. Slowly direct the breath down and back. The more you can relax the better. Although you can expect to feel a little uncomfortable and stiff, you should not feel any sharp pain. Focus on bringing the breath to wherever you feel tight or uncomfortable; try to consciously relax more on each exhalation. Pay particular attention to letting go of tension around the neck and shoulders; the lower back ribs; and the buttocks and pelvic floor. Remain here for about 3–5 minutes (up to 10 minutes).

4. Do not jump up quickly but roll onto your side and gather yourself.

Position B: This really opens the upper back and shoulders. Lie across the bolster with it under your mid/upper shoulder blades so that your nipples form the highest point. Your head falls back and will need to be suitably supported (Fig. 7.2d). The arms spread at right angles to your body, with shoulders barely touching the ground. Follow all the prompts for position A. Gradually work yourself up the bolster so that it creates opening through the lower rib cage. Here, you may be happy to go without head support. Whichever the position, always ensure your neck is comfortable and breathing is free.

Compensations: Upper chest breathing pattern; active holding patterns do not let go. (Be prepared to support the client's head, thighs or arms with blocks or cushions if they have pain or difficulty relaxing.)

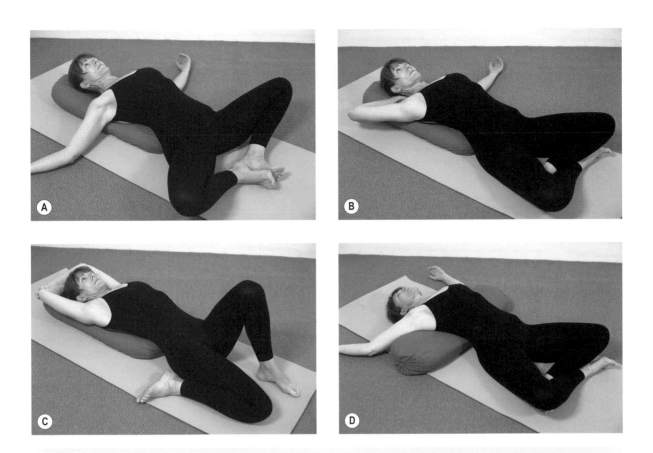

Figure 7.2
Constructive rest position: a),b) basic; c) advanced; d) more advanced.

3	**Sphinx**

(This is not advisable if you have neck or shoulder pain.)

Purpose: Improve passive extension, and also mobility of the spine and pelvis, while engaging the axial fundamental pattern plus the first head and shoulder patterns.

Benefits: This helps low back and pelvic pain and many lower limb pain disorders. Most of us lose flexibility into extension/back bending in the spine; 4-month-old babies have no problem doing this. This exercise helps you regain what you once had!

Position: Lie on your front supported by your elbows, which need to be directly under your shoulder joints, with your upper arm vertical, forearms in parallel, and the palms facing up (not shown in the photo). Relax the front top chest/shoulders and your buttocks, allowing the weight to fall back onto the pubic bone, and roll your heels out to the side (Fig. 7.3a).

Key moves in this exercise: Let your spine sag down between your shoulder blades.

1. Breathe down low into your body and, on the out breath, allow your whole spine to "hang loose" (think of softening and lengthening).

2. Lengthen the back of your neck, reaching the crown of your head – chin in – and engage the shoulder blades by bringing the points of the shoulders back and wide.

3. Gently explore micro-movements from either the points of the shoulders or rolling across your pubic bone. Expect to feel some stiffness and discomfort in the lower back here as, in general, your joints have been starved of this movement for a long time.

Try doing this exercise while reading the paper, playing with your toddler, etc.

Aim to eventually stay here for 10 minutes. To begin with you may only last a minute or so. It will become easier if you do it daily.

4. *Progression:* Spread the palms face down. Draw the points of the shoulders back and engage the muscles between your shoulder blades; as you sink the heel of your hand into the floor, float your elbows up and wide. The top of the breastbone moves forward and the collarbones widen as you soften and hang the spine down. The neck is soft and long, with the chin back. Gently draw the point of one shoulder back to bring your upper chest into a slight twist – and alternate (Fig. 7.3b).

Compensations: "Locking-in" with the shoulder inferior tethers blocks movement through the upper spine and feeds into the creation of a "dome" and thoracic stiffness. Hardening over the lower ribs with no expansion. The paucity of movement through the upper thorax creates neck tension and discomfort. (If there is a lot of low back discomfort, place a pillow under the pelvis.)

IMPORTANT: You are working into stiffness so you can expect to feel stiff and awkward coming out of the position. Do not jump up quickly (e.g., to answer the phone) but slowly come onto your side and work this stiffness out by doing Ex. 4: Rotation in side lying – on both sides for a least a couple of minutes each side.

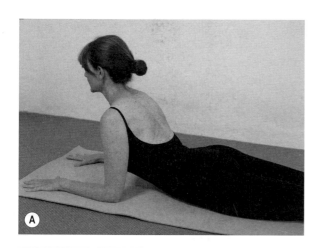
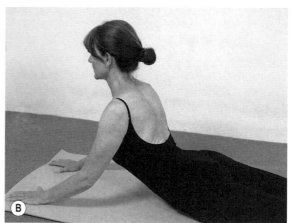

Figure 7.3

Sphinx: a) basic; b) progression.

4   Rotation in side lying

Purpose: To open the inferior tethers around the center, and the shoulder and pelvic girdles; increase rotation through the thorax while working the fourth axial fundamental pattern.

Benefits: This is a nice way to open up the body – even for someone in a lot of pain. It is also good to do first thing in the morning to "wake up" the spine.

It should be performed on both sides after the passive extension exercises (Ex. 2: Constructive rest position and Ex. 3: Sphinx) to ease out any expected stiffness.

Position: Lie on your side with both hips and knees bent to a right angle with a neutral spine. Here, think of creating a "pointy bottom" by widening your sit bones and reaching the tailbone long and back – without throwing the lower front ribs forward!

With the under arm at right angles to your body, wriggle it as far forward as possible – trying to maintain your neutral spine. Allow the point of the top shoulder to fall back. Your face will now point more toward the ceiling. Use a pillow under your head if your neck is uncomfortable. Gently drop your chin and lengthen the back neck.

Place your top hand on its pectoral muscle (Fig. 7.4a). This helps you monitor a correct breathing pattern (you don't want to feel it lift as you breathe in).

Place your bottom hand fingers over your lower tummy wall on the inside of your pelvic bone to monitor the activity here (not shown). Give your weight completely to the floor and relax.

Key moves in this exercise:

1. Begin by doing an exaggerated full exhalation so that your rib cage comes down and back. Your task now is to keep the rib cage in this position while simply letting the breath ebb and flow. You should be aware of the muscles engaging just above the groins

2. As you master this, gradually begin to also expand the lower rib cage sideways and backward. The lower rib cage now remains both down and back – and wider.

3. Maintaining this, on each exhalation allow your top shoulder to relax and drop back more toward the floor. Make sure you are not doing the movement by actively pulling back and "wringing" at your waist. That stops you breathing properly!

4. Ensure you breathe low down and slowly. If your tummy is a bit lazy, try blowing out more firmly and for longer through gently pursed lips.

5. Also allow the top sit bone to slide backward. You may well start to feel tight over the top hip – this is good! If this is very uncomfortable to start with or you have low back pain, place a pillow(s) between your knees.

About 3 minutes on each side allows time for the tissues to release here.

6. *Progression 1:* When you can manage all of the above you can also straighten the top elbow. If this is too much, place a block under your elbow. On exhalation, gently reach the hand wide and direct the point of the shoulder to drop back more while turning the head to look at that hand. Linger here as you deepen and widen the breath, and relax so that you feel a distinct stretch in the front shoulder and upper- and mid-back and pelvis (Fig. 7.4b).

7. *Progression 2:* Bend the top hip higher and drop the knee to the floor – hooking the top foot under the bottom knee (see Fig. 7.4b).

Compensations: Upper chest breathing with poor "inner unit" activity. CCPs dominate and the lower ribs stay up and forward. Waist wringing is apparent with poor opening in the thorax and shoulder girdle.

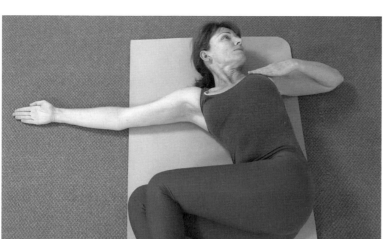

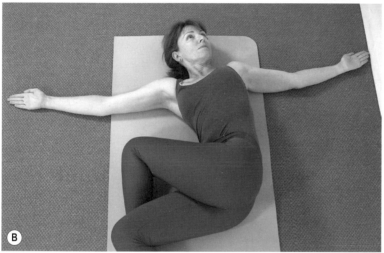

Figure 7.4
Rotation in side lying: a) basic;
b) progression.

Chapter 7

5 | Pinning the beetle

The basic pattern for correct "core control."

Purpose: Develop proficiency and endurance in the axial FP – coordinating intra-abdominal pressure and breathing.

Benefits: This is an important exercise for anyone with low back and pelvic pain and many lower limb pain disorders. Commonly there is underactivity in the deep muscles including core control. Reestablishing the correct action is practiced in lying to help reprogram the correct patterns without the influences of gravity on the postural system. For some, this can be a difficult exercise to achieve – it may take weeks.

Position: Lie on your back, supporting the head for comfort - and so that your chin is back. Bring your hips and knees to a right angle, thighs vertical, "standing" your heels on a chair or similar support. Relax your buttocks and legs. They should be "alert" to hold the position – but not tense. Place the tips of your index and middle fingers of one hand in the "valley" on the inside of the pelvic bone, just above your groin, to gently palpate your lower abdominals. The other hand rests on the upper chest to monitor that you do not lift the chest when breathing (not shown).

Key moves in this exercise:

1. Fully breathe out until you feel your lower ribs moving down and back onto (or toward) the support surface and notice a firming under your lower fingers. Imagine you are squashing a beetle under your lower back ribs. The task is to then to keep him pinned – while breathing low and slowly. Do not push with your feet and clench the buttocks! The action is ribs back – the pelvis will follow in a slight tip. When you can

both firm under your lower hand and regularly breathe down to it, you are properly engaging the core muscles – where the pelvic floor, deep tummy muscle and diaphragm work together (Fig. 7.5a).

2. Maintain the rib cage position and lower belly firming while simply allowing the breath to ebb and flow. On inhalation, ensure the breath goes down to meet your lower hand – and that it does not lift the chest under your top hand!

   If it is difficult to feel the muscles "setting" under your lower hand, purse your lips and deliberately blow all the air out as if to slowly blow out a candle. See how long you can keep doing this action. Or try breathing through a straw, focusing on exhalation. This should now activate the muscles.

3. When you can manage the above steps, widen the lower ribs while still keeping them back, and direct the breath here. When correct, you will notice a further increase in the "setting" under your lower hand. Your aim is to sustain the thorax position and wide lower ribs, and breathe easily – ideally for 3–5 minutes. Eventually, you should feel you could go to sleep while continuing to do this.

4. *Progression:* Challenges your ability to maintain the ribs down, back, and wide and maintain a regular breathing pattern while floating one foot off. If the ribs lift you have failed the test (Fig. 7.5b).

Compensations: Pushing with the feet, clenching the buttocks and tipping the pelvis back rather than bringing the ribs down and back. Lifting the chest to breathe in (resulting in loss of contact of the lower back ribs with the surface and poor generation of the core action). Sucking in the stomach and lifting the rib cage. Over-activity of the upper abdominal wall and over-approximation of the infrasternal angle. Abdominal "ballooning."

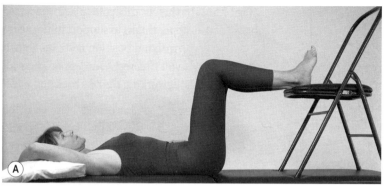

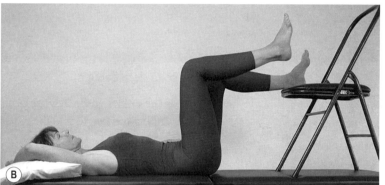

Figure 7.5
Pinning the beetle: a) basic;
b) progression.

7 First and second pelvic fundamental patterns

Purpose: To sense and develop intrapelvic control of anterior and posterior pelvic rotation.

Benefits: The pelvic patterns will help anyone with low back and pelvic pain and many lower limb pain disorders. Pelvic control is always deficient – first pattern in particular is commonly difficult, yet it is so important for spinal support. These foundation patterns help rebuild control.

Position: Lie on your back, head supported if more comfortable; knees bent, feet "standing" under your knees; heels wide; toes facing forward. Relax your legs and buttocks.

Place your middle finger tips in the valleys on the inside of each pelvic bone (not shown). Relax your shoulders and let your elbows rest on the floor. Imagining that you have headlights in your sit bones is useful (or maybe hooks).

First pattern

Key moves in this exercise:

1. Reach your sit bones long, widen them apart and point them back toward the floor. Your pelvis rotates forward and your very low back arches. You should also notice the muscles under your fingers and deep inside your pelvis "set" more. If you do not, focus more on the cues until you do. (Fig. 7.7a).

   You should also feel the muscles over your very low back activate and you may feel some stiffness and/or slight discomfort here. This is common at first as this pattern has usually been "lost" in function.

2. **IMPORTANT:** Make sure you do not tense over the lower back ribs and throw them forward.

This is a bad habit which increases if you try too hard. Try smarter, not harder.

3. You should also feel that as your sit bones spread and pelvis rotates forward, your fingers come slightly closer together, the groins deepen, the movement sequences through the spine, and your chin drops (see Fig. 7.7a). Maintain a regular diaphragmatic breathing pattern.

Compensations: Tensing the legs and poor initiation from the pelvis and core activation. The ribs initiate and throw forward. Holding the breath.

Second pattern

Key moves in this exercise:

1. Draw the sit bones together, tuck your tail and flatten the lower back without tensing your legs or buttocks. You want to feel the inner core muscles under your fingers doing the work. This is usually fairly easy to do, and so needs less practice.

2. As the sit bones come together your fingers will move further apart, the pelvis tips back, the movement sequences through, the spine and the chin protrudes (Fig. 7.7b).

Compensations: Poor "inner unit" activity, pushing with the feet, clenching the buttocks and inability to relax the legs. Coming onto the toes can help to inhibit leg overactivity.

Gently oscillate the movements back and forth emphasizing first pattern to subtly increase the reach and backward rotation of the tailbone, then hold this while continuing to breathe "low and slow," down, back, and wide over 4–5 breaths.

Stay relaxed. This skill is more brain than brawn: the less hard you try, the easier it is.

These patterns can also be practiced in other positions such as side lying with hips and knees bent.

The trick is to "bring your brain to your sit bones" and feel the movement start from them and the tailbone. Do not "go hard" in the center body, as that creates tension and disturbs the breath.

Your aim is to do this action naturally and easily so that you feel the vertebrae articulate, and the very low back and tummy muscles create the action. Remember: first pattern usually needs more emphasis.

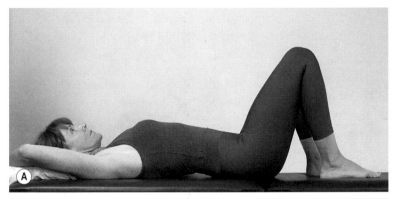

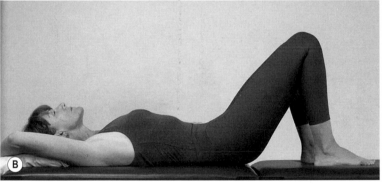

Figure 7.7
First and second pelvic patterns:
a) pelvic FP1; b) pelvic FP2.

8 | Third pelvic fundamental pattern

Purpose: To develop intrapelvic control of lateral pelvic rotation in the frontal plane.

Benefits: This exercise is helpful for anyone with low back and pelvic pain and many limb pains. Weak gluteals are considered a common problem. However, they need to be trained **with** the pelvic core muscles to effectively control the pelvis.

Position: Lie on your back, head supported if more comfortable; knees bent, feet "standing" under your knees; heels wide; toes facing forward. Place your middle finger tips in the valleys on the insides of each pelvic bone. Relax your buttocks, legs, and shoulders.

Key moves in this exercise: Imagining headlights or hooks at the end of your sit bones can help you sense the correct action.

1. Gently spread your sit bones apart and reach them long and back toward the floor. Your back will slightly arch. This brings your pelvis into the neutral position. Try to maintain this.

2. Notice that your weight is now centered on your sacrum. Keep it so while further reaching the (R) sit bone longer toward your (R) heel so that your (R) side waist lengthens and your (L) side waist shortens. Allow the ribs to move to the right while keeping them back and wide (Fig. 7.8).

   Here, you are actually swiveling on your sacrum while you keep your weight centered on it. The pelvis does not tip to one side. The kneecaps remain hip distance and pointing to the ceiling.

3. The movement sequences through your spine and the head gently turns/side bends.

When correctly performed, you will be aware of the muscles firming inside your pelvis, over your very low back, and under your fingers.

4. Repeat the same action on the other side – "growing" the (L) sit bone long, as above.

   Slowly alternate the movement, making it come more from very low down in the "basement of control" of your spine. Grow the movement gently, don't "throw" it!

   You may feel a slightly stiff discomfort with this, but you should not feel frank pain. If you do, your performance is incorrect.

Compensations: Inability to initiate the movement from the sit bone, and hardening the waist via central cinch patterns. The ribs pop forward, the breath is constricted, and movement does not sequence through the spine. Pushing with the legs and clenching the buttocks.

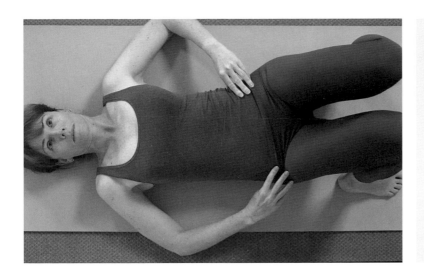

Figure 7.8
Third pelvic pattern.

Chapter 7

9 | **Fourth pelvic fundamental pattern**

Purpose: To develop intrapelvic control of intrapelvic rotation in the horizontal plane.

Benefits: This pattern is useful for anyone with low back and pelvic pain and many lower limb pain disorders. Pelvic rotation is important in functional movement, yet commonly lost in pain populations.

Position: Lie on your back, head supported if more comfortable; knees bent, feet standing under your knees; heels wide; toes facing forward. Place your index finger tip in the valleys on the inside of each pelvic bone with the middle finger on the actual bone (Fig. 7.9). Relax your buttocks, legs, and shoulders.

Key moves in this exercise: Imagine headlights in your sit bones. Also focus your attention on your front pelvic bone under your middle fingers. Further, imagine that your feet are on weighing scales to help you better sense not pushing through the feet.

1. Gently and slowly reach the (L) sit bone long, *back/down*, and away from you so that the knee reaches away, while at the same time think of drawing the (R) sit bone up and back to shorten the (R) knee toward you. The feet do not push and the kneecaps keep facing the ceiling.

   Notice that:

   ○ the pelvic bone under your left hand has moved slightly south while the right front pelvic bone has moved a little north (Fig. 7.9)

   ○ the left groin has deepened a fraction and you have rolled slightly to the right side of the sacrum and back of the right buttock (not the side).

2. The movement should sequence through the spine bringing it into rotation. You should also be aware of the left shoulder blade slightly lifting off the surface, and head roll.

3. Repeat the same action on the other side.

4. Slowly alternate the movement, refining its emanation from very low down, at the base of your spine. "Grow" the movement gently – don't "throw" it! It is a sensuous soft movement. Note how the movement of the sit bones results in your front pelvic bones doing a subtle yet distinct alternate north–south shuffle and the pelvis gently rocks from side to side. It is normal to feel a slightly stiff, albeit almost pleasurable, discomfort with this. You should not feel frank pain. If you do, your performance is incorrect.

Compensations: Poor pelvic "core" activity. Engaging the whole inferior posterolateral myofascial chain by pushing with the feet and clenching the buttocks to rotate the whole pelvis forward. (This is associated with wringing the waist and popping the lower ribs forward, which stops movement sequencing through the spine.) Breath holding.

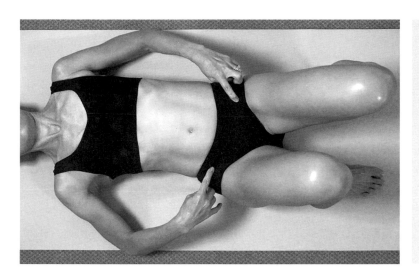

Figure 7.9
Fourth pelvic pattern.

Chapter 7

10 | Isolating hip flexion

Purpose: Engaging the first pelvic pattern to improve hip flexion with a neutral pelvis.

Benefits: This exercise helps anyone with low back and pelvic pain and many lower limb pain disorders. Commonly, flexing the hip results in the lower back being pulled into flexion, which bothers it over time. This seemingly simple movement is invariably difficult to perform properly, yet it is an important pattern of movement in many basic daily actions.

Position: Lie on your back with your (L) leg extended and the (R) bent so that you are standing on the (R) foot.

Key moves in this exercise: You really will need to "bring your brain to your sit bones" here.

1. Reach them long, back and wide so that you roll down on your sacrum toward your tailbone – notice how your pelvis has rotated forward and the very low back arches. Most people experience slight discomfort with this because they have lost the arch and are stiff here.

   It is IMPORTANT that you are creating the arch low down by bringing the sit bones back and wide – not by pushing the ribs forward.

2. Maintain this arch and slide the fingers of only the (L) hand into the space created (I call it a cubby house) (not shown). This helps you monitor your ability to maintain the arch, which is important for the next movement.

3. Lift the (R) leg so that the kneecap faces the ceiling without the lower back flattening onto your hand. To help achieve this, think: keep bringing both sit bones back and wide, particularly the

(R) as the (R) kneecap comes up and forward (Fig. 7.10).

- In the correct action, the foot does not lift but dangles. The large front thigh muscles are inactive. You should feel a folding in the groin, and "inner" muscle engagement.

- The (R) knee may want to roll out. Try to limit this and point it toward your breast so that it, the heel, and sit bone are in line with each other.

- Ensure that you are not working too high, throwing your ribs forward, and holding your breath. The breath remains low and slow and the rest of the body is relaxed.

   Repeat a number of times, and also practice sustaining the action. The art is to be able to isolate the action without creating tension. Practice more on the most difficult and stiff side. And repeat on the other side

Compensations: Poor pelvic core initiation and control results in little anterior pelvic rotation and the lower ribs thrusting forward when attempting a neutral pelvis. The large superficial hip flexors are dominant rather than iliopsoas – evidenced by tension in the front thigh and the knee being held at 90° flexion rather than in full flexion with a dangling foot.

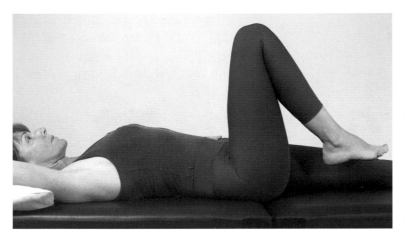

Figure 7.10
Isolating hip flexion.

11 Head pattern 1 – and eye movements

Purpose: Improve head pattern 1 – isolated nodding of the head on the neck. Improve head and eye movement coordination and lessen neck tension.

Benefits: This is helpful for anyone with head, neck, and arm pain syndromes. Work and leisure pursuits commonly involve us constantly looking down and forward, which is detrimental to posture and the important coactivity between our eyes and the neck muscles. When this coordination becomes rusty it can contribute to neck pain disorders and affect balance.

Position: Lie on your back with knees bent and your head well supported for comfort (a spiky pod is ideal). Place your hands on your lower belly and be aware of the breath coming down to them. Relax your shoulders and let them drop down and back.

Isolated head nodding

Try to move the head rather than the neck. This involves the deep front "core" neck muscles (the big front neck muscles remain relaxed).

Key moves in this exercise: Reach your sit bones long and wide, and point them back slightly to the floor. This creates a slight arch in your low back which helps the head movement.

1. Look down and feel the chin come back, the back neck lengthen, and the space at the base of the skull "open." Feel the muscles firm at the front of your throat under your jaw. You should feel as though you have three double chins! This is good. Sustain this over a number of breaths (Fig. 7.11).

2. *Progression:* Maintain the above action, but just lighten the weight of the head on the support.

Do not lift off the surface – this is a subtle action. IMPORTANT: the forehead leads the movement, not the chin. Attempt to increasingly sustain this while continuing to breathe down (not up).

These movements usually feel hard work, but you should not feel any pain with either step.

Compensations: Poor deep muscle activity and overactivity of superficial neck flexors (sternomastoids and scalene) make the chin protrude. Flexion of the whole neck rather than the head on the neck. Poor abdominal action in bringing the lower ribs back on unweighting the head.

Head and eye movement integration

Benefits: (Useful because working at computers can rob us of good eye function.) The eyes can move with or against the direction of head movement. We can keep a stable gaze while the head moves – or move the eyes without the head moving.

Key moves in this exercise:

a) Keeping your head still:

1. Roll your eyes fully: down and up; side to side; diagonally; in circles clockwise and anticlockwise. These are rotations of the eyeball in the socket.

2. Place a finger close in front of your nose and focus upon it, and then focus upon something in the far distance. Keep alternating your focus back and forth.

If you start to feel dizzy, giddy or a bit nauseous: pause, close your eyes, and take a few deep breaths. Gently and slowly begin to repeat the sequences one at a time, pausing as necessary. Take it slowly; with practice you will develop more tolerance.

b) Allowing your head to move:

3. Eyes and head move in the same direction: Repeat all four movements described in a)1.

    Ensure you really look with the eyes and allow your head to move so you can "see further." Explore the extremes of the movement. Do you move equally each way?

4. Eyes move in the opposite direction to the head: Take this slowly, particularly if you have noticed a tendency to be at all dizzy. Do the same four eye movements while moving the head in the opposite direction.

5. End up by fixing your gaze at a certain spot and then circle your head in both directions.

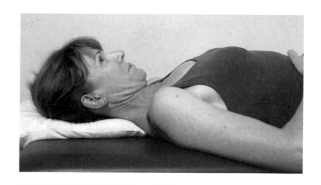

Figure 7.11

Head pattern 1 – and eye movements.

12 | Rag doll

Purpose: Increase thorax mobility by engaging axial fundamental pattern 1 to stabilize the lower thorax while initiating movement in the upper thorax through shoulder pattern 3.

Benefits: This helps all spinal pain problems – particularly head, neck, and arm pain syndromes. It helps loosen the upper chest and back, open the shoulders, and relax the neck. Think of yourself as a rag doll: remain loose and floppy (i.e., do not tense up by trying too hard).

Position: Lie down with your knees bent and feet flat on the floor, arms spread as close to a right angle to the body as you can, palms facing up. If your upper back/shoulders are very stiff, place a small cushion under your head for comfort. If you would like and are able, bend both knees to the chest and cross your shins (Fig. 7.12A) – otherwise keep your feet resting on the floor.

Key moves in this exercise: Give the weight of your body to the floor.

1. Sink the lower back ribs into the floor and widen them so that you feel your core switch on. Try to sustain this action and the rib position – and breathe naturally.

2. With heavy arms, gently, slowly and lazily "grow" the (R) arm longer and reach as far as you can without tensing, allowing the head to roll to the (R) and the (L) arm to "shorten" (Fig. 7.12b). Imagine someone pulling you by your (R) hand and give in to it.

   You should feel a nice stretch through your upper back and shoulders. Hover here and breathe deeply, letting go on the exhale.

3. Repeat to the (L) allowing the head to rotate to the (L); both palms face up and the (R) arm "shortens."

4. Slowly alternate the movement, making it languorous.

Compensations: Tensing the muscles of the low back ribs and holding the breath. Tensing the neck, front chest and arm muscles, which restricts the movement. (Remember: less tension = more movement.)

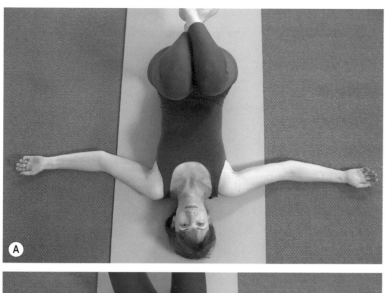

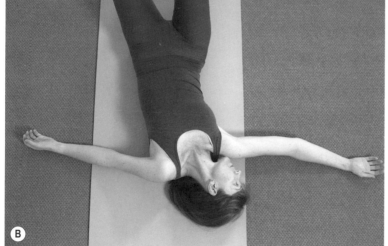

Figure 7.12
Rag doll.

13 | "Temperature check" rotation

Purpose: To improve upper spinal mobility and open the upper chest and shoulders by reconnecting head, neck, and shoulder movements via fourth shoulder and head patterns.

Benefits: This is helpful in all spinal pain problems – particularly head, neck, and arm pain syndromes. Common to all is stiffness in the thorax and shoulder girdle which compromises neck function. This exercise improves flexibility and eases neck tension and pain.

Position: Lie down on your (R) side with your hips bent to 90° and your spine in a neutral position; the tailbone points behind (not tucked under). The (R) arm lies forward perpendicular to the body. Place the palm of your (L) hand in contact on your forehead and keep it so. Sink the underside of the body into the floor (Fig. 7.13a).

Key moves in this exercise: Imagine a headlight in the point of your (L) elbow searching wide.

1. Gently reach the (L) elbow forward as far as you can and then slowly back and wide as far as you can. Visualize the movement being led back from the front point of the (L) shoulder – the shoulder blade rolls back around the chest wall (Fig. 7.13b).

2. Focus upon widening the (L) elbow and letting it drop further back each time you go back. Notice the opening in the top front chest muscles and a stretch in the top of your back. There should be no tension or effort. The neck should be heavy and relaxed. Do not lose hand contact with your forehead.

3. Linger in the elbow "back" position and explore bringing the breath down and back with a gentle (though extended) exhalation. Feel your stomach muscles engage more, and the simultaneous greater stretch in the shoulder/top back – which is the aim.

Do not harden over the lower back ribs. The "center" body remains soft and open and the breath freely travels down and back. Picture yourself as relaxed as a rag doll.

4. *Progression 1:* In the "back position" extend the elbow. If it does not touch the floor, place a support under it for comfort – and continue to let the shoulder fall back while breathing down and back (Fig. 7.13c).

5. *Progression 2:* Sweep the (L) hand on the floor in a 180° arc over your head to touch the (R) fingers. Sweep the arm back and forward like a windscreen wiper. If possible, keep the elbow straight and the hand in contact with the floor (Fig. 7.13d).

Compensations: Leading the movement from the elbow rather than the point of the shoulder; loss of contact palm to forehead; excess neck and arm tension; breath holding; "waist wringing."

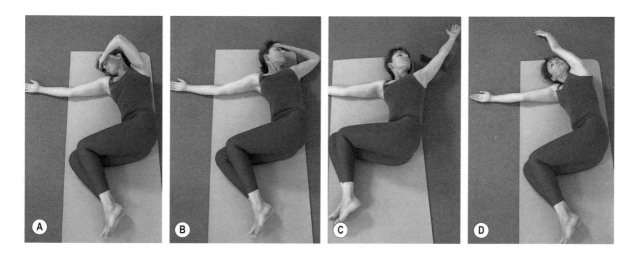

Figure 7.13

"Temperature check" rotation: a),b) basic; c) progression 1; d) progression 2.

Chapter 7

14 | Prayer stretch: connecting breath, core and pelvic patterns

Purpose: This stretch helps improve inner awareness and core control, and also its functional interconnection with the pelvic floor. It involves engaging the axial FP and first shoulder patterns.

Benefits: This is helpful for all spinal pain problems – particularly head, neck, and arm pain syndromes. Moving coarsely with excess effort and tension is common and makes it difficult to "connect" with the "inner" muscle system. Focusing upon the breath and "core" activity (without the stretch) is nice to do with someone in acute pain.

Position: Lie on your stomach, placing your arms above your head – elbows as close as you can get them – and slide them further away. Bring your hands into a prayer position and rest your forehead on your upper arms. If your neck and shoulders are very stiff, place a pillow under your chest (or lower if your low back is sore) and place your arms where you can get them. Relax your legs and buttocks, and allow the heels to roll out.

Key moves in this exercise: Surrender your whole body into the floor. In particular, consciously relax your shoulders through the whole sequence:

1. Inhale so that your lower ribs widen and lift and you notice the lower belly muscles gently firm – and that your tailbone has slightly dropped. This is because the diaphragm descent reflexly activates the deep transversus abdominis and the pelvic floor muscles.

2. Gently and actively exhale through pursed lips, noticing more firming low "down under" and that your sit bones widen and lift allowing the tailbone to slightly rise. The pelvic floor and transversus work together to push the air out; the diaphragm ascends and relaxes. Quietly explore the breath cycle and enhance this motion of your sit bones and tailbone. You will not feel this if you are clenching your buttocks.

3. Further, now sustain the expanded lower rib position and the lower belly firmness while allowing the breath to freely come and go – low and slow. Try to extend the out breath and notice even more lower belly firming as the pelvic floor and transversus work harder to push the air out. There should be no neck or shoulder tension (Fig. 7.14a).

4. Further, keeping the arms soft, draw the front point of one shoulder back, away from the floor. There will not be much movement but you should feel more stretch in the shoulder. Repeat with the other, exploring the stretch while working the core with the breath.

5. *Progression 1:* While maintaining an open center, float the head back and forward keeping the chin back and neck long. Ensure the lower ribs remain back and wide as you do this (Fig. 7.14b).

6. To deepen the shoulder stretch, place your elbows on blocks (see Fig. 7.14b).

Compensations: Poor core and pelvic floor muscle activity and no/little expansion of the lower rib cage. Inability to maintain the expansion through the breath cycle. Increased breathing rate or shortening exhalation so as not lose the lower belly firmness. Neck tension and upper chest breathing, and fixing the front shoulder girdle rather than release. Clenching the buttocks.

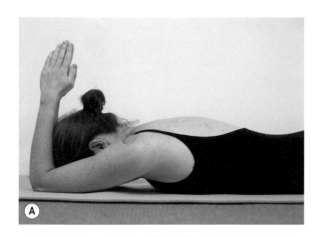
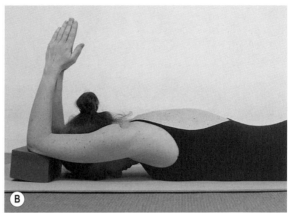

Figure 7.14
Prayer stretch.

15 | Windscreen wipers

Purpose: 1. To stabilize the pelvis, isolate hip movement, and increase hip rotation range by engaging the pelvic patterns. 2. To connect pelvic/hip rotation to spinal movement.

Benefits: This is helpful in all low back and pelvic pain disorders, and many hip, knee, and leg pain problems. It helps address the common problem of stiff hips and a "spatially unstable" pelvis.

Position: Lie on your stomach, placing one hand comfortably above your head. Bring the other to palpate the front pelvic bone and also to monitor sustained lower abdominal and pelvic floor activity (not shown).

Isolating movement to the hip only

Key moves in this exercise: With your thighs parallel, bend both knees to a right angle:

1. Drop your feet apart. Gently firm your lower stomach muscles and keep your pelvis stable (both front pelvic bones equally in contact with the floor) (Fig. 7.15a) and (L) foot still while slowly moving the (R) foot as far as you can to the right and left, like a windscreen wiper. As the foot moves to the right, the left pelvis will want to lift, and vice versa. Do not let it. You will probably feel that it is easier to go to one side.

   Expect to feel stiff discomfort in your hip sockets. In fact, you are chasing this feeling. Slowly repeat the movement back and forth, attempting both to gradually increase the hip movement without the pelvis moving and improve any difference between swinging the foot to (L) and (R) – and between sides.

Compensations: Poor inner pelvic control and an unstable pelvis, plus an inability to relax/lengthen the hip/thigh myofascia.

Allowing pelvic rotation

Key moves in this exercise: Bring both arms loosely up above your head.

1. Keeping both knees in contact with the floor, swing both feet to the (R) trying to touch them to the floor – the pelvis now moves, following the hip (Fig. 7.15b).

   You should sense activity in the lower belly and groins. Ensure you do not harden over the lower back ribs. Note how the sit bone follows the heel and that your whole spine has gone into a twist. Allow the head to roll (not shown). Explore the movement to each side – and also with your head turned to either side.

2. *Progression 1:* Glue the knees together as you bring the feet to the floor to the (R) – and then explore this to either side. Keep the shoulders relaxed and feel a bigger twist through the spine (Fig. 7.15c).

Compensations: Cinching at the waist with no "inner unit" activity and poor articulation through the mid and upper spine. Fixing with the shoulders which blocks movement through the spine.

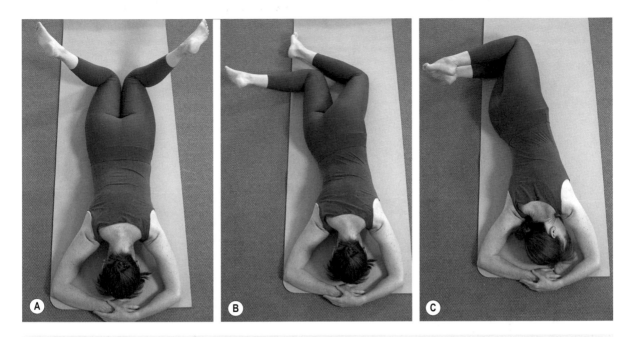

Figure 7.15

Windscreen wipers: a) isolating movement to the hip only; b) allowing pelvic rotation; c) progression.

Chapter 7

16	**Backward pelvic rotation**

Purpose: To initiate pelvic and spinal rotation in extension via the first and fourth pelvic patterns.

Benefits: This helps low back and pelvic pain disorders and many hip, knee, and leg pain syndromes. Movement initiation from the pelvis is commonly difficult and this helps redress it.

Position: Lie on your stomach, placing your arms loosely above your head and elbows about level with your ears. Place a pillow under your chest if your neck/shoulders are very stiff. Turn your face to the (R). If this is uncomfortable, take the weight of your head on your forehead/ bridge of your nose. Completely relax your neck, shoulders, buttocks, and legs.

Key moves in this exercise: Focus upon gently expanding the lower ribs sideways and back, and breathe down into your pelvis.

1. Gently reach your (R) sit bone long, up, and back toward the (L) and the ceiling (as though someone were pulling it back with a string). Your weight will roll to the left side of your pelvis and your right inner groin will deepen and "firm" – and the (R) hip and knee will softly bend all on their own. Your head will roll slightly more to the right.

   IMPORTANT: you must feel a firming over your lower tummy and back, and within your pelvis – **not** around your waist and lower ribs. Thinking about "going long and back with the tailbone" helps (Fig. 7.16).

2. Allow the movement to sequence right up through your spine. Can you feel it as high as your neck and shoulders? If not, try relaxing more as you do the movement.

3. Repeat the same sequence with the head turned (L), reaching the (L) sit bone back. Then alternate to each side with the head centered yet free to turn.

It should feel easy and pleasant.

Compensations: Poor "inner unit" activity with poor pelvic rotation and "hip hiking," hardening over the lower ribs, and little or no movement into the thorax. Stiffening of the legs and tensing the shoulders, which blocks the movement.

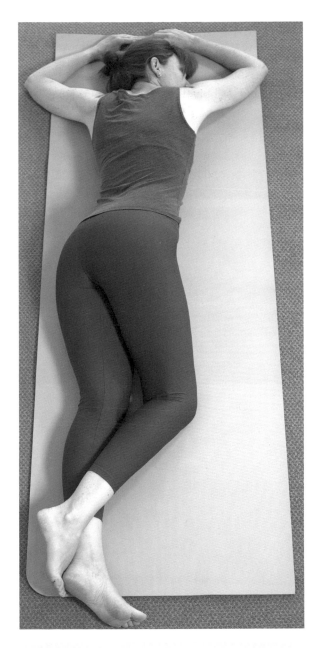

Figure 7.16

Backward pelvic rotation.

Chapter 7

18 | Praying mantis

Purpose: To mobilize the upper thorax and cervicothoracic junction; and to release myofascial restrictions between the shoulder and upper chest by engaging shoulder patterns 1, 3 and 4.

Benefits: This helps all spinal pain problems – particularly head, neck, and arm pain syndromes. Lazy upper back and shoulder blade muscles and thorax stiffness is common. This exercise mobilizes the upper thoracic spine and improves shoulder girdle control.

Position: Lie on your stomach and rest on your forehead and the bridge of your nose. Place your hands so that they are **at** shoulder level and wide apart, your forearms are vertical, and your fingers point to the wall above your head. Spread your fingers, ensuring that all four corners of the hand are contacting the floor– particularly the heel. Check that your neck is "long" and relaxed, and allow the backs of the legs, buttocks, and waist to relax as well.

Key moves in this exercise: Imagine that you have a searchlight in the points of each elbow.

1. Soften and gently sink your hands into the floor and draw the front points of your shoulders back and wide, shining your elbow lights toward the ceiling and wide apart. You should notice that the muscles between your shoulder blades have now "engaged."

2. Relax the muscles over your lower back ribs then push them back and wide to engage your core (and make space for the breath). Sustain this, allowing the breath to come and go for a minute or so to give you time to correctly perceive this (Fig. 7.18a).

3. Being mindful of the above cues, now draw the front point of the (R) shoulder further back so that the shoulder blade moves diagonally down and back toward your spine and waist, while keeping your elbow light pointing up and out. Your neck should lengthen further, and turn slightly to the right. Your weight will shift more onto the left breast, and also the (L) pelvis, though to a lesser extent (Fig. 7.18b).

   IMPORTANT: Relax your pectoral muscles at the front of your shoulders and do not push your hands into the floor – simply let them sink. Expect to feel both a combined front shoulder stretch and muscles being activated in the spine between your shoulder blades.

4. Repeat a few times on each side and then alternate the movement, feeling your shoulder blades "swiveling around and over your back." It should feel free and pleasing.

5. *Progression:* When this action is going well, you can also "look" either under or over the moving shoulder – still ensuring that the back/down movement of the shoulder blade leads the movement.

Compensations: Pushing with the hands and tensing the anterior chest/shoulder muscles blocks the movement. Tensing the lower ribs and wringing the waist disturbs breathing; dropping the elbows and tightening the back armpit muscles also blocks the scapula and spinal movement, creating neck tension.

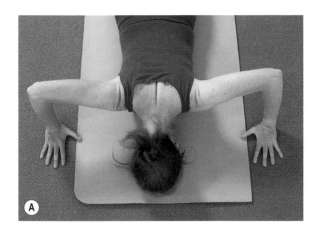
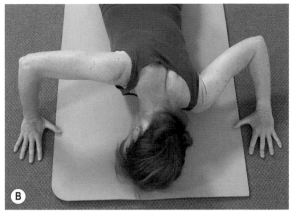

Figure 7.18

Praying mantis.

19 | **Wide wings**

Purpose: Rebalance thoracic and shoulder girdle myofascia length/tension relationships via improving first and fourth shoulder pattern control with the glenohumeral joint in internal rotation.

Benefits: This helps all spinal pain problems – particularly head, neck, and arm pain syndromes. Our lifestyles can lead to lazy upper back and shoulder muscles, as well as poor rotator cuff balance. This not only contributes to poor posture but also to shoulder and neck pain. Doing this exercise tones them up.

Position: Lie down on your stomach, resting on your forehead, with your hands by your side, all finger tips under your front pelvic bones (not fully shown), palms facing the ceiling and elbows well bent so that they resemble a pair of wings. Place a pillow under your chest if you are very stiff or uncomfortable (Fig. 7.19a).

Key moves in this exercise: Inhale and widen the lower back ribs. Maintain the expansion and breathe regularly. Aim to maintain the wings wide in the movement.

1. Keeping your arms completely relaxed, draw the front point of your (L) shoulder back – away from the floor and your ear so that the shoulder blade draws in toward your spine. The elbow reaches wide yet hangs forward. Imagine your arm is a soft wide wing. The work is between the shoulder blade and the spine - the hand does not push (Fig. 7.19b).

2. The weight shifts over the (R) breast and the head turns slightly to the (L). The neck should lengthen and remain relaxed. There should be no pain.

3. Keep expanding and pushing wide over the lower back ribs, and try to sustain the action for 3+ slow breaths. You will feel your whole back working.

4. Repeat on the (R) – and then alternate.

5. *Progression:* Maintain the above position and unweight the hand to hover it just above the surface – without losing the scapular stability where the point of the shoulder falls forward.

Compensations: Poor initiation with the point of the shoulder causing "locking-in" over the lower ribs. The elbows lead and the "wide wings" are lost with tensing and shortening of the neck; tensing the arm and the back armpit with little scapular movement. Breath holding.

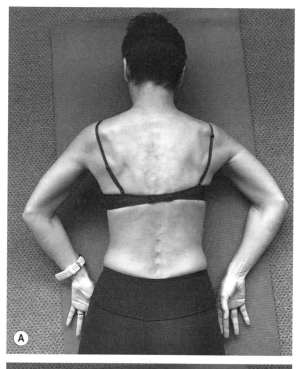

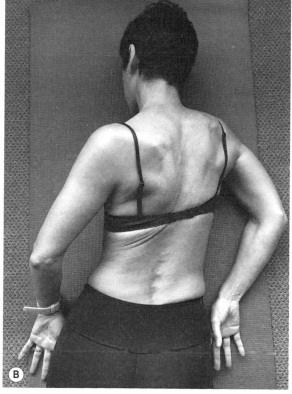

Figure 7.19
Wide wings.

20 Half Sphinx to Amphibian

Purpose: Initiate upper spinal rotation in extension by engaging shoulder patterns 1 and 4.

Benefits: This helps all spinal pain problems – particularly head, neck, and arm pain syndromes. Most of our waking hours involve us with our head and shoulders forward one way or another, so the spine and shoulders lose their suppleness. This exercise gently mobilizes the whole spine.

Position: Lie down on your stomach, resting on your elbows ensuring that they are directly under your shoulders, that your forearms are parallel, and your fingers face forward.

Key moves in this exercise: Stand the (R) hand under your (R) shoulder – the elbow should be bent and the palm and fingers spread. Let go any tension.

1. Without pressing the hand, draw the front point of your (R) shoulder back. The elbow straightens but does not lock or drop (the arm remains soft (Fig. 7.20a).

   Notice that you have rolled onto your (L) pelvis and your (R) hip and knee have bent – and that your head has turned to the right to look over your shoulder. Can you see your (R) foot and that the (L) hand has swung in to point to the (R) hand (Fig. 7.20b)?

2. Now let the point of the (R) shoulder fall forward and notice that your (R) elbow has bent and the (L) hand has swung back to face forward; the weight has fallen to your (R) pelvis – and you now look over your (L) shoulder (not shown).

3. Oscillate the movement back and forward – emphasizing the shoulder back phase – allowing your spine to soften and lengthen as it rotates back and forward. Make it light and sensual. Expect an agreeable stiffness in your spine.

4. Repeat on the (L).

Compensations: Pushing with the hand and tensing the arm not only locks the shoulder girdle, it limits spinal and pelvic movement as well as weight shift and rotation.

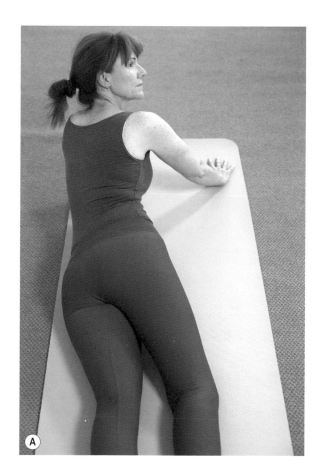

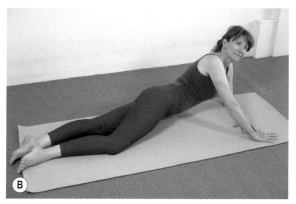

Figure 7.20
Half Sphinx to Amphibian.

Chapter 7

21 Cat/Camel

Purpose: To animate the first and second pelvic patterns to explore the relationship between the secondary and primary curves and improve proprioception and spinal mobility.

Benefits: Good pelvic control is the basis for a healthy spine. People with spinal pain commonly lose mobility and control of the secondary spinal curves – in particular the lumbar lordosis. Their spine resembles a long C curve more typical of the primitive infant spine.

Position: Assume an all fours position, knees hip width apart, with hands forward of your shoulders and your (R) hand and knee slightly in front of your (L) (not shown). Open the palms and spread the fingers. Keep your elbows soft and wide.

Key moves in this exercise: Imagine that you have headlights in your sit bones.

1. Reach them long, back and wide and shine/point them up toward the ceiling. Notice your weight shifts back, your spine/tailbone lengthens, and that you probably inhaled.

2. Drawing your shoulder blades back, lift your head to look up. The movement starts at the sit bones and sequences through your spine to your head. Try to widen the lower ribs as you breathe in and the spine lengthens. This is Cat – initiated from the first pelvic pattern (Fig. 7.21a).

3. Now draw the sit bones together and tuck your tailbone under – your spine rounds and your head then drops to look between your knees. Notice that your weight shifts slightly forward. *Focus upon really expanding and rounding the lower rib cage.* Your belly works! Keep the hands

light, elbows pointing sideways and the front top chest soft. This is Camel, initiated from the second pelvic pattern (Fig. 7.21b).

4. Repeat the sequence reaching the tailbone back, long and up on the inhale – in Cat; dropping it and curling the mid/lower back on the exhale in Camel. You should be aware of the lower belly working in both patterns. Focus more on the first one (the Cat).

5. Repeat the same sequencing with the (L) hand and knee slightly forward of the (R).

Compensations: *Cat:* Poor initiation from the first pelvic pattern is associated with poor backward weight shift and anterior pelvic rotation; "throwing the lower ribs forward"; poor action in shoulders coming back to assist head lift.

Camel: Dominance of glutei over pelvic FP2; pressing into the floor, locking the elbows and over engagement of the front shoulders into second shoulder pattern, which reinforces a "dome" and increased upper thoracic flexion (with poor thoracolumbar flexion). Poor posterolateral expansion of the lower rib cage.

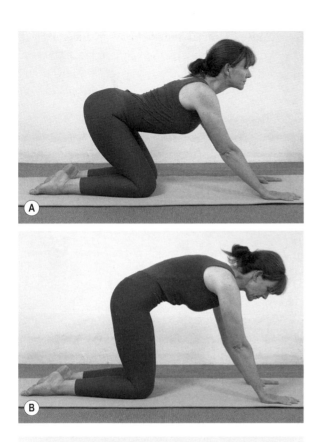

Figure 7.21
Cat/Camel: a) Cat; b) Camel.

Chapter 7

<table>
<tr><td>

22

</td><td>

Supplicant pose

</td></tr>
</table>

Purpose: To open the hips and shoulders, and align the spine by engaging all the first patterns of the axis. Movement is initiated from the pelvis.

Benefits: This helps all spinal pain syndromes. It not only stretches stiff hips, shoulders, and the upper/mid back but also lengthens the spine while focusing on coordinating core control.

Position: Kneel forward on the floor with your forearms and elbows resting loosely above your head as shown in Fig. 7.22a. Walk your knees back and wide and bring your big toes together. Let your forehead and nose rest on the floor behind your forearms. If your head does not touch the floor, place a small support under the forehead.

Key moves in this exercise: Imagining that you have headlights in your sit bones is helpful – particularly in moving them wide and up into "high beam."

1. Sink your knees heavily into the floor and relax your buttocks.

2. Reach your sit bones *long, wide and up* (Fig. 7.22a–c) so that the tailbone floats long and lifts. Feel how the lower belly engages. If you cannot feel this, soften the legs more and work more decisively with the sit bones. Your weight will shift further back over your legs.

3. Soften the muscles around your lower ribs and expand them so that you feel you open the center body sideways and back – the front ribs draw back. Sustain this while allowing the breath to quietly come and go.

4. Refocus on the tailbone and reach it further back and up to lengthen the spine from its base – still keeping an "open center" (Fig. 7.22a–c).

5. You should now be feeling a decent stretch in your shoulders. This is good. Try not to tense against the discomfort, but breathe into it and "let go" on the out breath. Keep the head heavy on the ground, the neck relaxed as you "stay in it" – quietly breathing, softening, and lengthening. While your brain is working to control this pose properly, it should feel restorative.

6. *Progression 1:* Swing the hands apart so that the forearms are parallel, then repeat the same actions.

7. *Progression 2:* Straighten your arms, carefully placing your hand with fingers spread – and the weight is evenly spread across your knuckles and the heel of the hand (Fig. 7.22b,c). Repeat the actions described above.

8. *Variations:* Explore growing one sit bone longer and higher, or growing one arm longer. The rib cage moves to the lengthening side in both but should remain aligned and "open" – and back.

Compensations: Clenching the buttocks stops the weight shifting back and the sit bones/tailbone lifting. Moving the weight too far back and collapsing the pelvis down – the tailbone drops rather than lifts. "Cinching" over the lower ribs prevents the thorax aligning with the pelvis and disturbs core control, so the spine cannot fully lengthen. Tensing the shoulders prevents them opening and encourages upper chest breathing and breath holding.

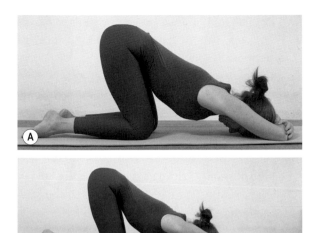

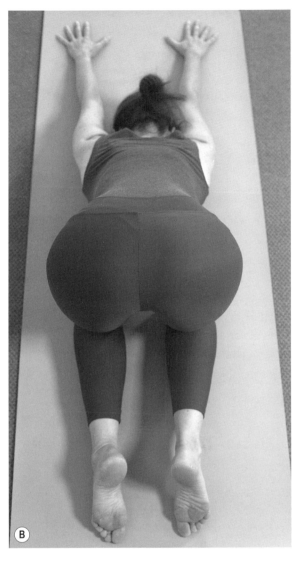

Figure 7.22

Supplicant pose.

<table>
<tr><td>**23**</td><td>**Healthy sitting**</td></tr>
</table>

Purpose: Strengthen core and proximal limb girdle control by engaging the first FPs in ideal postural alignment.

Benefits: This helps ALL spinal problems. We know that most people cannot sit properly, and that this is a potent contributor to spinal pain. Changing bad sitting habits involves being mindful of *how* you choose to sit and focusing upon the correct way to do so. Good sitting habits involve actively balancing on the sit bones. This naturally activates part of the core.

Position: Sit on a chair with a firm flat seat. The sit bones are rocker shaped and most of us have a bad habit of rolling back on these – the weight falls onto the buttocks and the tailbone tucks under. The spine collapses. This is unhealthy (Fig. 7.23a).

Sitting up correctly

Key moves in this exercise: Bring your sit bones back and wide on the seat and ensure that you are balancing on the top front part of them.

1. Actively widen them and allow your tailbone to point back. Be aware of feeling your lower belly muscles doing this action by monitoring the firming just above your groins. Your front pelvis rolls forward. Notice your spine lift. (Fig. 7.23b).

2. When you first attempt to "sit up," you'll predictably throw your front ribs forward, tensing the neck and the back muscles above your belt line. This inhibits the core, is hard on your spine, and stops you breathing properly!

   To counteract this reflex action place your hands around the lower rib cage, soften the muscles under your hands (Fig. 7.23c) and expand and widen the lower ribs under your hands. Feel the lower belly muscles contract more. This is the core working naturally. Aim to sustain this action and breathe normally (Fig. 7.23c).

3. Further, still balancing on the top front of the sit bones, gently press them down into the chair. Notice how this promotes a further "inner lift" and your breathing becomes easier. Also notice as your spine lifts: the neck lengthens, your chin drops, and the crown of your head floats tall.

4. If you meditate, ensure that you adopt a correct sitting position and breathe low and slow for a great natural core workout. The spine lengthens – the center is open.

Compensations: Poor pelvic and core activity with excess muscle tension and "cinching" around the lower ribs. This is tiring – hence reverting to slump is predictable.

Mini pelvic rolls: recharging the "correct sitting action"

Key moves in this exercise:

1. Roll back on your sit bones and notice your whole spine slumps, your neck shortens, your chin pokes forward, and your shoulders slouch forward. Feel familiar?

2. Now slowly roll up onto the top front inside of your sit bones, repeating all the steps above. The tailbone initiates the movement by coming back – movement sequences through the spine vertebra by vertebra. The spine lengthens without obstruction around the "center"; the front chest and shoulders open; and the head floats tall.

3. Ensure you can sense the movement being initiated from your tailbone not your ribs. Practice being aware of "sitting up from below" as often as you can till it becomes a habit.

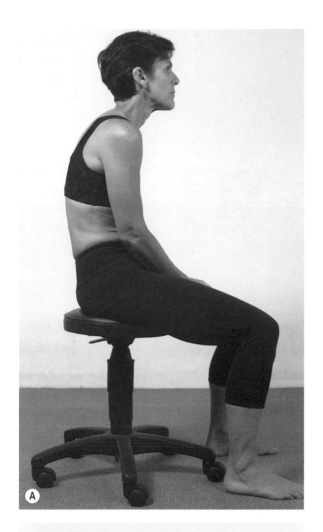

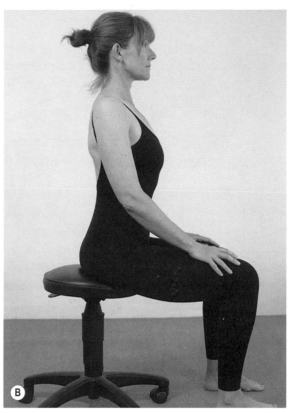

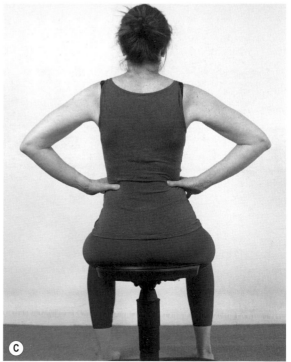

Figure 7.23
Healthy sitting.

24 "Opening the center"

Purpose: To build core capacity by engaging the axial fundamental pattern when upright and active.

Benefits: This helps all spinal problems. Postural collapse switches off the core and stops you breathing effectively. Do this exercise frequently throughout the day when sitting and standing (properly!) It naturally gives your core a great workout and better supports your spine. Muscle tension melts away. The following describes the action in sitting.

Position: Sit with your pelvis in neutral – on the tops of your sit bones – and maintain this position.

Key moves in this exercise:

1. Place your hands to softly encircle your lower rib cage – thumbs pointing behind.

2. Drop your shoulders, "present" the top of your breastbone, and draw the front points of the shoulders back, keeping the elbows wide. The shoulder blades come closer together.

3. Breathing down, gently widen the lower ribs sideways and back into your thumb webs. Imagine that you are creating an internal "roundness" of the lower rib cage. Some of you will need to widen more across the front ribs. You should feel the back muscles under your thumbs soften as you do this – while you feel your lower pelvic core firming – it has to in order to create widening of the lower rib cage.

4. Aim to keep the "center open" like this as you continue to breathe down and back – regularly and slowly (Fig. 7.24). Maintain this action for increasing periods of time during the day to build endurance and it becomes automatic, whatever you are doing.

Compensations: Lifting the chest and shoulders, with poor core activation and widening. Tensing under the thumbs and throwing the lower ribs forward (and probably holding the breath). Inability to sustain the opening while breathing regularly. Ballooning the belly.

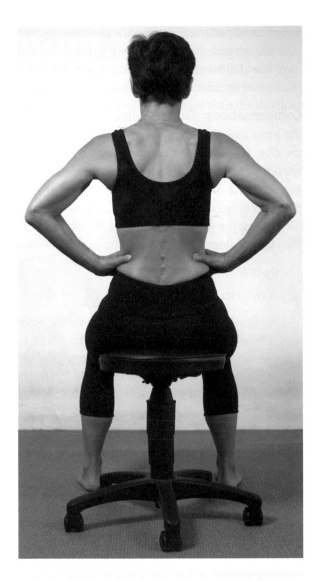

Figure 7.24
Opening the center.

26 | Head fundamental patterns

Purpose: To improve head and neck posturo-movement control by engaging the head patterns when upright to mobilize and fine tune movements of the head on the neck. These are discrete micro-movements which only move the head on the top neck vertebrae.

Benefits: These help all head and neck pain, and upper limb pain syndromes. Ideally the head is poised on top of a flexible upright spine and free to move and orient the senses. Its control suffers when posture is poor (slump sitting is common). Be mindful of doing these patterns as "pause gymnastics" through the day, e.g., at the computer.

Position: Sit with a neutral spine (with your weight on the front of the sit bones and the feet). "Float your head" tall and ensure the back of your neck is soft and long.

First and second patterns

Key moves in the exercises: Do not hold tension around your lower ribs – expand and widen them and breathe easily.

1. *First pattern:* "Present" the top of your breastbone as if you were opening your heart, and draw the points of the shoulders back and wide. Notice that this lengthens the neck. Gently sustain this action.

2. Softly drop the chin and glide your head backward as you keep looking straight ahead. The back of your skull lifts. You will feel you have a "double chin" and should feel the muscles working under your chin and between the shoulder blades. Keep floating the head tall. In the "back

position," see if you can add a gentle discrete nodding movement of the head **only**, as in gesturing "yes" (Fig. 7.26a).

3. *Second pattern:* Simply relax the first pattern. This usually results in you being in second pattern, where the chin pokes forward. Explore moving from this into the first pattern – which requires more emphasis (not shown).

Compensations: Overworking the mid neck (because of poor alignment of the spine and shoulders). Over-engaging the superficial neck muscles, and increasing neck and shoulder tension. Tensing over the lower back ribs.

Third pattern

Key moves in this exercise: Maintaining the positional "cues" for the first pattern and the head erect:

- Gently slide your (L) ear to the left, and tip it up as though wanting to hear more clearly. The (R) ear drops. Gently repeat each side. Try and feel the skull rotating side to side while the neck remains tall (Fig. 7.26b).

Compensations: Poor isolated movement of the head (the whole neck side bends). Poor control of upright "neutral" and sustaining first pattern (the chin moves forward).

Fourth pattern

Key moves in this exercise: Maintaining the positional cues for the first pattern:

- Turn your eyes to the right, letting the head follow but not the whole neck. Only expect to achieve about 40–45° turning here at best – as in the gesture of saying "no – no" (Fig. 7.26c).

Compensations: Poor control of upright neutral and sustaining first pattern – the chin moves forward – and the whole neck turns.

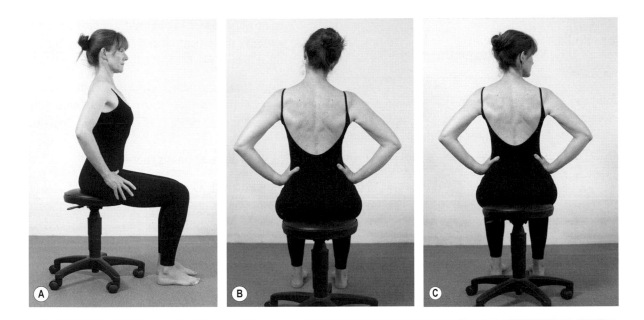

Figure 7.26

Head fundamental patterns: a) head FP1; b) head FP3; c) head FP4.

27 | Shoulder shrug and slide

Purpose: To improve upper thoracic and scapular mobility, and its three-dimensional control on the chest wall, by engaging shoulder patterns 1, 3 and 4.

Benefits: This helps head, neck, shoulder, and upper limb pain syndromes. A common finding is increased tension over the front chest and shoulder accompanied by poor scapular control. This exercise is easy to do during the day – especially when at the computer.

It can also be done in side lying, which is nice for someone with acute shoulder pain.

Position: Sit with a neutral spine: weight on the front of your sit bones, feeling the spine lift (where the neck is soft and long and the head can "float tall").

Rest your (R) open palm on the top of your head without disturbing a neutral neck posture. Float your head into your palm and drop your chin slightly. Relax your shoulders and arms.

Do not hold tension around your lower ribs. Breathe easily.

Key moves in this exercise: Imagine that you have a searchlight in the (R) elbow point.

1. Soften both your hand and whole arm; float the elbow wide. Maintain this while reaching the front point of your (R) shoulder up in a "shrug" to point your elbow light to the ceiling, letting your ribs move to the right – and the weight shift more onto the (R) sit bone. The head will tilt left, but the neck is relaxed. Keep the lower ribs soft and wide (Fig. 7.27a).

2. Slowly draw the front point of the (R) shoulder back and down so that the elbow light shines down and back – and the scapula slides down and back toward the spine. Your weight shifts more onto your (L) sit bone, the upper ribs move slightly (L) and turn slightly to the (R) with the head (not shown) (Fig. 7.27b).

3. Gently oscillate back and forth, fine-tuning the point of the shoulder leading the diagonal slide of the scapula.

Compensations: Gripping the hand and tensing the arm (which also tenses and shortens the neck – and the back of the armpit). The scapula does not slide freely over the chest wall and there is little movement through the upper thorax and shoulder girdle – particularly into retraction.

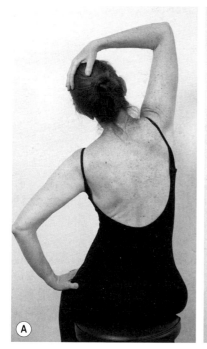

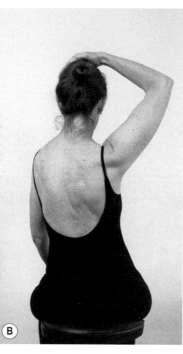

Figure 7.27
Shoulder shrug and slide.

28 | Windmills

Purpose: To improve neutral postural control of the upper thorax and shoulder girdle, and control of arm elevation by engaging first and third shoulder patterns integrated with the axial FP.

Benefits: Useful in all spinal pain problems – particularly head, neck, and arm pain syndromes. Most of us hang our shoulders forward, which limits how easily and well we can lift our arms. Try it! Then compare the movement in this exercise, which wakes up lazy shoulder girdle control.

Position: Sit or stand "tall" though relaxed, arms loosely by your side.

Key moves in this exercise: Drop your shoulders, widen the lower rib cage until you lower belly firms – and maintain this.

1. Gently float your arms out to about 30° as you turn your palms up to face the ceiling.

2. Float the top of your breastbone forward and draw the front points of shoulders back. The hands move slightly forward (Fig. 7.28a).

   [Notice: how this makes it easier for you to turn the palms up; that the muscles between your shoulder blades are working. Can you point your thumbs behind you?]

3. Continue to engage the shoulder blades and bring the arms up to the horizontal, reaching the fingers wide – palms still facing up.

4. Turn your head right to look at the (R) upturned palm – as you reach out to the right – while allowing the (L) palm to face down (Fig. 7.28b). Repeat the same action looking left. And alter-nate. There is a "skewing" action between your top shoulder blades.

5. Reengage the top breastbone forward, points of shoulders back and palms up. Look at your (R) palm as you bring it up to the vertical, allowing the top of your breastbone to come further forward. The (L) hand drops and the top rib cage moves to the right. Stay soft, back, and wide over the lower back ribs (Fig. 7.28c).

6. Repeat the exercises side to side, carefully attending to each step.

Compensations: Inadequate achievement of the steps as prompted – the hands draw back more than the point of the shoulders (leading to excessive tension over the back armpit, poor "neutral" upper spinal alignment, and neck tension as the arms lift). Inadequate core control – with tension over the back ribs, which lift and "pop forward."

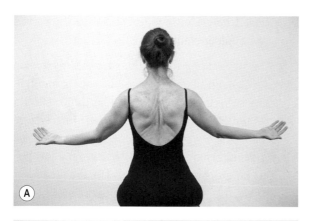

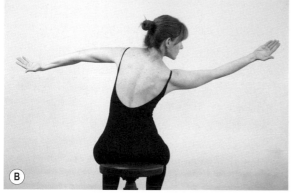

Figure 7.28

Windmills.

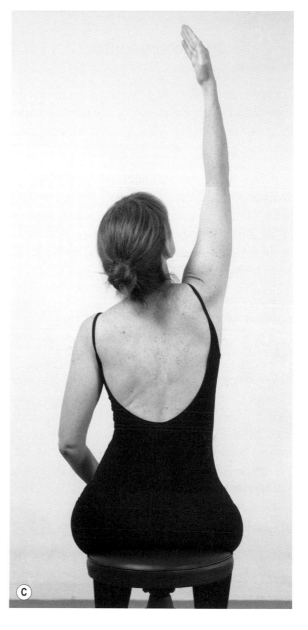

29 Pelvic dancing in sitting

Purpose: To mobilize the pelvis and lower spine, and strengthen the core by activating the pelvic patterns with the axial fundamental pattern in functional postures.

Benefits: This helps all spinal pain problems, particularly low back and pelvic pain and lower limb pains. Most of us collapse in sitting, which switches off the core and bothers the back. These movements mobilize the pelvis and lower spine and reactivate the "core" and spinal muscles.

Position: Sit on the front of a firm flat seat with your sit bones back and wide so that you are balanced right on the top of them. Imagine each of them as the pointy base of a spinning top.

Key moves in these exercises: Wearing a Key Moves Core Retrainer Belt helps you activate your "primary core" while doing these movements from your "pelvic core." Expand and widen your lower ribs into the belt (or hands) so that you lower belly firms. Try to sustain this action during the movements. The legs remain relaxed and do not contribute to the actions.

1. Sink your sit bones gently into the seat as you spread them wider and roll right onto the front of them. Your tailbone will come back and your body will incline slightly forward. The movement sequences up through your spine and your top front chest and shoulders open. Be aware of your lower belly firming even more (Fig. 7.29a). Then allow the weight to fall back so that you roll onto the back of the sit bones and the tailbone rolls under – and the spine curls back down (Fig. 7.29b). Slowly repeat the sequence, paying particular attention to the first action.

2. Come onto the top of the sit bones, as above, and remain there while sinking the (L) and lifting the (R). Let your ribs and head move to the (L) so that your head is over your (L) leg. Notice that the lower pelvic core is nicely firm. Keep widening into your Core Belt as you allow the breath to come and go, and feel the lift in the spine from below. Repeat coming onto the (R) sit bone. Alternate the action from side to side (Fig. 7.29c).

3. Come onto the (R) sit bone, as above, and remain there while now drawing the lifted (L) sit bone back and shortening your (L) knee. Notice your (L) groin deepens and your body and head have rotated back to the left – and that your pelvic core is engaged. Keep the (L) sit bone lifted and now bring it forward so that the (L) knee lengthens. Think of your (L) sit bone like a brush painting the seat in a back/forward motion. Pay particular attention to the backward reaching phase. Repeat the same sequence on the (L) sit bone (Fig. 7.29d).

The pelvic core is the active driver in all these movements led by the sit bones. The rest of the spine is lifted, yet relaxed and free to move in a sensuous and fluid way.

Compensations: Inadequate primary and pelvic core activity lead to poor initiation from the sit bones and movements being initiated by "cinching" around the center body: the ribs lift and/or throw forward. This prevents the spine moving freely and constricts the breath.

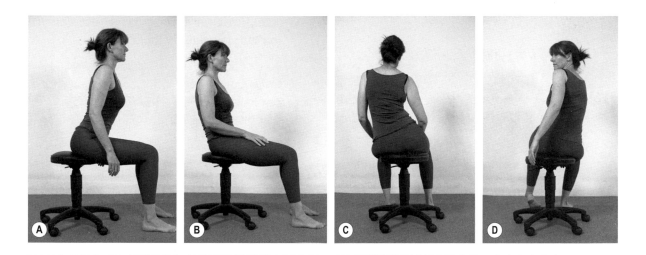

Figure 7.29
Pelvic dancing in sitting.

30 | Sit to stand

Purpose: To improve core integration and pelvic pattern 1 strength through functional movements.

Benefits: This helps all spinal pain problems: particularly low back and pelvic pain. We all move from sitting to standing to sitting countless times a day. Yet we usually do not do it well initiated from the pelvis, which is the ideal powerhouse of the body. Instead, the head leads and we often push down with our hands. By being mindful of doing this differently, simple everyday activities can become a great workout for your core strength.

Position: Sit on your sit bones at the front of a chair with a firm seat. If you know you are weak, use a higher chair. Stand your feet with the heels back close to/against the front chair legs if possible – toes pointing forward.

Key moves in this exercise: Make sure that the weight is distributed evenly over your feet – particularly the heels. Relax the legs. Expand the lower ribs and feel your core engage.

1. Sink your sit bones down into the seat as you roll onto the *very front of them* while also bringing them wide so the tailbone moves back. Continue the action until your trunk inclines forward so that your head is over/in front of your knees. Your spine remains aligned and you should be aware of your "pelvic core" working (Fig. 7.30a).

2. Push down through your feet particularly the heels and lift your sit bones **up** off the seat. You are literally "pushing down to come up" to standing. Trust in your legs rather than pushing with your hands – they will work if they are asked to. (Also great for cellulite!)

3. Then, straighten up by bringing your sit bones together, forward, and up to stand.

4. To sit down, reverse the action. Initiating from the sit bones, reach them back, wide, and **up** as you lower your pelvis to hover it over the seat (Fig. 7.30b). Gently lower to the seat.

5. Repeat.

Compensations: The head and shoulders lead the movement (due to inadequate control of the first pelvic pattern and poor weight shift initiated in the pelvis) – creating neck tension. Poor grounding and base of support in the feet. Spinal alignment is lost – a flexed spine is indicative of this.

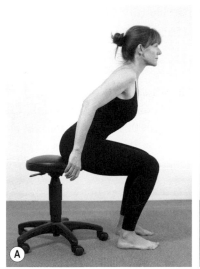

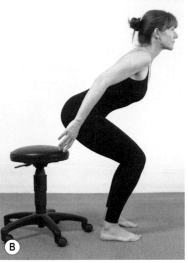

Figure 7.30
Sit to stand.

Chapter 7

31	**Healthy standing**

Purpose: To develop postural strength by activating the first and third pelvic patterns in standing.

Benefits: This will help anyone with spinal pain problems. Despite the fact that we are up against gravity for most of the day, most of us do not do this in an energy efficient way. Adopting healthy habits of "uprightness" automatically switches on our core muscles; yet insidious bad habits can develop that switch these off. We either "prop" on one leg and hang, or stand with feet apart and toes turned out, tucking the tail and clenching the buttocks. Instead, try to be mindful about "active standing."

Position: Stand with your feet only narrow hip-width apart and toes facing forward. Imagine that you are standing on narrow railway tracks and want full foot support.

Key moves in this exercise: Sense your weight being distributed evenly over your feet – in a tripod of support between the heel and the balls of the big and little toes. Soften your ankles and knees – think of a micro bend. Imagine your kneecaps pointing slightly outwards.

Place your hands on your pelvis; use the middle finger to palpate the lower belly inside the pelvis. Widen the lower ribs and keep directing the breath down.

1. Bring your pelvis into "neutral" by softening the buttocks and allowing your sit bones to float slightly apart and back until you feel your pelvic core automatically switch on. This action is subtle though definite. Your tailbone points back rather than under (Fig. 7.31a). (Do not "poke your bottom out" or throw the ribs forward!)

2. Sustain this action (the first pelvic pattern). Notice that if you gently "sink" your feet into the floor, your pelvic core firms more, and the spine subtly "lifts."

3. Sustain first pattern and now activate the third pattern: sink and press your (L) foot into the ground. Your weight will move over your (L) leg and your (R) pelvis and heel will lift (Fig. 7.31b). Your pelvic core will firm even more.

   Sustain this action and lighten the weight through the (R) front foot *without the (R) pelvis dropping* (or the (R) knee bending, or the (L) knee locking).

4. *Progression:* Further challenge your core by maintaining the above prompts and tapping the (R) foot without the (R) pelvis dropping.

5. Repeat the same sequence on the (R) leg.

6. Be mindful of *how* you stand during the day and practice this standing sequence whenever you can (e.g., when waiting for a lift, at traffic lights, in a queue).

Compensations: Poor "grounding" of the feet is associated with the pelvis being poorly active and/or it does not initiate the third pattern movement – with "cinching" of the waist and poor lateral weight shift and spinal alignment. Inability to maintain the lift of the (R) pelvis. Stiffening of the weight-bearing leg.

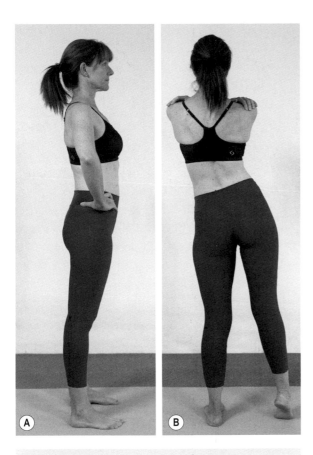

Figure 7.31
Healthy standing.

Chapter 7

32 | Forward bend pattern

Purpose: To master pelvic pattern 1 and "core control" in loaded functional activities.

Benefits: This will help all spinal pain problems. The way you habitually perform simple everyday activities like bending forward more often than not robs your core muscles of a decent workout. When our movement patterns are healthy, these muscles naturally work all the time and protect the spine.

Every time you need to bend forward (e.g., when picking something up off the floor or unloading the dishwasher), concentrate on doing it this way where your core is active and your low back is protected. Simply getting good at this does wonders for your back and firms your buttocks and thighs.

Position: Stand in front of a mirror with feet parallel, facing forward, and more than hip width apart.

Key moves in this exercise: Widen the lower ribs to engage your core – and sustain this.

Place your hands on your sit bones to help encourage a good action from them.

1. "Sink into" your feet (particularly the heels) and bend the knees forward, tracking them in line with your second toe. Keep looking at yourself in the mirror.

2. Reach the sit bones *well back, wide, and up* – and go long from the tailbone. Notice how you naturally bend forward – from the hips and not your back. When correct, you will notice your pelvic core really working.

3. The spine lengthens; the lower back ribs stay wide, and the chest and shoulders open.

   Put simply: the sit bones lead the movement back and up when you bend forward and down.

4. Keep actively pushing the action of the sit bones. The buttock muscles need to learn to "play out" to allow the sit bones to lead the movement. This actually gives your buttock muscles a great workout (Fig. 7.32a).

If the action is correct you should also feel a good stretch in your hamstrings.

This same action is required and much further developed in order to be able to bend forward like this yogi. Note the grounded feet, soft knees and the lift in the well aligned spine, the sit bones which eventually creates more length in the posterior hip and leg tissues and allows the spine to drape forward (Fig. 7.32b).

Compensations: Flexing the spine (because of stiffening the knees) and clenching the buttocks (which blocks the pelvis driving the movement) means there is neither core workout nor hamstring lengthening – and the low back is more vulnerable.

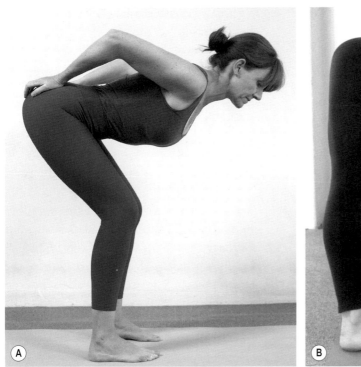
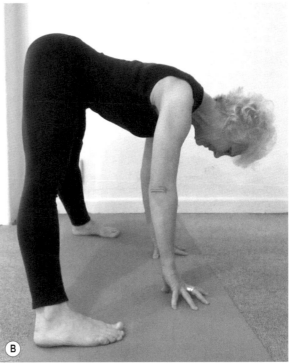

Figure 7.32
Forward bend pattern.

<table>
<tr><td>**33**</td><td>**Basic abdominal exercises for a healthy spine**</td></tr>
</table>

Purpose: To train the abdominal group in control of the thorax on a spatially stable pelvis. This also involves the axial FP in postural control, countering appropriate limb load challenge.

Benefits: This will help all spinal pain problems: particularly low back, pelvic, and lower limb pains.

There are many myths and conflicting messages as to which abdominal exercises are best. Crunches, curls, sit-ups, and "plank" can place a lot of stress on the disk and joints in the lower back and contribute toward stiffness in the mid/upper back.

Pulling in the stomach hampers healthy breathing and postural control patterns.

The abdominal muscles attach to the pelvis and rib cage – and control their relationship. Most people find it difficult to keep a "neutral" pelvis while bringing the rib cage down and back. This is IMPORTANT in correctly activating the core.

Position: Lie on your back with your heels resting on a chair or similar support – or standing as shown.

Key moves in the exercises: Place a middle finger inside the pelvic bone to palpate core activity. Rest the other hand on your chest to monitor your breathing (not shown).

1. Exhale fully and bring the lower rib cage down, back, and wide to make contact with the surface – without moving the pelvis.

   Maintain this position (and note the firming of the core under your lower hand) while continuing to breathe down, back, and wide – not up and forward. Keep your neck and shoulders relaxed.

2. When you can comfortably and correctly sustain the above, you can progress by challenging the effectiveness of this control: lift one foot off the support – with the foot, knee, and ankle at a right angle – *without the ribs lifting*. Sustain the lift for 10 seconds, progressing up to about 30 seconds. You should be aware of an increased firming under your lower hand (Fig. 7.33a).

   Repeat with the other leg, slowly alternating (while maintaining the ribs back and wide).

   If you start to lose control – either the firming under your lower hand and/or throwing the lower ribs forward and/or losing a regular breathing pattern – STOP and rest. Go back and get better at doing the correct basic pattern better and for longer. With repetition, your ability and endurance will improve sufficiently not to lose control when you lift a limb.

   Real functional strength requires this underlying pattern of "deep core" control.

3. Alternative core challenges (beware of over-challenge where the core control is lost):

   ○ Elevate one arm – and alternate with the other

   ○ Lower the lifted leg to the ground to stand and return (if the feet are on a chair)

   ○ Lift opposite leg and arm (see Fig. 7.33a)

   ○ "Push away" with the foot of the lifting leg, keeping the shin horizontal

   ○ Straighten the lifted leg and lower it to the floor. WARNING – this is very challenging! (Fig. 7.33b). Initially it is easier if the non-moving leg is standing as shown in Fig. 7.33a.

Compensations: Failed challenge: cinching around the lower ribs, which lift and "pop forward" – axial stability is lost. Holding the breath; increased neck tension.

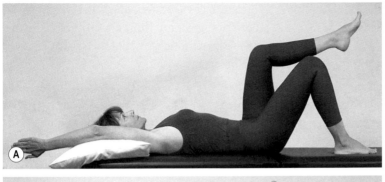

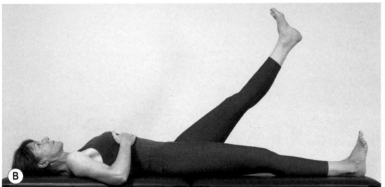

Figure 7.33
Basic abdominal exercises for a healthy spine.

Chapter 7

<table>
<tr><td>## 34</td><td>### Pelvic reach and roll</td></tr>
</table>

Purpose: To mobilize the pelvis and spine, and the joints and myofascia of the upper thorax and shoulders through the fourth pelvic and axial patterns.

Benefits: This will aid all spinal pain problems. This exercise demonstrates the integrated function of the spine and the continuity of the fascial web – and how we can work one part of the body to affect another further away.

Position: Lie on your back with your arms straight above your head or hands clasped behind your head. Reach your elbows wide and let them fall back. If your shoulders are too stiff and sore for this, place appropriate support behind your elbows for comfort or lie your arms out straight from (better) or by your side (Fig. 7.34a).

Bend both hips and knees so that your feet are "standing" – but do not push down with them.

Key moves in this exercise: Relax and sink the whole body completely into the ground. Without lifting your shoulders, gently widen the lower ribs to engage your "core"– try to sustain this.

1. Reach the (L) sit bone *long, wide, and* back; feel the weight roll slightly to your (R) pelvis and your pelvic core switch on. The (L) knee will grow long and away. Your (R) knee will shorten. When correct, the knees keep facing the ceiling and the chin drops.

   Also notice the (R) shoulder blade now bears more weight – and that there is a stretch in the (L) shoulder and upper back. The whole spine has lengthened and gently rotated to the (R) (Fig. 7.34b).

2. Ensure that the movement begins from the sit bone and tailbone. This naturally activates your core. The movement should then sequence right up through your spine.

3. Repeat, reaching the (R) sit bone, and gently explore the movement from side to side. The movement should feel calming and sensuous, with an agreeable stretch in the shoulders and top body. Keep chasing this!

Compensations: Clenching the buttocks and pushing with the feet (the result of poor pelvic initiation – the whole pelvis gets locked in rotation). The ribs "cinch" and throw forward, and there is "waist wind." The thorax does not follow the pelvis – nor is there movement through it to the head.

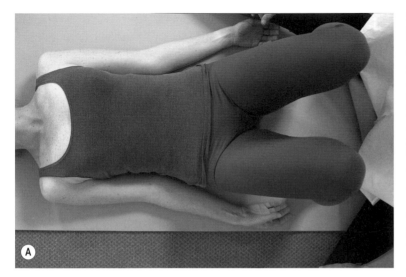

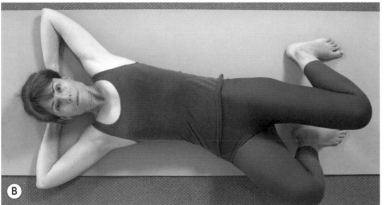

Figure 7.34
Pelvic reach and roll.

35 | Pelvic hovercraft

Purpose: To develop competency in the first pelvic pattern (and third in the progression) and ability in stabilizing the pelvis and lumbar spine in "neutral" under load. This is important basic control for "bridging."

Benefits: This can help all spinal pain problems: particularly low back and pelvic pain, and lower limb pains. Bridging is a popular exercise although it is usually taught in posterior tilt, which is disadvantageous for healthy lumbopelvic function. Most people have poor intrapelvic control and stiffness as well as difficulty in controlling anterior pelvic rotation and stabilizing the lumbar spine in neutral. This is important in initiating a bridge. This exercise addresses this.

Position: Lie on your back with your knees bent, heels in line with your sit bones and toes facing forward. Place the middle finger of the (L) hand on the inside of your pelvic bone to monitor "pelvic core" activity (not shown).

Key moves in this exercise: Without lifting your shoulders, gently widen the lower ribs to engage your core- try and sustain this

1. Activate the first pelvic pattern as follows: reach your sit bones long, wide and point them back down toward the floor. Notice the firming under your finger, and of the muscles over your very low back (which has rolled into an arch). Slide just the fingers of your (R) hand under this arch to provide feedback as to your ability to sustain it.

   Really keep your attention on the sit bones – they need to keep working into first pattern to maintain the **low** arch and allow the tailbone to reach long and back.

2. Maintaining the arch, sink your heels into the floor and *just unweight* your pelvis so it is like a hovercraft; i.e., there is only a thin film of air between your buttocks and the floor.

3. At the same, time ensure that you are not gripping over the lower back ribs – push them wide, directing the breath down and back. Relax the neck and shoulders (Fig. 7.35a).

4. With your pelvis still lightly brushing the surface, breathe low and slow. Try to sustain the action for at least 30 seconds. Repeat.

5. *Progression:* This adds in the third pelvic pattern. Maintaining the pelvic hovercraft, gently brush the buttocks from side to side across the surface without losing contact with either buttock (Fig. 7.35b). This action is led by the sit bones and the movement occurs in the hip sockets (the weight also shifts through your shoulder blades and the ipsilateral side waist lengthens).

Compensations: Poor intrapelvic control, and lifting the pelvis up high to enable "locking in" with the legs. Here, dominant activity of the whole posteroinferior myofascial chain, particularly of the glutei and hamstrings, pulls the pelvis into posterior tilt. This is easily apparent as the lumbar spine will lose its arch and hovering becomes difficult. In the progression, the sit bones do not lead the movement and there is "cinching" through the center.

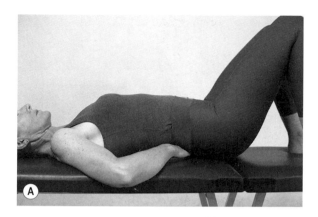

Figure 7.35
Pelvic hovercraft: a) basic; b) progression.

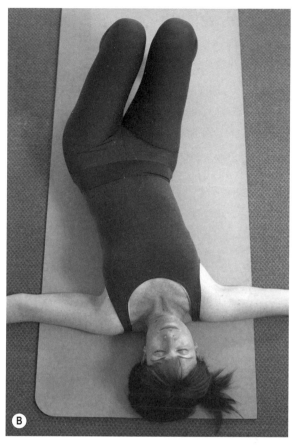

36 | Advanced abdominal exercise for a healthy spine

Purpose: To develop integrated control between the axial FP and the abdominals in stabilizing the lower thorax in a "neutral" position; this is particularly indicated in the posterior PXS client.

Benefits: Many myths abound as to which abdominal exercises are the best. Most do not correctly activate the core but do bother the spine. Some people have too much abdominal activity – others not enough. Getting your "core control" right will usually sort out these group differences.

A common fault is difficulty bringing the rib cage down and back and keeping a neutral pelvis. This exercise wakes up the abdominal control of the thorax, integrates the core, mobilizes the thorax, and does not bother the lower back.

Position: Lie on the floor with your legs straight and hands clasped behind your head.

Key moves in this exercise: Draw your elbows wide and relax your head back into your hands.

1. Point your toes strongly, noting that your pelvis rotates forward and your very low back arches. Keep it like that.

2. Inhale back and wide into the lower ribs – and on the exhale curl forward trying to round out the lower back ribs and bring them in contact with the floor. The elbows remain wide and the head falls back. The work is in the center (Fig. 7.36a).

3. Try and remain here for an increasing number of slow breaths – growing the ribs wider on each inhale – and curling the ribs back more on the exhale. Ensure you do not fall back on the inhale.

Perhaps imagine reading a book held between your feet!

Try to build up your endurance by sustaining the above for about six or more breaths.

4. *Progression 1:* If you are able, cross your forearms behind your head, taking hold of the upper arms over the deltoid muscles so that your head is cradled and rests back on the forearms as in Fig. 7.36b. Repeat as above.

5. *Progression 2:* Repeat the above while holding one hip flexed to 90° (see Fig. 7.36b). Keep pointing the toes and extending the knee of the straight leg.

Compensations: Loss of pelvic position through clenching the buttocks. Falling back on the inhale (indicates an upper chest breathing pattern and poor abdominal/core integration). Elbows coming forward and excess shoulder and neck tension (because of upper chest breathing and/or compensating for weak abdominals).

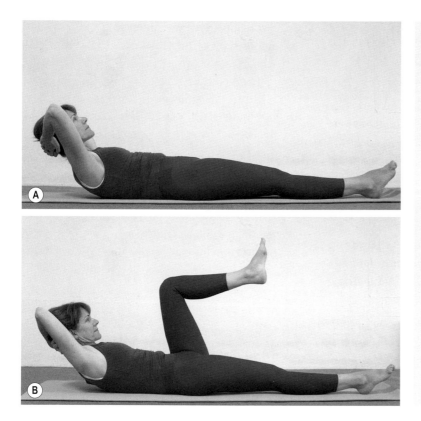

Figure 7.36
Advanced abdominal exercise for a healthy spine: a) basic; b) progression.

37 | **Smart hamstring stretch**

Purpose: To release the hamstrings and posterior myofascial chain while engaging the first pelvic pattern to control and stabilize the pelvis in "neutral" and protect the lower back.

Benefits: This is helpful for all spinal pain problems: particularly low back, pelvic, and lower limb pains. Tight, overactive hamstrings are common. This is a sign of poor lumbopelvic control. Many hamstring stretches chronically stress and irritate the lower back, further perpetuating the hamstrings tightness and various pain disorders. A vicious cycle ensues.

As the hamstrings attach to the sit bones, we need to stabilize them to achieve effective hamstring lengthening. This exercise establishes a better brain connection between the "pelvic core" and the hamstrings, helping them to "let go" neurophysiologically.

Position: Lie down on the floor with a support under your head and both legs extended.

Key moves in this exercise: Point the toes and reach them long. This helps to engage the first pelvic pattern, where the sit bones reach long, back, and wide. Your lower back assumes its natural arch. Ensure that you have **not** thrown the ribs forward.

1. Place your (L) hand in the "cubby house" of the lumbar arch so you can check you are maintaining this space. This is IMPORTANT!

2. Guide or lift the (R) thigh to vertical – or further, without losing the arch. You will really need to work the sit bones back, wide, and long to achieve this – particularly the (R) as the knee comes up and forward. If this is difficult, place a belt behind your thigh – still keeping the (R) arm controlled as described below. Do not tense your shoulders or arm.

3. Place your (R) elbow on the floor and your hand just in front of the (R) thigh. It must assume a "fixed point in space" (as in Fig. 7.37a). Ensure that you both keep the thigh vertical (or more) and touching the hand. Maintain this and the lower back arch while you perform the following…

4. Float the (R) foot toward the ceiling feeling that the heel lifts up against the sit bone, working down and back. Think of your lower leg like a "pump handle" – it moves up and down while the thigh remains still. Sustain the heel lift and breathe into the stretch. Imagine you were "kicking" that foot over your head. You should feel your "pelvic core" working a lot to maintain the stable pelvic position and your thigh vertical (see Fig. 7.37a).

5. If your hamstrings are tight you will not get the foot very high. Do not be ambitious and "end gain" – what is important is not how far you go but how well you control it. If you lose the lumbar arch or the vertical thigh, you have defeated the point of the exercise and risk stressing the lower back (Fig. 7.37b). This is incorrect.

6. Ensure you maintain a regular and slow abdominal breathing pattern. Shoulders and neck should be completely relaxed.

7. *Progression:* Flex the foot back and forward in the heel raised position.

Repeat on the other side

Compensations: Poor control of the first pelvic pattern leads to an unstable pelvic position, flattening of the lower back, the thigh pumping away from the fingertip touch (or the fingers chasing the moving thigh), together with overworking the arms and tensing of the neck (see Fig. 7.37b).

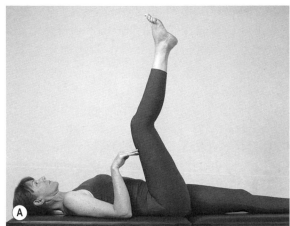

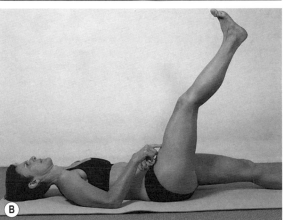

Figure 7.37
Smart hamstrings stretch.

38 Brainy buttock release

Purpose: To release the inferior posterolateral myofascial chain and the posterior hips while engaging the pelvic patterns as key points of control in maintaining a "neutral" spine.

Benefits: If correct, this helps all spinal pain problems, particularly low back and pelvic pain and lower limb pains. Tight buttocks generally mean that you have poor "pelvic core" control and a bothered spine. Most common buttock stretches are passive and compromise the lower back – leading to further buttock tightness. Instead, activating your pelvic core muscles protects the lower back.

This exercise helps "get your brain into your butt." It is tricky to do well, so carefully follow the prompts.

Position: Lie down on a firm surface with support under your head, standing your feet with half-bent knees (shins at a 45° angle). Have a block handy.

Key moves in this exercise: Place your (R) ankle over your (L) knee; (L) middle finger over the inside of the (L) pelvic bone to monitor core activity, and your (R) hand fingers under your very low back (not shown). Bring the lower ribs back and wide to make space for the breath; maintain this.

1. Imagining you have headlights in your sit bones, reach them *long, wide, and back* to point their headlights down toward the floor – so that you create an arch in your low back. Your (R) hand monitors your ability to maintain this arch. This is IMPORTANT!

2. Let the (R) knee fall out and further focus upon your sit bones: are they equally long? (this will be reflected in the length of your side waist – the (L) will tend to shorten). Are they equally wide?

Do they both shine their light equally back toward the floor? Keep fine-tuning these actions (Fig. 7.38a).

3. You should now be feeling your pelvic core working and a considerable stretch over the back of your (R) buttock – and probably into the thigh. *Note:* how manipulating the sit bones alters the stretch. Explore this to find the best vector to stretch. Ensure you do not tense over the lower back ribs.

4. *Progression 1:* Provided that you are equalizing the three-dimensional sit bone action – and maintaining the arch – you can increase the stretch by sliding the (L) foot closer to its sit bone.

5. *Progression 2:* Provided that you can still maintain the sit bones back and the arch – try coming onto your (L) toes or place your (L) foot on a block (Fig. 7.38b).

6. Repeat the same sequence on the other side. Spend 1–3 minutes in the pose.

One side will generally be tighter, so spend more time here ensuring that you bring the breath to the stretch.

Compensations: Loss of neutral spine and pelvis; poor "core control" and buttock release; lifting or throwing the lower ribs forward; tensing the legs and not initiating from the pelvis; upper body tension.

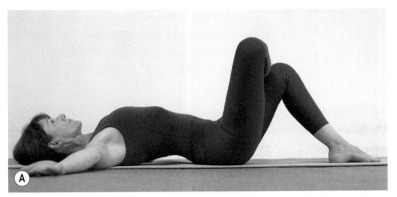

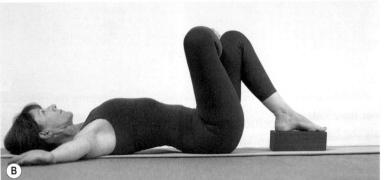

Figure 7.38
Brainy buttock release: a) basic;
b) progression 2.

40 | Half baby to Cross-over

Purpose: To mobilize the pelvic and hip joints and release the inferior posteromedial/lateral myofascial chains by activating the FPs.

Benefits: This is helpful in all spinal pain problems: particularly low back, pelvic, and lower limb pains.

Poor "core" activity and compensatory patterns of control lead to joint and myofascial restrictions around the pelvis and hips which disturb the mechanics of the lower back. This exercise can be a strong stretch to the sacroiliac joint and hips, so take it carefully.

Position: Lie on the floor with a small head support and, in case you need one, a rigid belt handy.

Key moves in the exercises:

1. Bend your (L) hip and knee, then take hold of the outer side of your foot – with your (L) arm to the inside of your (L) knee (Fig. 7.40a). If this is difficult, loop a belt over your foot. Let the pelvis fall heavily back into the floor – tailbone pointing back to the floor. The (R) arm is spread out to the side, palm up.

2. Draw the (L) point of the shoulder back, keeping the arm straight and relaxed. Imagine it falling back into the floor from the shoulder blade.

3. Allow your (L) knee to fall back and wide toward your (L) shoulder – and your foot to point to the ceiling. Your weight will have fallen slightly more over your (L) pelvic bone.

4. Now focus on the (R) leg: point the toes and bring the back of the knee toward the floor, and recharge pointing your tailbone long and back to the floor. Your (R) low back will arch slightly.

5. Maintaining the above, give your whole body weight heavily to the floor. Direct the breath down, back, and wide, and open the center – giving in to the stretch on the exhale.

6. **Cross-over:** Now cup the (R) hand over the (L) heel, bringing it toward your (R) breast and high – while sinking the (L) buttock heavily into the floor.

7. Spread the (L) arm out to the side. Draw the front (R) shoulder back but keep the arm soft and the shoulder engaged (Fig. 7.40b). Breathe down into the stretch over the back (L) hip and let go.

8. Repeat on the (R). Spend 1–3 minutes in the pose.

Compensations: Holding excess tension, particularly in the shoulders and arms. Excess pelvic movement into posterior tilt with poor (L) hip opening (because of poor (R) leg action) – the tailbone does not point long and back, and the lumbar spine risks being more stretched than the hips.

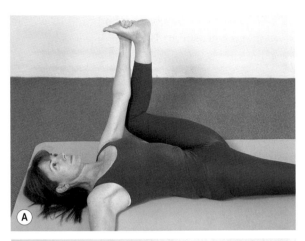

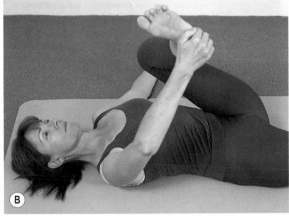

Figure 7.40
Half baby to Cross-over: a) Half baby; b) Cross-over.

42   Shoulder pattern combo

Purpose: To improve control of the upper spine and shoulder girdle by developing coordination and endurance of the posterior shoulder girdle stabilizers through shoulder patterns 1, 3 and 4 integrated with the axial FP.

Benefits: This will help all upper spinal pain problems: head, neck, and (especially) shoulder and arm pain syndromes. Stiffness of the upper back – and weakness of the posterior shoulder girdle and upper spine – is common. This helps wake up the "dead zone" over the upper back.

Position: Lie on the floor resting on your forehead. If your shoulders are very stiff, place a pillow under your chest and rest your forehead on a "spiky pod" or similar height support. Place your arms "half up" with the elbows bent and slightly above the shoulders; the hands are above the head, open and relaxed.

Key moves in this exercise: Focus on breathing down to gently expand and widen the lower back ribs – "opening the center." Sustain this, allowing the breath to freely oscillate while keeping the neck soft and long (Fig. 7.42a).

1. Draw the front point of the (R) shoulder back and wide away from the floor to float the elbow off the floor. (The hand retains soft contact with the floor.) The sequencing is IMPORTANT: the point of the shoulder initiates and the elbow follows. The arm remains relaxed and the hand does not push down (Fig. 7.42b).

2. Gently explore reaching the point of the shoulder up and then back and down such that the floating elbow points up toward the wall above your head and then back toward your feet. You want to feel the action coming from between your shoulder blades while the elbow remains somewhat forward and wide, and the back of the armpit stays soft.

3. Also focus on staying soft over the lower back ribs and on breathing down and back. There should be no neck tension or pain. Play the movement back and forth, maintaining all of the above steps.

4. Repeat the same on the (L) side. Alternate the action between sides.

5. *Progression:* Continue the actions as above, and float the hand off so it just hovers.

Compensations: Poor initiation from the point of the shoulder leads to poor scapular control accompanied by excessive glenohumeral, arm, neck, and waist tension plus breath holding. This will be made worse by poor core activation and opening the center with disturbed breathing.

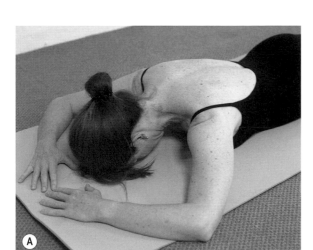

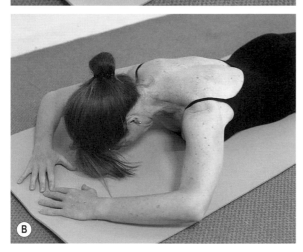

Figure 7.42
Shoulder pattern combo.

<table>
<tr><td>**43**</td><td>**Double arm triangles**</td></tr>
</table>

Purpose: To mobilize and build control and endurance in the upper back and shoulder girdle by engaging first shoulder pattern integrated with the core.

Benefits: The upper back and shoulders are frequently a functional "dead zone," which has repercussions in the shoulders and through the whole spine. This exercise reawakens and tones this region.

Position: Lie on the floor on your stomach, resting on your forehead with your chin tucked. If you are stiff, place a pillow under your chest and a support under your forehead.

Key moves in this exercise: Place your (R) hand on your head and your (L) hand behind your back so that your forearm rests over your lower back ribs. Expand the lower ribs so they gently lift your (L) arm/hand (Fig. 7.43a). Maintain this and breathe regularly.

1. Draw the front points of both shoulders back *away* from the floor; reach the elbows wide as they float back. Sustain this while continuing to breathe down and back under your (L) hand for five or so breaths. You should feel strong work in the muscles between your shoulder blades – but the neck should be soft and long. Let the weight fall heavily through your pubic bone (Fig. 7.43b). Repeat a number of times.

   Expect to feel all the back muscles working – yet the "core" muscles are also working hard to widen the lower ribs.

2. *Progression:* Without dropping the points of the shoulders or the elbows, slowly turn your head side to side with your (R) hand. As you roll across your forehead the chin remains tucked and the upper body weight shifts slightly from side to side. The challenge is to work the shoulder blades and center but remain flexible and allow the head and neck movement (see Fig. 7.43b).

3. *Variations:* The basic exercise can be done during the day when sitting at a computer.

Compensations: Poor initiation from the shoulder blades with poor coactivity in the core leads to poor support in the upper back and shoulders, with hardening of the back armpit, neck tension, and "locking in" over the lower ribs – and breath disturbance. There is also loss of spinal alignment in sitting.

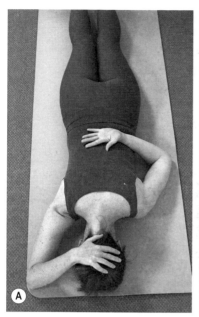 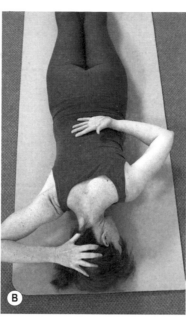

Figure 7.43
Double arm triangles.

44 | Spreadeagle

Purpose: To mobilize the upper back and improve shoulder girdle control via shoulder patterns 1, 3 and 4 integrated with "core" control.

Benefits: This helps all spinal pain problems, particularly head, neck, shoulder, and arm pain syndromes. Stiffness and weakness through the upper back and shoulder contributes to neck and shoulder pain – and low back problems. This exercise tunes up the upper back and shoulders and also challenges control and coordination with the core.

Position: Lie on your stomach, resting on your forehead with your arms out level with your shoulders, palms face down, and fingers spread out (Fig. 7.44a). If this is uncomfortable, or you are very stiff, place a pillow under your chest and a support under your forehead.

Key moves in this exercise: Widen the lower ribs and keep them so while you do the following:

1. Without bending the elbow, shorten the (R) arm by drawing the front point of the (R) shoulder back so that the (R) shoulder blade moves closer to the spine. Do not lose the right-angle position of your arm. The open hand slides lightly across the floor (Fig. 7.44b).

   Notice that your weight has shifted more over your (L) breast and pelvis and that your head has rolled to look at your (R) hand. Sustain the action, keeping the lower ribs wide and breathing softly for a number of breaths. The neck is soft, long – and comfortable.

2. Repeat on the (L) side. Slowly and gently oscillate the movement from side to side.

3. *Progression:* Push the lower back ribs wider and sustain this while continuing to draw the point of the (R) shoulder back until you *just unweight the hand* and it hovers no more than 1 mm off the floor. The whole back is working, but there should be no neck tension or pain; and the breath is low and slow.

Compensations: Poor initiation and control from the shoulder blade leads to hardening over the back armpit and little movement of the shoulder blade and through the top back. The movement is attempted by "cinching" over the lower rib cage rather than the shoulders – breathing and core control are compromised. On unweighting, the point of the shoulder falls forward and the hand is lifted too high, thus creating tension over the neck, back armpit, and lower back ribs as well as neck discomfort.

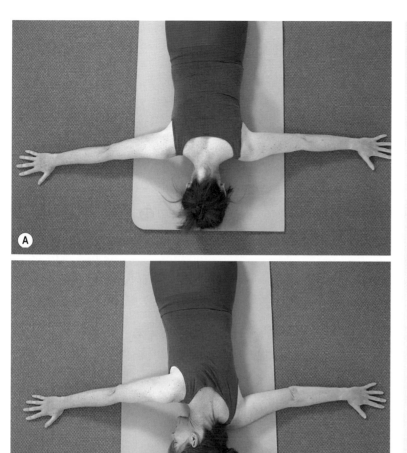

Figure 7.44
Spreadeagle.

Chapter 7

45 Slow heel kicks

Purpose: To improve pelvic and core control via activation of the first pelvic and axial pattern so as to control anterior pelvic rotation, stabilize the spine, and better support hip extension.

Benefits: This helps all spinal pain problems, particularly low back, pelvic, and lower limb pains. Because we sit a lot, our lower back and "core" muscles weaken, as do those that bring the pelvis and leg back. In this exercise you should not feel tense while working the back muscles. It can be done in lying or standing.

Position A: Lie on your stomach with a firm pillow under it if you feel you need it. Place the (L) hand loosely up beside your head while the (R) palpates the lower belly (clear of the pelvic bone) to monitor your ability to sustain a "firming" here [not shown]. Allow the pelvis to fall heavily into the support surface.

Key moves in these exercises: Expand the lower back ribs wide and maintain this while breathing slowly and regularly down to your (R) hand. You should feel the muscles gently firm.

1. With your knees close together, bend the (R) knee to a right angle, reach the tailbone long and spread the sit bones back and wide – the muscles should firm further under your (R) hand. Draw the point of the (L) shoulder gently back and sustain this so that the (L) forearm is light and the neck remains relaxed.

2. With the (R) sit bone leading, float the (R) knee, reaching the heel toward the ceiling. Try to "push" it straight up without the heel rolling in or out. Your very low back will arch and you should also feel the muscles working over both your sacrum and your lower belly (Fig. 7.45a).

3. Keep pushing the lower ribs wide to make space for the breath, and hold the lift for 5 breaths. Repeat 3 times. Then do three sets of 5 repeated lifts, being mindful of all the above cues see (see Fig. 7.45a).

4. Repeat on the other side.

5. *Progression 1:* Lift the (R) leg as described while also floating the (L) arm off the support (not the hand) – ensuring the point of the shoulder draws back and that the neck is soft and long (the center is open and breathing is free).

6. *Progression 2:* Lift the leg with a straight knee (Fig. 7.45b).

Position B: Stand in front of a table or kitchen bench (or a chair as shown), with the edge in your groin, and bend forwards so the hip forms a right angle. Bend the (R) knee and repeat the exercise for position A through a larger range. Keep the standing knee slightly bent (Fig. 7.45c).

Position C: Stand close to, and facing, a wall (or a chair, as shown) with your feet close together and knees soft. Bring both sit bones back and wide and also lift the (R). Sustain this and do a slow kick back with the (R) heel leading from the (R) sit bone (keeping the knee straight). Repeat and sustain all the cues for position A (Fig. 7.45d).

Compensations: Poor core support and control of the first pelvic pattern leads to pushing down with the arms, "cinching" over the lower ribs, holding the breath, and poor anterior pelvic rotation. Dominance of the external rotators and gluteus maximus leads to the heel falling in and the thigh going wide. Tightness of the front thigh makes it difficult to bend the knee to a right angle.

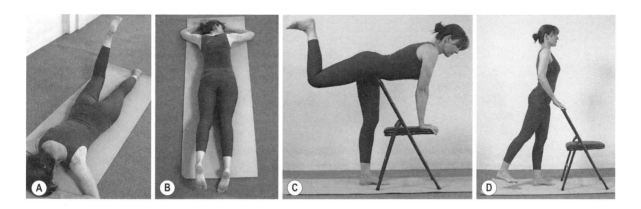

Figure 7.45
Slow heel kicks: a) position A, b) progression 2; c) position B; d) position C.

Chapter 7

46 Shoulder and pelvic backward rotation in lying

Purpose: Rotation through the axis initiated by either shoulder or pelvic patterns 1 and 4.

Benefits: These are great for all spinal pain problems. Stiffness in the upper back and shoulders and/or the pelvis/hips diminishes the rotation through the spine that is important for its health and movement freedom (e.g., energy-efficient walking and sports). Backward rotation of the limb girdles particularly suffers. Here, it is initiated either from the shoulder or the pelvis.

Shoulder initiation

Position: Lie on your stomach with your (L) arm straight up beside your head, touching your ear, and palm up. Place your (R) arm behind your back and resting over your lower ribs (Fig. 7.46a). In this exercise, imagine that the only parts of your body that work are your shoulders.

Key moves in these exercises: Gently widen the lower back ribs and feel your "core" switch on; maintain this.

1. Bring your brain to the (R) front point of the shoulder. Draw it back, keeping the arm relaxed – and keep doing so until your weight falls to the left, your head turns, your pelvis has rotated back, and the hip and knee have bent of their own accord, and you are now lying on your left side (Fig. 7.46b).

2. Roll back onto your stomach by bringing the point of the shoulder forward.

3. Repeat the action back and forward – keeping the rest of the body completely heavy and relaxed. Remember, the only movement is the shoulder blade drawing back.

4. Repeat the movements with the (R) arm up instead, and initiating from the (L) shoulder.

Compensations: Hardening over the lower back ribs, stiffening of the legs, and poor rotation and roll (caused by the shoulder blade failing to effectively initiate the movement).

Pelvic initiation

Position: Now bring the (R) arm up beside your head as well, with the elbow slightly bent and the palm and fingers spread. Bend the (R) knee.

Key moves in the exercises: Keep the arms soft and relaxed, do not push down, and imagine here that only your pelvis works.

1. Bring your brain to the (R) sit bone and, initiating from there, reach the (R) heel up and scoop it back and behind (Fig. 7.46c) to stand it on the floor behind you. As the pelvis rotates back you roll onto your left side (Fig. 7.46d).

2. Rotate the pelvis forward to lift the foot and roll back onto your stomach.

3. Repeat the action back and forward, keeping the rest of the body completely heavy and relaxed. Remember: the only thing working is the pelvis/sit bone drawing back.

4. Repeat the moves with the (R) arm up beside the ear and initiating from the (L) sit bone instead.

Compensations: Hardening over the lower back ribs, using the arm to push, and poor backward rotation and hip extension (caused by the pelvis failing to effectively initiate the movement).

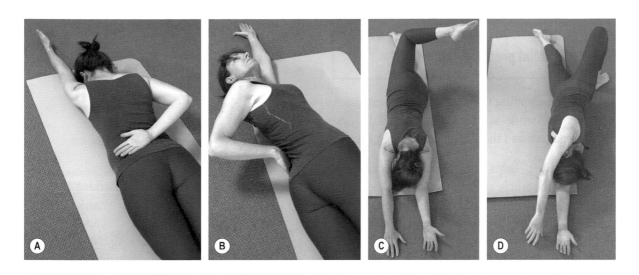

Figure 7.46
Shoulder and pelvic backward rotation in lying: a),b) shoulder initiation; c),d) pelvic initiation.

48   "Core" challenge in sitting

Purpose: To challenge axial FP ability in stabilizing a "neutral" spine while moving a leg or an arm.

Benefits: This will help *all* spinal musculoskeletal pain disorders. Common to all is deficient control of the deep myofascial system that makes it difficult to sit erect without tension.

Correct "core" action provides internal support and stabilizes the spine against internal and external loads. This exercise refines this control.

Position: Sit on a firm surface on the top of your sit bones, then widen them to create an "active pelvic base of support." Your feet should be flat on the floor with toes facing forward.

Encircle your hands around your lower rib cage, thumbs pointing behind (Fig. 7.48a).

Key moves in this exercise:

1. Drop your shoulders and expand the lower ribs sideways and back under your hand (particularly under your thumbs). When this "opening the center" is correct, this will firm your lower belly and bring the rib cage over the pelvis. And your spine is erect.

2. Maintain this action and allow the breath to cycle naturally – topping up the expansion on the inhale and trying to maintain the expansion on the exhale. Picture your torso as an open cylinder (see Fig. 7.48a).

3. *Progression 1:* When you can sustain the above without tension, slowly peel the heel of one foot off the ground without losing spinal alignment, the openness under your hands or the firming over your lower belly.

4. *Progression 2:* All going well, fully unweight the foot while maintaining spinal lift, opening the center, and soft, low, slow breathing. Initially the foot should hover just off the floor. The model has excellent function and is able to lift the foot higher without losing control. Do not be in a hurry to perform steps 3 and 4 before you have quality core control. Repeat the action with either leg (Fig. 7.48b).

Compensations: Improper or inadequate core activation – and ability to coordinate this with breathing. This inability to generate enough internal support to stabilize the pelvis and spine in an upright "neutral" position on limb load causes the shoulders to lift, the spine "jerks" – or the person leans back or to the side and/or throws the lower ribs forward).

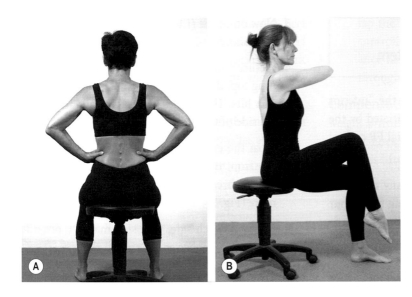

Figure 7.48
"Core" challenge in sitting.

50 Hamstring releases in sitting

Purpose: To increase hamstring myofascial slide and extensibility by controlling pelvic pattern 1.

Benefits: This is helpful in all spinal pain problems: particularly low back, pelvic, and lower limb pains. Hamstring tightness is common; however, many hamstring stretches bother the spine and create more tightness. A vicious cycle ensues. Done correctly, this exercise works your "core" muscles and releases the hamstrings while protecting your back.

Position: Sit bringing your sit bones right to the back of a chair or high plinth, so you are on the top of them and your thighs are in contact with the seat/support. On a chair, you may need to slide the foot forward.

Key moves in these exercises: Place your hands on your pelvis so your thumbs are palpating over the dimples (Fig. 7.50a). Be mindful of expanding and widening the lower back ribs to activate your core. Sustain this.

1. Sink your sit bones into the seat while rolling right onto the top/front of them as you also widen them. When correct, you will be aware of firming in your pelvic core and your thumbs moving slightly up and forward. The body inclines forward without losing alignment, and the hips are well flexed. Remain exactly here while you...

2. Yield the weight of your (R) thigh into the support surface. Slowly start to lift the (R) foot while ensuring that there is **no pushback** under your (R) thumb. You really need to bring your brain to your (R) sit bone to keep it working back, wide, and up so your pelvis remains completely stable. As the hamstrings attach to the sit bone, their tightness pulls the sit bone under and forward

unless counteracted by good pelvic core control. Explore floating the foot up and down with no pelvic movement (Fig. 7.50b). Repeat on the (L).

3. *Progression 1:* Continue exactly as above but add alternate toe/heel pointing to the lifted foot. Expect discomfort.

4. *Progression 2:* This requires you to be sitting on a chair/stool on castors. Bring your sit bones to the front of the seat. Walk your feet forward so the knees are semiflexed, big toes facing forward. Roll onto the very front of the sit bones as you push them wide and lift your tailbone back – angling your body further forward from your hips. When the action is correct, the spine is aligned, you core works, and you feel a hamstrings stretch (Fig. 7.50c). Increase the stretch by pushing the chair further back using your sit bones – the knees move toward straightening.

Compensations: Poor pelvic initiation and stability leads to poor forward bending at the hips: when lifting the foot, the pelvis tips back, and brings stress into the lower back – and the hamstrings do not lengthen. Excess holding around the lower rib cage (when primary core control is inadequate). Loss of pelvic initiation and spinal alignment during the second progression.

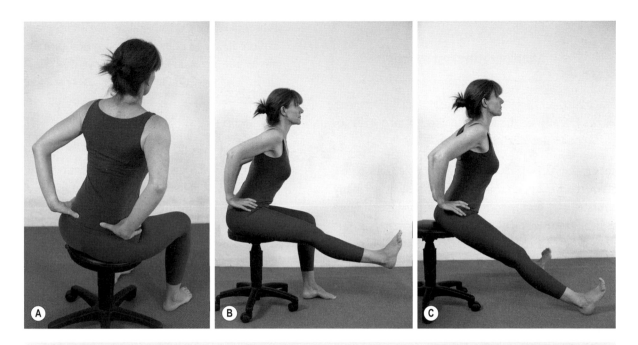

Figure 7.50
Hamstring releases sitting a),b) basic; c) progression 2.

51 Shoulder and chest opener

Purpose: To mobilize the upper thorax and shoulders by engaging the first shoulder pattern with the axial fundamental pattern.

Benefits: This helps all upper spinal pain problems: head, neck, shoulder, and arm pain (and stiffness). Most of us spend many hours a day at work and play using our arms down in front of our body, so our head and shoulders come forward. In time, they begin to stay there. This exercise counteracts poor upper body posture. Do it throughout the day – particularly if working at a computer a lot. It can be done in sitting or standing – or prone.

Position: Sit up nicely on the top of your sit bones, creating an "active pelvic base of support." Clasp your hands behind your back, interlocking your fingers and keeping elbows soft and wide.

Key moves in this exercise:

1. Widen the lower ribs and feel your "core" engage; sustain this with the ribs remaining down/back.

2. Gently "present" the top of your breastbone forward and draw the front points of the shoulders back and wide. Feel the muscles work between the shoulder blades, which come closer together and sightly drop. The arms should remain relaxed.

3. Allow the head to float tall – with the chin tucked (Fig. 7.51a).

4. Maintaining the above action and soft arms, see how far you can straighten the elbows *without the front shoulder tips narrowing, dropping or coming forward.* The top breastbone moves forward as the points of the shoulders move back.

5. *Progression:* Maintaining the above prompts, explore reaching your hands back and up. You might not move far if control is correct. Think "head back; shoulders back; ribs back; breathe down and back" – the only thing coming forward is the top of your breastbone. Chase the feeling of stretch in the shoulders and upper back (Fig. 7.51b).

Note: You may only get as far as step 3 to start with. That's OK – just keep working at it and in time you will get to steps 4 and 5. Remember, quality is more important than quantity.

Compensations: Incorrect activation of shoulder pattern 1 (there is no extension through the upper thorax and movement of the scapula into retraction). Inadequate core control and poor stability of the lower thorax, with "cinching" over the lower back ribs and loss of spinal alignment. Neck tension and breath holding.

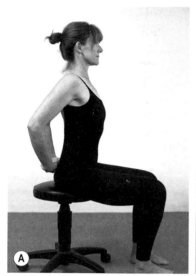

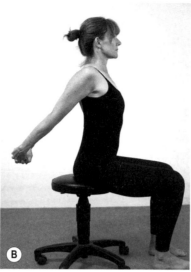

Figure 7.51
Shoulder and chest opener a) basic;
b) progression.

Chapter 7

| **52** | **Pelvic rock and roll in side sitting** |

Purpose: To improve pelvic/hip mobility and spinal weight shift and lift via training the pelvic patterns in asymmetrical postures which also inhibits the "inferior tethers."

Benefits: Correctly performed, this helps low back and pelvic pain, and many lower limb pains. Common to all is inadequate pelvic control in providing an adaptable base of support for the spine – further compounded by stiff hips. This helps you find your pelvic core and brings an oilcan to your hips.

Position: Side sit on the floor with your hips and knees bent – knees wide and pointing (L), feet to the (R) – and ideally free (Fig. 7.52a). If you are very stiff or have difficulty bringing your spine erect, place a small support under the top third of your (L) thigh bone, ensuring the sit bone is free [not shown]. Try to yield and sink your (L) mid/lower thigh into the floor. Take the weight on your (L) hand – palm open and fingers spread. If needs be, also place it on a block. Keep the arm and shoulder soft, and allow your (L) shoulder to move up toward your ear and your lower rib cage to shift to the (L). Your spine will tilt to the (L).

Key moves in these exercises:

Movement is driven from the sit bones – and the spine follows. The lower ribs stay soft.

1. Palpate both sit bones so you know where they are. Your tailbone is between them. Then place your (R) hand on your pelvis (not shown), the middle finger palpating the lower belly.

2. Give your weight completely to the V formed by your (L) leg. Expand and widen the lower ribs – particularly on the (L) – and note the firming in your low belly. Sustain this.

3. Reach your (L) sit bone long, back, and wide so that your pelvis and (R) hand tip forward, your tailbone lifts, and your feel your core working even more. This is pelvic pattern 1. Your spine inclines forward, but it does not collapse (see Fig. 7.52a).

4. Now allow the weight to fall back so that the tailbone rolls under, your spine flexes, the head and shoulders fall forward, and the (L) knee lifts. Note how easy this is! (not shown)

5. Now repeat step 3 – emphasizing this as you oscillate back and forward. You will roll over your hip. Your brain really needs to be with your sit bones and lower back ribs.

6. Activate step 3 to bring your spine upright and then fully lift your (R) sit bone. Notice how your body weight, rib cage and head shifted further over to the (L) over your hand (Fig. 7.52b). This is the third pelvic pattern.

7. Now drive the (R) sit bone down as though it were a piston. Your spine will move to the (R) and fall back slightly. Repeat the movement a number of times, emphasizing step 6. Note how your head and spine shift sideways in space to the (L) and (R)

8. Now bring your (R) sit bone fully up and forward so that your (R) hand and pelvis rotate to the (L) – the whole spine and head follow. How far back can you see to the left? (Fig. 7.52c). This is the fourth pelvic pattern.

9. Now bring the (R) sit bone back and down so that your (R) hand and pelvis rotate to the (R) – and the spine follows. Oscillate back and forward, emphasizing step 8.

Compensations: Poor grounding in the (L) leg and initiation from the sit bone (leads to poor pelvic movement, poor spinal alignment and movement, and holding excess body tension). The client is unwilling to weight bear through the heel of an open hand (the ribs do not shift over to the (L) and/or the shoulder girdle is held in depression). Lower rib "cinch" dominates in all three patterns.

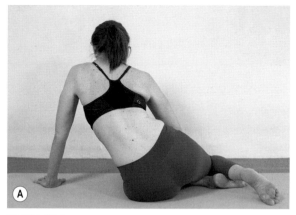

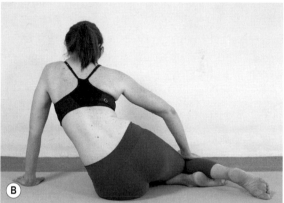

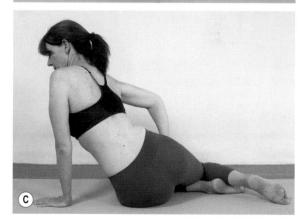

Figure 7.52
Pelvic rock and roll in side sitting.

<table>
<tr><td>**53**</td><td>**V to Z hip stretch**</td></tr>
</table>

Purpose: To open the inferior posterolateral myofascia by engaging the pelvic and axial patterns.

Benefits: This helps low back and pelvic pain, and many lower limb pains – particularly iliotibial band problems. The stretch can really open the hips and legs provided that you carefully follow the prompts. Expect to feel some hip and thigh discomfort with this, but **not** in the lower back.

It can be challenging on the knees. If so, try placing a small block or support under the upper third of the weight-bearing thigh (ensure the sit bone is free).

Position: Sit on the floor with your knees facing (L) and feet (R), bringing your knees as wide as possible so your (L) foot is free. *Your (L) leg forms a V.* Lean on your (L) open hand and allow your lower ribs to move to the (L) and the (L) shoulder to move up toward your ear (Fig. 7.53a).

Key moves in these exercises:

Let your weight fall to the (L) and forward, yielding your weight completely into your (L) front thigh – melt! Relax your (L) shoulder. Lengthen your spine.

1. Open the lower ribs back and wide, particularly on the (L), and feel your core switch on – sustain this. Some of you will already feel a stretch here. Bring your breath to it.

2. Draw the (L) sit bone *long, back, and wide*, and feel your pelvic core switch on more. Keep sinking the thigh and reaching the sit bone back to engage the stretch. Your body will incline forward from the hips, not the head. The tailbone reaches long, back and lifts.

   Gently experiment with the movement, being mindful of breathing slowly and deeply.

3. *Progression 1:* Provided you keep moving from your sit bones and maintain alignment, you can place the (R) hand forward on the floor to deepen the stretch (Fig. 7.53b).

4. *Progression 2:* **Moving to Z:** Walk your (L) heel further forward so that your leg now looks like a Z. Do not be too ambitious. With correct practice you will increase range.

5. Reach the (L) heel long; try to feel the outside shin also sinking. Continue with the previous prompts – surrendering the thigh, actioning the sit bone, and softening and lengthening the spine (Fig. 7.53c).

6. Further *Progression:* Bring the (R) leg behind as shown in Fig. 7.53c.

7. Hold the stretch for 60 seconds or more each time if you can.

8. Repeat on the other side.

Compensations: Difficulty allowing the weight to fall to the (L) – weight is taken on the (L) finger tips instead of the heel of the hand – associated with increased tension around the center, neck, and shoulders. (If your client complains of back pain, this is usually what is happening.) Inability to yield the (L) leg and initiate the action from the sit bones results in poor spinal alignment and opening of the myofascial tissues of the posterolateral pelvis and thigh. Disturbed breathing.

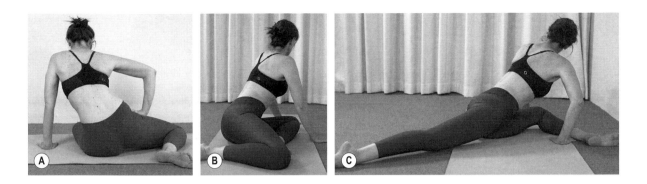

Figure 7.53

V to Z hip stretch a) basic; b) progression 1; c) progression 2.

54 Butt booster on all fours

Purpose: To strengthen the pelvic core and buttock muscles, enabling them to control the anterior pelvic rotary force couple in the sagittal plane.

Benefits: This is helpful in low back and pelvic pain, and many lower limb pains. The common problem is poor control of the pelvis on the leg. Many "glute" exercises "lock-in" the pelvis and hip – and, too often, people doing squats simply do not have adequate pelvic control, so their spine suffers.

This exercise works the glutei in outer range with the pelvic core muscles. Together they have to work hard to maintain correct control. Getting it right is quite tricky.

Position: Come into all fours with knees together, aligning your spine so that the head and tailbone are in line and reaching away from each other.

Key moves in this exercise: Gently draw the shoulders back. Imagine that you have two big search lights in your sit bones.

1. Breathe down and back to "open the center" by bringing the ribs back and wide. Sustain this.

2. Reach your sit bones *back, wide, and up*. How far can you shift back without your searchlights dropping to low beam? The groins deepen. Repeat this a number of times; note that the further you go back, the less weight is taken through the arms (Fig. 7.54a).

3. *Stay back* and now slide the (R) leg back as far as you can – headlights still on high beam.

4. Reach the (R) leg further back and lift the heel high to the ceiling – big toe facing the floor. Watch that your weight does not shift forward.

The (L) sit bone in particular has to keep working up, back, and wide. Ensure that you maintain your headlights level and up. Your "core" and (L) buttocks should be really working (Fig. 7.54b).

5. *Progression:* By this stage, if the action is correct, your arms are barely taking any weight. Gently unweight the (L) arm – sustaining the reach and lift of the (R) leg. Breathe easily (not shown).

6. Repeat on the opposite side. Aim to sustain the action with low, slow, easy breathing.

Compensations: The arms overwork, bringing tension to the shoulders and neck (caused by inadequate pelvic control – the weight does not shift back). Locking the hips into external rotation – the pelvis tilts posteriorly, the (R) pelvis lifts, and the big toe faces out to the side.

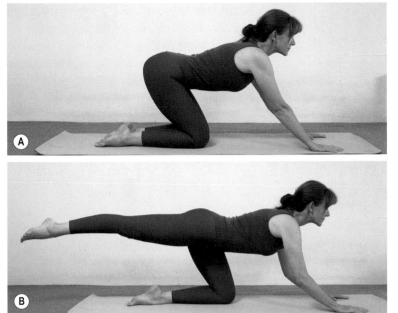

Figure 7.54
Butt booster all fours.

55 | Rebooting your iliopsoas and core

Purpose: To lengthen the hip flexor and open the torso by integrating the FPs.

Benefits: Helps all low back and pelvic pain disorders and many hip, knee, and leg pain syndromes. Iliopsoas is intimately involved with both primary and pelvic "core" function in supporting and stabilizing the pelvis and spine. It can either underwork or overwork (where it becomes tight and short, limiting hip movement). This exercise helps rebalance iliopsoas function – working it on one side while elongating the other – as it contributes to core control at the same time.

Position: Kneel on the floor, close to the wall or a support in case you need it. Bring the (L) foot up and forward so the (L) shin and the (R) thigh are both vertical. If your knees are sore, kneel on a firm flat cushion with your kneecap free.

Key moves in this exercise: Place your hands on your head. Drop your shoulders and draw the points of the shoulders back/wide. Keep 85% of your weight on the (R) back leg and the lower ribs expanded back and wide. Sustain this and breathe naturally.

1. Bring the (R) sit bone forward and underneath you, and lift the (L) sit bone. Watch you do not throw the belly and lower ribs forward – (the ribs should come back at the same time). Your stomach and (R) buttock need to work with the pelvic core here.

2. The aim is to feel a stretch over the (R) front hip and thigh. Chase this, bringing the breath down and back, and relax a bit more into it on each out breath. Ensure the (R) thigh remains vertical and the body is aligned over the (R) leg (Fig. 7.55a).

3. *Progression:* Maintain all the above cues and reach the (R) elbow toward the ceiling. The rib cage moves more to the right, but stays back and wide – and the whole side body lengthens. Keep bringing the breath down and back, particularly to the right (Fig. 7.55b; Note: unfortunately this shows the action when kneeling on the (L) leg).

4. Repeat three times, holding the stretch for 30 seconds or more. Repeat on the other side (shown in Fig. 7.55b).

Compensations: Inadequate core/pelvic control and abdominal activity, and overworking around the center back, the neck, and shoulders. There is loss of alignment in the axis and/or thigh and poor opening over the front hip and thigh.

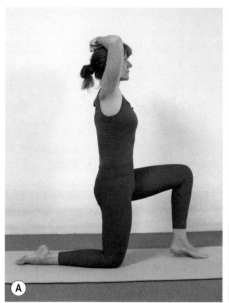 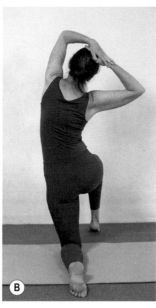

Figure 7.55
Rebooting your iliopsoas and core:
a) basic; b) progression.

56 | "Distorsion" progressing to Crescent stretch

Purpose: To open the pelvis, hips, and thighs while maintaining spinal alignment. This stretch brings the pelvis into "distorsion" and releases tight pelvic and leg myofascia.

Benefits: Helps all low back and pelvic pain disorders, and many hip, knee, and leg pain syndromes. The pelvis commonly lacks spatial control but is stiff within it – losing elasticity and pliability.

Associated hip/leg stiffness means that the spine has to compensate and is further compromised.

IMPORTANT: Aim to give your weight to the legs as much as possible, and relax the upper body. If you know you are very stiff, have two blocks handy in case you need them.

Position: Come into half kneeling on the floor – placing your (L) heel forward so that your shin is at a 45° angle. Align your foot so that the outer border is in a straight line forward – and the weight is distributed evenly between the heel and the balls of the little and big toes.

Slide the (R) leg behind you as much as you can. If using blocks, place them either side of your (L) foot.

Key moves in these exercises:

1. Sink your weight into your (L) foot – *ensuring firm pressure through the heel*. If you cannot feel this – move the foot further forward.

2. Bring your (L) knee forward and drop the (L) sit bone down as close as you can to your (L) heel.

3. Allow your torso to lie along your (L) thigh and bring your hands to the ground. If you are stiff in the hips, the arms will feel "too short" – so place your open hands on the blocks. This is not to encourage taking a lot of weight through the arms. Rather, it helps you to draw the points of the shoulders back – and keep the arms light – and bring the head back in line with the tailbone.

4. Focus on the center – expanding the lower back ribs and allowing the breath to freely cycle. Focus on softening and lengthening the spine from the crown of the head to the tailbone (Fig. 7.56a).

5. Yield your weight fully to your legs and let go on the exhale. Expect to feel a strong stretch over the back (L) buttock and thigh – and particularly over the (R) front groin and thigh. Try and "stay in it" for 5 breaths plus. Repeat on the other side.

6. *Progression:* Continuing all the above cues, tuck your (R) toes under and raise the (R) knee **without** raising the pelvis and (L) sit bone away from the (L) heel (Fig. 7.56b).

7. *Advanced progression into Crescent:* Stand your (R) hand beside your (L) foot (on a block if it is easier). Allow the point of your (R) shoulder to lift as you place your (L) hand on your pelvis and draw your (L) shoulder back, look back and "hang" your (R) side body down between your (R) arm and (L) pelvis. Soften and breathe into the stretch so your body hangs in a crescent shape (Fig. 7.56c).

These are strong stretches and you may notice some tenderness around the hips for a few days. However, if you take it easy and keep at it, you will improve.

Compensations: Poor grounding and centration of the foot and heel/sit bone connection – the pelvis/hips do not release and the top of spine and head are hyperflexed as tension is created in the front shoulders and around the center. The top of the body overworks trying to hold itself up rather than sinking down into the stretch.

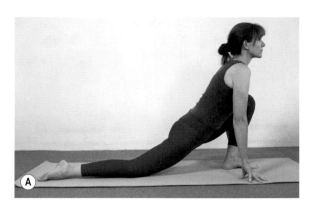

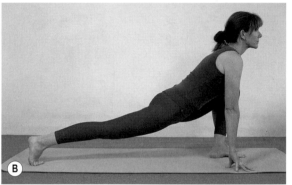

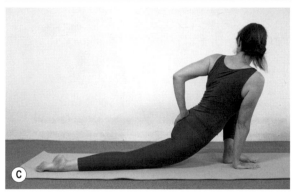

Figure 7.56

"Distorsion" progressing to Crescent stretch: a) basic
distorsion; b) progression; c) advanced progression into
Crescent.

57 | Prone piriformis stretch

Purpose: To open the posterior inferior pelvis, hip, and thigh by engaging the pelvic patterns.

Benefits: Helps all low back and pelvic pain disorders and many hip, knee, and leg pain syndromes. Tightness of the posterior inferior myofascial chain limits anterior rotation of the pelvis on the femur and hip flexion. Done correctly, this stretch both activates the pelvic core and releases tight buttocks while protecting the back. If you have knee problems, you may find it difficult to do. Begin with version (A); you may or may not be able to progress to version (B).

Position: Come onto all fours. Bring the (R) knee forward and the (R) sit bone to sit on the (R) heel. Slide the (L) leg back as far as you can. Place your hands either side of your (R) knee, palms open and centered. Draw the points of the shoulders back and widen the elbows.

Key moves in this exercise: Widen the lower ribs and engage your "core" – sustain this and breathe naturally.

1. Sink down into your (R) shin and draw both sit bones long, back, and wide so that your spine lengthens and the tailbone reaches back and lifts (Fig. 7.57a).

2. Explore moving your (R) sit bone either side of your (R) heel. Your body will rotate from side to side (not shown).

3. *Progression:* Swing your (R) foot across so that the heel is under the (L) groin. Let your (R) knee and shin sink into the floor and let the (L) groin drop down over the (R) heel.

4. Now drop down onto parallel forearms – palms facing up – and widen the points of the shoulders drawing them back. Keep the center open and reach the tailbone long (Fig. 7.57b).

5. Draw the tailbone long and both sit bones back, wide, and up – particularly the (R) to chase the stretch over the (R) buttock and thigh. Keep reaching the (L) foot back. Ensure the (R) sit bone does not drop (Fig. 7.57c) – it needs to really actively lift. If this is difficult, support the (R) upper thigh on a block (Fig. 7.57d). Do not passively collapse onto this.

6. Continue to "ground" the (R) shin/knee. Focus on the sit bones and "true them up" so that they are equally long, wide, and level (even if your thigh is on a block). The (R) sit bone needs to work very smartly in lifting and widening and reaching back in order to effectively access the myofascial restrictions.

   Stay in the stretch for 30 seconds or more using the breath to aid the release.

7. Repeat on the other side.

Compensations: Passive collapse with poor grounding in the (R) leg and pelvic initiation – the (R) sit bone drops and the weight falls to the (R) with shortening of the (R) waist. The pelvic core is disengaged. The lumbar spine is pulled into flexion and there is excessive flexion and tension in the upper spine and particularly over the anterior shoulders.

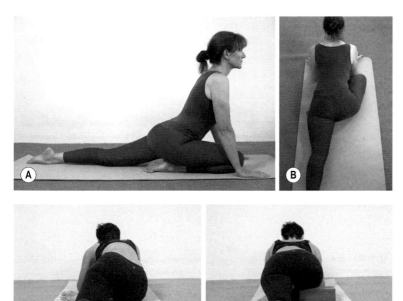

Figure 7.57

Prone piriformis stretch: a) basic;

b) progression – c) incorrect; d) assisted.

58 | Foot exercises

Purpose: To mobilize the foot arches and activate the intrinsic foot muscles.

Benefits: The feet are commonly overlooked, yet they are so important in providing a dynamic but stable base of support for the legs and contribute a rich stream of sensory information to the postural system. They act as both propulsive props and shock absorbers as we walk. Rather than being dexterous and pliable, the feet of many people I see have such poor flexibility they resemble paddles. We address the feet passively and actively.

Know your foot: The foot has many bones contributing to the arches which give it flexibility. Ideal weight bearing forms a tripod between the heel (A), and the balls of the little toes (B) and big toe (C). The mid-foot arch is point D (Fig. 7.58a). Try to go barefoot as often as you can.

Position: Sit on a chair to begin with then progress to doing these exercises in standing.

Use either a firm small ball or, better, a Mini Blackroll (Fig. 7.58b)

Key moves in these exercises:

1. *Mobilizing:* Place the roll (or ball) under –

   ○ the forefoot between points B and C (Fig. 7.58b)

   ○ over the mid foot (point D)

   ○ just in front of your heel (point A).

   Yield as much weight to your foot as you can bear while micro-rolling your foot and curling your toes over. Expect to feel sweet pain!

2. *Doming:* Center your heel (A); spread the toes and, keeping the toe nails visible and the toes all in contact with the floor, draw the front foot

(points B and C) back toward the heel (A). Note how the small arch muscles work. Repeat this whenever you think about it (Fig. 7.58c). If it is difficult to achieve good toe pressure (particularly the big toe), place a common highlight marker under points B and C and work toward making toe contact with the floor. If this is difficult, lift the heel to make toe contact and try and maintain while lowering the heel again.

3. *Foot sweeps:* Slide your foot away so the knee is semiflexed. The knee does not move.

   ○ Center the weight back on your heel and (without losing this) spread the toes. Keeping them all in contact with the floor, sweep the forefoot inwards. Focus upon leading this with the big toe and maintaining its contact (Fig. 7.58d). Then sweep out, as far as you can without losing the heel position. Notice how the arches work.

   ○ Center the forefoot, spreading the toes with the weight equal between points B and C and maintain this while sweeping your heel in and out. The arches work differently.

Compensations: Poor flexibility in the foot makes isolated activity difficult at first. With focus and enough practice, flexibility and control improve.

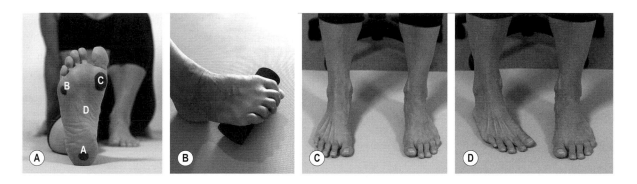

Figure 7.58

Foot exercises: a) know your foot; b)mobilizing; c) doming; d) foot sweeps.

59 | Calf stretches in standing

Purpose: To release the posterior leg myofascia while controlling the foot position.

Benefits: Helps all low back and pelvic pain disorders, and many hip, knee, and leg pain syndromes. Tightness in the posterior inferior myofascial chain limits the ankle, knee, and hip movement necessary for the pelvis to freely move back and anteriorly rotate, which is important for function. IMPORTANT: As with all stretching, you need to maintain a correct alignment, breathe regularly, and surrender to the stretch for at least 30 seconds, and repeat a number of times.

Each calf stretch is in two parts and targets: (A) the deep, and (B) the superficial calf muscles.

Position A: Face a wall or other suitable support for your hands (but do not rely on them).

Place your (R) foot forward with the big toe about 10 centimeters (4 inches) from the wall, ensuring that you align your foot correctly so that its outside border at right angles to the wall. You will invariably need to bring your heel wide to achieve this position. The big toe points slightly in. The (L) foot stands behind, lightly taking weight through the forefoot.

Key moves in the exercises:

1. Distribute your weight evenly through the center of the (R) heel and between the balls of the little and big toes. Ensure the heel is "well grounded."

2. Maintain this foot position and bring most of your weight onto the (R) foot, moving your knee toward the wall – in line with your second toe – until you feel a stretch in your (R) low calf (Fig. 7.59a).

Compensations: Losing foot alignment and pronation; the knee rolls in; losing heel pressure.

Position B: Still maintaining this position, focus now upon your (L) foot behind you, ensuring that you align it properly (as above). Pay particular attention to bring your heel wide – and maintain good pressure down through it and the outside foot. Do not lose this!

Key moves in the exercises: Recheck that your body is well aligned and maintain this.

1. Bring most of your body weight back down through the (L) leg into the heel.

2. At the same time, bring the (L) knee back and the pelvis forward.

3. Angle your body forward from the ankle. Picture a straight line from your (L) heel to your head. Chase the feeling of stretch in your (L) top calf and the back of the knee (Fig. 7.59b).

4. *Progression:* Sweep the big toe further in and repeat as above, exploring the differing vectors of stretch.

Repeat both exercises on the other side – with the (L) foot forward

Compensations: Loss of foot position – particularly the heel – and pronation. Inability to extend both the knee and the hip. Loss of torso alignment.

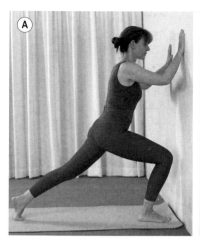

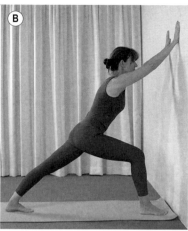

Figure 7.59
Calf stretches in standing: a) position A;
b) position B.

Chapter 7

60 Table-top stretches

Purpose: To control spinal alignment and open the hips, shoulders, and posterior inferior myofascial chains by engaging the first patterns.

Benefits: This is a great stretch no matter what your problems are – provided you are mindful of all the cues. All of us lose some – if not a great deal – of flexibility in the hips, legs, spine, and shoulders. This stretch gets into everything. It can be done with your hands spread on the seat of a chair, a kitchen bench or the wall.

Position: Stand facing a flat-seated chair and place your hands on the seat with fingers spread and palms open. Walk your feet back, bringing them in line with the chair legs and so that the outside border is roughly parallel (with your big toes pointing slightly in) and knees bent.

Key moves in the exercises: Ensure the heels of the hands and the finger knuckles are in contact with the surface (particularly the index). Drop your shoulders and draw the points of the shoulders slightly back. Widen the lower ribs to engage your core. Maintain this.

1. Bring your weight so that it is evenly distributed over your feet between the balls of the little and big toes and your heel in a "tripod of support." Focus upon the weight falling more through the little toe ball and outer heel. Maintain this.

2. Sink your heels into the floor and *scoop the sit bones back, wide, and up* – keeping the knees bent. The heels push down and the sit bones lift. Your pelvic "core" has to work to do this. And you should feel it in your hamstrings.

3. At the same time, reach the crown of your head long (chin tucked in) and reach the tailbone away and up, while also ensuring that you bring your lower ribs back and wide and that the breath is free to cycle. You should be feeling your core "on" and a strong stretch in your shoulders and particularly your hamstrings – without unnecessary tension (Fig. 7.60a).

4. Keep cycling your attention to adjusting the body through all the cues mentioned above. You will tend to initially find that when you correct one, you lose another. Hold for over 60 seconds if you can, to deepen the stretch.

   ○ *Progression 1:* Bring the feet together. Continue with the above prompts. Ensure that both sit bones remain equally high and wide and that your pelvis remains level. Lift the (R) leg up and long, with the big toe facing the floor. The neck and hands are soft (Fig. 7.60b).

   ○ *Progression 2:* Go to a wall – hands at hip height. You have "got it" when you can make connections with all the cues at once (and look like the model in Fig. 7.60c). Lift the leg as described above, if so inclined.

Compensations: Poor grounding of the feet and pushing the knees back rather than lifting the sit bones – the heel/sit bone connection is not made. Knees and feet roll in. Poor grounding of the hands and connecting to the shoulder blades results in excess neck tension and shortening. Inability to lengthen the spine and open the center. Breath holding. Lifting the leg in external rotation – the knee and foot point out to the side.

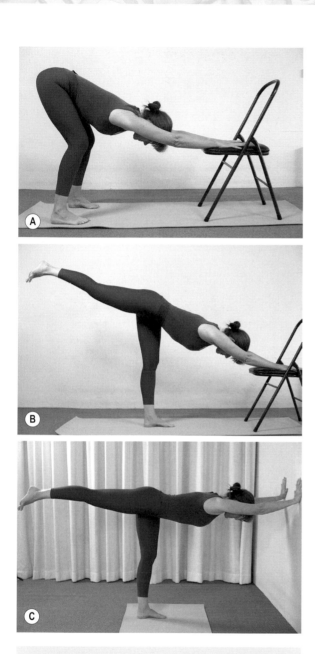

Figure 7.60
Table top stretches: a) basic; b) progression 1;
c) progression 2.

Chapter 7

Which exercises for which conditions?

The Key Moves is a whole person approach to therapeutic exercise and movement. While each exercise proffered targets a particular aspect of torso function, the effect is never completely local but regional – and it affects the whole movement system one way or another.

This method sees that the spine, head, and proximal limb girdles form a functionally integrated movement system: control in one part influences the whole system. It also adopts an integrated systems approach (the nervous, myofascial, and joint systems are functionally interdependent so changed function in one will affect the others).

The Key Moves appreciates the functional body as a "biotensegrity" system and exploits the advantages of the fascial system. By initiating and controlling movements from "key points," we can influence the architecture of the whole tensegrity system, contribute directly or indirectly to movement and/or stability, and improve spinal and limb girdle control and flexibility.

As a quick reference, and to assist your exercise prescription skills in the early stages of working with this model, I have also grouped the exercises differently to the inventory at the front of this chapter.

Those with upper and lower quadrant problems will also benefit from many of the exercises in the general section. Many of your clients will have pain problems in both upper and lower quadrants.

A. General application

These influence the whole torso and will benefit all your clients one way or another. Bear in mind that the axial and limb girdle FPs are always active.

1. Diaphragmatic breathing

2. Constructive rest position

3. Sphinx

4. Rotation in side lying

5. Pinning the beetle

6. Baby pose: Building further "core control"

22. Supplicant pose

23. Healthy sitting

24. Opening the center

30. Sit to stand

31. Healthy standing

32. Forward bend pattern

33. Basic abdominal exercises for a healthy spine

34. Pelvic reach and roll

39. Windswept pose B

41. Twister

46. Shoulder and pelvic backward rotation in lying

47. Mini press to Seal

48. "Core" challenge in sitting

49. Lateral weight shift pattern

60. Table-top stretches

B. Lower quadrant pain disorders

5. Pinning the beetle

7. First and second pelvic patterns

8. Third pelvic pattern

9. Fourth pelvic pattern

10. Isolating hip flexion

15. Windscreen wipers

16. Backward pelvic rotation

21. Cat/Camel

29. Pelvic dancing in sitting

35. Pelvic hovercraft

36. Advanced abdominal exercise for a healthy spine

37. Smart hamstring stretch

38. Brainy buttock release

39. Windswept pose A

40. Half baby to Cross-over

45. Slow heel kicks

50. Hamstring releases in sitting

52. Pelvic rock and roll in side sitting

53. V to Z hip stretch

54. Butt booster on all fours

55. Rebooting your iliopsoas and core

56. "Distorsion" progressing to Crescent stretch

57. Prone piriformis stretch

58. Foot exercises

59. Calf stretches in standing

C. Upper quadrant pain disorders

11. Head fundamental pattern 1 and eye movements

12. Rag doll

13. "Temperature check" rotation

14. Prayer stretch: connecting breath, core and pelvic patterns

17. Happy neck exercise

18. Praying mantis

19. Wide wings

20. Half Sphinx to Amphibian

25. Shoulder fundamental patterns

26. Head fundamental patterns

27. Shoulder shrug and slide

28. Windmills

42. Shoulder pattern combo

43. Double arm triangles

44. Spreadeagle

51. Shoulder and chest opener

Key Moves® Functional assessment summary and exercise prescription inventory

Date: ....

Name: ....

Occupation: ....

Phone: .... Age: ....

Referrer: ....

Diagnosis: ....

Associated problems: ....
....

Aggravating postures/activities: ....
....

Past treatment including exercise regimens: ....
....
....

Weekend activities/sports/hobbies: ....
....
....

Mark in all your client's signs and symptoms
0–10 numeric pain scale

Nil   Moderate   Severe

Functional diagnosis (clinical syndromes): ....
....

Patient specific functional scale (if appropriate): ....

Client's goals: ....

Principal functional deficits which you aim to redress with exercise therapy:
(Initially, prioritise the 2–3 most basic functional deficits, e.g. lack of extension; poor AFP control)

1. ....   2. ....

3. ....   4. ....

5. ....   6. ....

7. ....   8. ....

9. ....   10. ....

Date	Aim of the exercise	Prescribed exercise	Progress/comments

Patient-Specific Functional Scale

This useful questionnaire can be used to quantify activity limitation and measure functional outcome for patients with any orthopaedic condition

Clinician to read and fill in below: Complete at the end of the history and prior to physical examination

Initial assessment

I am going to ask you to identify up to three important activities that you are unable to do or are having difficulty with as a result of your _____ problem. Today, are there any activities that you are unable to door having difficulty with because of your _____ problem? (Clinician: show scale to patient and have the patient rate each activity.)

Follow-up assessments

When I assessed you on (state previous assessment date), you told me that you had difficulty with (read all activities from list at a time). Today, do you still have difficulty with: (read and have patient score each item in the list)?

Patient-specific activity scoring scheme (point to one number)

0	1	2	3	4	5	6	7	8	9	10

Unable to
perform
activity

Able to perform
activity at same level as
before injury or problem

(Date and score)

Activity	Initial						
1							
2							
3							
4							
5							
Additional							
Additional							

Total score = sum of the activity scores/number of activities
Minimum detectable change (90%CI) for average score = 2 points
Minimum detectable change (90%CI) for single activity score = 3 points

PSFS developed by: Stratford, P., Gill, C., Westaway, M., Binkley, J. (1995). Assessing disability and change on individual patient: a report of a patient specific measure. Physiotherapy Canada, 47, 258–263.

The preceding chapter offered a suite of exercises in basic motor control aimed at improving performance of the FPs, releasing tight myofascia, and mobilizing joints.

When the FPs have been "found" we can incorporate them into more dynamic actions and movements. We want them to be more accomplished and automatic so that they become reestablished into the movement repertoire and the spine can enjoy better health. For this, supervised small group classes provide an ideal learning situation. Here, various further important aspects of control are considered.

Breathing

The breath underlies everything. We always look for breathing that is regular, low down in the body, and slow – no matter what the activity. It is important that breathing is not made to be hard work, because that only creates tension. Rather, we observe and make space for the breath via the axial fundamental pattern – and simply allow it to come and go. This is "deepening the breath."

While we do not "make" the breath, we can modulate its various aspects: slowing it; sending it here or there. And extending exhalation, and the pause after it, aids relaxation.

Playing with positive expiratory patterns

In the early stages of training these can help wake up and give the client a better sense of LPU "deep core" activity. Gently blowing out fully through pursed lips specifically engages the pelvic floor and lower transversus abdominis. It is initiated in the lower rather than upper abdominal wall. Fogging a mirror or breathing through a straw also helps this action.

We can further train the basic core response by activating the axial FP in sustained postural control – maintaining a well-aligned, "open center" while asking for other expiratory patterns: talking, singing, humming, chanting, blowing, whistling, laughing, etc. The wise yogis knew about this. So do professional singers. Blowing up a balloon significantly challenges control.

The posterior PXS client can have a lot of difficulty bringing the lower thorax down into alignment with the pelvis, but this is necessary for achieving control of the basic axial FP. Tipping the pelvis into posterior tilt is a common compensation. To circumvent this, a strong active exhalation such as "Sshhh" can help wake up the whole abdominal wall to bring the thorax down and back – and stabilize the LPT in a more neutral alignment with the pelvis. The client's task is then to keep it there – and breathe – particularly with a long exhalation. Breathing through a straw can help this.

We can also use exhalation in movement where we want better abdominal activity and core stability in anticipation of limb load challenge (e.g., lowering a leg to the ground in lying – particularly if it is straight).

Using the Key Moves Core Retrainer Belt

It is important to establish ability in the axial FP when recumbent with gravity eliminated (see Ch. 4: Controlling the center). Challenging correct control of this pattern with limb load tunes it up for upright control. If people cannot gain adequate basic pattern control here, they are unlikely to do so when dealing with gravity and moving about.

Even with reasonable control in lying, the axial FP can be hard to "find" when upright and focusing upon other aspects of control. To help overcome this, each of our students wears our specially developed Key Moves Core Retrainer Belt in class to facilitate axial FP control during all poses and movement. The belt also helps maintain core activity during sustained postural activities such as sitting working at a computer (see Fig. 3.34b) and when walking.

The belt acts as an aide memoire, reminding the wearer to focus their attention on control of the center – to let go of any superficial muscle tension and engage the axial FP by expanding into the belt sideways (and back in a posterior PXS client). You cannot do this properly unless you are correctly engaging your core.

It is important that the belt has "Goldilocks' s tension" (i.e., not too tight and not too loose). You should be able to put your hand down under it. The belt is designed to act as a proprioceptive cue to help the person "know where to go" and what to do. If it is too tight it will constrict the lower ribs, which we do not want (and the anterior PXS group are already doing that to themselves). If it is too loose there is no sensory feedback.

The posterior PXS group find posterior basal breathing particularly difficult. To help facilitate this I place "buttons" (actually Velcro-backed bottle tops) in the lower posterior part of the belt so that they rest over the lateral end of the 12th rib (Fig. 8.1). My cue in class might be "fill back into your buttons" – or, perhaps "push back and wide into the (L) button" with lateral weight shift to the left in Ex. 49 (see Ch. 7).

Working the center

We initially work the center to reestablish a neutral axis, which itself facilitates inner core support.

Establishing sagittal control of the axis

Control of the basic axial FP brings the thorax and pelvis into alignment and provides internal support, which allows for minimal superficial torso muscle activity. This is the basis of a flexible "neutral" upright spine. Reestablishing this can take work because many people lack control of the lower thorax in essentially two ways:

- The posterior PXS can't bring the spine into neutral (i.e., align the thorax with the pelvis). Core mechanisms and spinal alignment suffer. To help this we work the center more into flexion: by bringing the ribs back without tipping the pelvis back to assist core control (see Exs 5, 6, 33, and 36). This helps the client's journey toward achieving a better upright posture.

- In the anterior PXS group the thorax is over-anchored by tight/overactive upper abdominal myofascia. Again core mechanisms and alignment suffer (see Ch. 3, The clinical syndromes). Here we work the center by asking for more "opening" : engaging the axial FP to "push" the lower ribs wide – and keep them so while breathing and holding a pose. The core

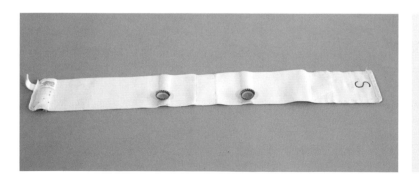

Figure 8.1

The Key Moves Core Retrainer Belt has been opened out to show the "buttons" attached to the bottom of the Velcro strips on the inside.

engagement helps inhibit the upper abdominal wall hyperactivity, even during forward curling.

- When good sagittal alignment is achieved, maintaining this can be challenged in sitting via the basic core challenge (see Ex. 48) and further challenge asks for maintaining correct alignment and an open center during forward weight shift (see Ex. 29, Fig. 7.29a) or backward tilts (Fig. 8.2). All these moves challenge integration of iliopsoas with the core.

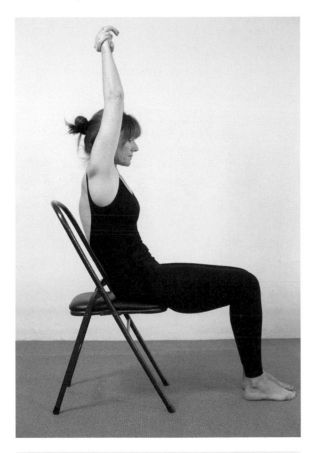

Figure 8.2
Sitting backward pelvic tilts maintaining sagittal alignment. This is different to axial FP2, which asks for backward curling of the lower pole of the thorax (see Fig. 5.18a). Also ensure that "jacking" does not occur (see Fig. 5.18b).

Controlling the axial FP in three-dimensional movement

The center actually initiates spinal movement in that the core response is a pre-movement postural reflex that occurs before movement to support and stabilize the spine. It is this response that we have to work to reestablish in our clients.

With able control of the center in neutral, we look for its control in movement. Most actual spinal movements are initiated from either the head, or the pelvic or shoulder girdles, and the center should be free to adaptively follow while maintaining its alignment and internal support. To smarten up this role we can also actively work the center.

We work into the axial fundamental patterns AFP1–AFP4: either flexion/extension, lateral shift, rotation – or combinations thereof (see Ch. 4: Controlling the center). Pelvic dancing in sitting (see Ex. 29) is useful here. Incidentally, posterior PXS clients will have more difficulty controlling the second axial pattern (see Figs 5.18a,b).

To promote more elasticity in the thorax, we use passive poses, such as over a bolster in supine and side lying (Ex. 2) or Sphinx (Ex. 3). Engaging the axial FP in these various passive poses in different planes helps both improve its adaptable control and mobilize the thorax and spine.

Shape change of the torso can be further augmented by assistance from the breath, as in the lateral weight shift pattern (Ex. 49) where we direct the breath more down, back, and wide into the lower thorax of the weight-bearing side.

More advanced moves involve controlling the axial FP through more challenging movement; for example, curling forward from a passive backbend over a bolster or Rolla which is placed under the thoracic dome helps improve core competency as well as rib cage and thoracic spinal mobility and control (Fig. 8.3a,b). Here it is important that the pelvis remains stable.

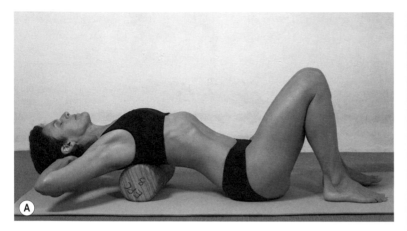

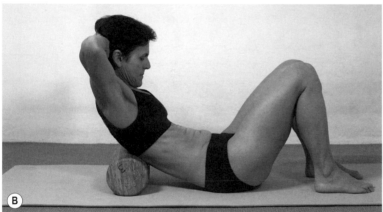

Figure 8.3

a) Backbend over a Rolla, which is placed over the "dome" or dorsal hinge region. b) During the curl forward, the pelvis should remain stable.

When the spine enjoys this adaptable internal support it is buoyant and moves more freely.

The head–tailbone connection

The head and tailbone, being at the top and bottom of the spine, are always in a changing functional relationship with each other. Either can initiate spinal movement – which is then followed by and reflected in the other, however subtle.

In an ideal upright spinal posture, the posterior head and tailbone are behind the gravitational line of force (see Fig. 2.1). The chin and front pelvis are in front of it and drop slightly. The head and pelvis are in ideal (neutral) balance. Spinal elongation and "lift" occurs when the tailbone reaches down and slightly back and the head reaches up. We look for this relationship in all the poses, exercises and movements.

When we adopt a fetal position with the tailbone tucked under, the head goes forward. This is a common spinal configuration and posture. When the tailbone moves back, ideally so does the head – and vice versa. This automatic relationship is often missing in our clients. They may have lost the ability and sense of initiating movement back from the tailbone (or head), or even when they can do this, the head does not necessarily follow; this is largely due to stiffness in the upper thorax and shoulders. When the tailbone moves to the side, so should the head; when the sacrum rotates back, so does the head. Again, stiffness in the pelvis/hips and thorax limits this.

Spinal segmental articulation

The function of the spine, a flexible column which is both stable and mobile, is to support the head and limbs and promote their freedom to move. The ability to sequence movement through the spine becomes diminished through lack of movement (and its variety), poor postural habits, and age. We become stiff and painful.

Relearning to initiate movement from the FPs is basic to this approach. Wherever movement begins, we look to encouraging its sequencing through each spinal segment. This is particularly so in the thorax, whether it be flexion, extension, side bending or rotation. As ribs are attached to each of the thoracic vertebrae, directing the breath is a valuable adjunct.

In particular, look for segmental sequencing in Exs 4, 7–9, 12, 13, 15b and c, 16, 18–21, 25, 27, 29, 34, 41, 42, 46, 47, 49 and 52. Nice segmental movement can also be encouraged in supine "wiggly worm" : "walking" up and down the mat through the sit bones/buttocks and shoulder blades; the ribs stay soft and wide.

There is also "Body wave rock" : via rhythmical plantar flexion in supine with legs extended. Watch for no rib thrust or butt clench – dominant dorsiflexion activity is related to butt clench!

Getting movement into the thorax and shoulders

It is important to recognize that while the spine is stiff, some regions are stiffer than others. Control of the FPs allows us to better align the spine and work more specifically into the regional "blocks" or areas of stiffness (e.g., the thoracic dome and shoulders) while protecting the "hinges" or areas of relative flexibility, which are the weak links (e.g., neck and low back).

Fundamental to getting movement into the thorax is adequate control of the center and the axial FP, which aligns and stabilizes the LPT as we work the shoulder patterns in order to gain movement into the upper pole of the thorax, dome, and shoulder girdle. The following exercises address this in various ways: # 2, 4, 12–14, 17–22, 25, 27, 28, 34, 41–44, 46, 47, 49, 51, and 60.

The shoulder patterns are also practiced in various body and arm postures, such as on all fours or side sitting. An important functional pattern in the shoulder is that of a forward arm with scapula retraction. This can be practiced sitting or standing with the hands shoulder height on the wall and the elbows soft (Fig. 8.4), or behind the wheel of the car when stationary at the lights.

Getting movement into the pelvis and hips

The lumbar spine becomes problematic when the pelvic and hip joints become stiff and their related myofascia loses flexibility and slide. Disorganized motor control is the root cause. While the pelvis as a whole suffers from lack of spatial stability, intrapelvic and

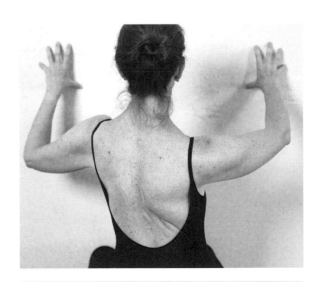

Figure 8.4

Working the shoulder FPs hands on wall. The shoulder FP4 is shown – helping to "re-groove" the important functional pattern of forward arm flexion with scapular retraction. The center should remain active and open.

hip mobility is lost. Fundamental to gaining mobility in the pelvis and hips, and protecting the lower back, is control of the pelvic patterns – coordinated with the axial FP. Opening the hips/pelvis and their control is addressed one way or another in Exs 2, 4, 7–10, 15, 16, 21–24, 29, 30–32, 34, 35, 37, 38, 39a, 40, 41, 45, 46, 49, 50, 52–57 and 60.

Heel–sit bone and hand–shoulder blade connections in functional movement

The feet and hands contain a rich density of sensory receptors which contribute important information to the CNS for regulating postural control and organizing movement. Many reflex neuromuscular chains have their origin in the feet and hands, particularly when they are the base of support. When the hands and feet are "well grounded," and the body weight is evenly distributed through them, the associated limb myofascia is freer to let go and allow more adaptable movement of the proximal segments. Good grounding also facilitates a better functional connection with fundamental pattern control of the proximal limb girdles. Pressure through the heel of either is particularly important in achieving this. This grounding of the base of support together with proximal limb girdle control frees the spine.

Tight, bound limb myofascia, however, can pull the foot or hand off-center and hamper grounding; hence we really need to focus on cueing correct foot or hand positions prior to a movement.

This is particularly important in first pattern control of important functional movements (e.g., Exs 30 and 31), closed-chain hip flexion in the forward bend pattern (e.g., Exs 32 and 60), and shoulder girdle retraction with the arm forward (e.g., Exs 18, 21, 22, 47, 52–54, 57, and 60).

The current fashion of wearing thick-soled trainers deprives the sensory motor feedback loop and stops the foot making flexible contact with the earth. Posture and lumbopelvic movement control are more compromised. Hence in class we always work in bare feet, aiming for correct foot position and active arches – and adaptively maintaining these through the activity.

Lengthening the sides

Lateral weight shift and "lengthening the sides" are important aspects of functional movement which become detuned in spinal pain populations. The inferior tethers create spinal stiffness and bound myofascia, thus limiting movement freedom.

Lengthening the sides is initiated by the third pelvic or shoulder FPs with third axial FP control. The head is also involved. Lengthening the sides is important for both effective load transfer through the pelvis and balance (standing on one leg, walking up or down stairs, etc.) – and for increasing spatial reach of the upper limb. Many falls in the elderly can be attributed to poor spinopelvic mobility and control of lateral weight shift.

We can work on increasing frontal plane flexibility and third pattern control in a number of ways. As an example, during exercise we can alternately lengthen (Fig. 8.5a) and shorten (Fig. 8.5b) the top side body. Whichever way we work the frontal plane, it is important to also aim for maintaining the sagittal alignment and to cue corrections when alignment is lost (Fig. 8.5c) – even though the range of movement may appear to be less.

Breaking up the holding patterns: working off-center

We also work in the frontal plane to relieve the spine from the shackles of "central fixing" by the crude inferior tether strategies and thereby help bring the client out of their sagittal fix. This aids lateral opening of the spine, thorax, and proximal limb girdles; helps inhibit CCP activity; and improves adaptable control of the axial FP and proximal limb girdle FP control.

The base of support can be off-center, such as in side sitting (see Exs 52 and 53) – or we can ask for

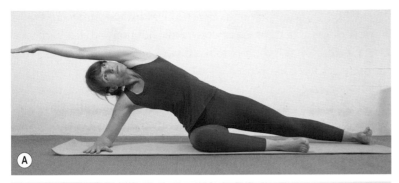

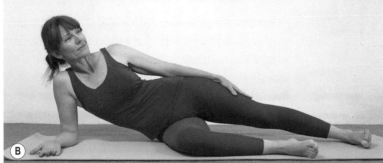

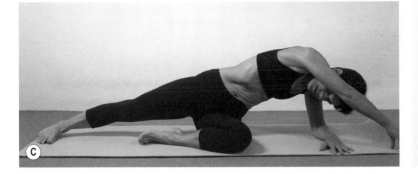

Figure 8.5
Lengthening the sides in side-lying elbow support. a) Lengthening the topside: the topside lateral rib cage lifts and opens as the foot and hand reach away while also controlling sagittal alignment. b) Shortening the topside: the underside rib cage drops and laterally opens. c) Poor lengthening with loss of sagittal alignment.

actively sustaining an off-center base posture, such as by maintaining the third pelvic pattern and adding movement (see Exs 49 and 55). This helps lengthen the sides.

Again here, we also aim for sagittal alignment; for example, in side sitting, inadequate pelvic control and axial stiffness results in the common fault of collapsing into flexion with poor axial FP control (Fig. 8.6a). Similarly, in upright sitting, with poor axial FP control, the lower ribs throw forward and lift (see Fig. 5.18b).

When working in side sitting it is important to cue your patient out of the inferior tethers. These hamper achieving a good pelvic base of support and result in a falling back into spinal flexion, which is usually associated with holding around the center, shoulder depression, and trying to bear weight through the fingertips (see Fig. 8.6a). The weight does not shift laterally. For contrast, see Figs 7.52 and 7.53, where you will note that there is good grounding through the (L) thigh and control of pelvic FP1; the spine has lift; the ribs have shifted to the (L); and the (L) shoulder is elevated and free to move. We can assist opening of the side body, including the proximal limb girdles, by "hanging" from a stick while working the center and moving forward and to the right – initiating the movement from the pelvis (Fig. 8.6b) This is a precursor to being able to be self-supporting and raise the weight-bearing arm (Fig. 8.6c).

Rotation

Habitual sagittal collapse and inferior tether activity result in poor lateral weight shift and rotation in movement. In healthy control, with good sagittal alignment, rotation primarily occurs in the pelvic/hip girdle, head, thorax, and shoulder girdle. Rotation creates weight shifts. Lateral weight shifts facilitate rotation and limb movements.

When upright, rotating to (say) the right is freer when the weight shifts to the left. Try it yourself: Sit on a chair with a firm seat; now collapse and see how far you can see to the right. Now sit **up** on your sit bones and turn to the (R). Can you see further? Now also come onto the (L) sit bone and turn right. Notice that you see a lot further when the weight shifts to the opposite sit bone, because this allows the pelvis to rotate back – and the spine, shoulder girdle, and head follow. Also notice that forward rotation has occurred on the (L) weight-bearing side. The better the sagittal alignment, the better and more easily do these movements occur.

One of the potential problems of doing "twists" in yoga is that prior elongation of the spine and subtle weight shifts through the pelvic base of support are usually not encouraged. Neither is the rotary contribution from the proximal limb girdles and opening the center (Fig. 8.7a). Consequently, rotation is not free to occur where it ideally should. What we see instead is "wringing the waist" and CCP reinforcement, with

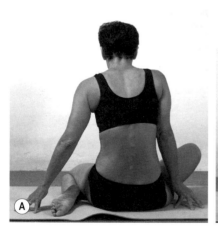 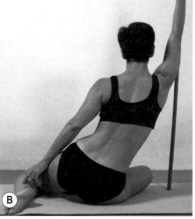 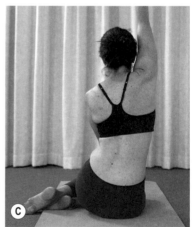

Figure 8.6

Working in side sitting. a) Sagittal collapse begins in the pelvis. The client has to sufficiently work the pelvic FPs against the effects of the inferior tethers. A poor pelvic base of support and trying to "hold oneself up" by central cinch pattern (CCP) strategies results in the client trying to hold the spine centrally and being disinclined to let the bodyweight and thorax move laterally and be supported by the ipsilateral arm in elevated shoulder FP3 (see Fig. 7.52a). This model's function is too good, however – she is not showing any CCP activity. b) Using a stick, ensuring the arm is relaxed and the body hangs, is a nice way to lengthen the shoulder and axial inferior tethers and work for better pelvic and sagittal control in frontal plane movement c) ... all of which is a precursor to being able to raise the arm in free side sitting.

excess anterior shoulder tension making the neck and lower back vulnerable. Spinal lift, subtle lateral weight shift, backward rotation in the pelvic and shoulder girdles – together with controlling axial FP4 and an open center – should be the prime focus. Watch the body open more (Fig. 8.7b).

Using rotation in movement is also a nice way of breaking up the holding patterns. It is important that it is initiated from the head and proximal limb girdles, and that there is no central disconnect because of poor axial FP activity. Rotation is pleasurable movement. There seems to be a deeply embedded archetypal link between rotation and the limbic system in the CNS. Get your clients doing rotary movement and they will just keep going until you ask them to stop! We can work rotation more passively (Exs 4, 39a, and 41) or more actively (Exs 13, 15b,c, 16, 20, 34 and 46).

Bilateral/symmetrical vs single/asymmetrical limb movements

Bilateral, symmetrical limb movements are reflexly linked with more "total pattern" control. For example, lifting both arms up and out is associated with spinal extension, pulling them into the body with spinal flexion. In healthy control, effective control of the center and proximal limb girdles is automatically integrated into these movements.

In someone struggling with sagittal plane control, bilateral limb movements easily trigger and reinforce coarse patterns of control in the form of inferior tether activity and further sagittal fixing.

Most functional activities do not usually involve both limbs in symmetrical limb postures and movements – even in weight bearing on all fours – yet many exercise streams adopt an approach that uses bilateral, symmetrical limbs in weight-bearing postures and movements.

Unilateral limb movements facilitate improved deep system patterns of control and help counter inferior tether control strategies, and their reinforcement. When initiated by the proximal limb girdle FPs, they bring about subtle or overt weight shifts and rotation through the axis, and engage the diagonal vector, thereby creating tensions and counter-tensions through the myofascial system.

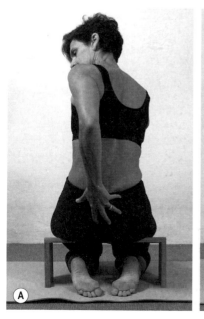
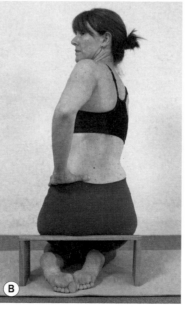

Figure 8.7

Rotation. a) Poor rotation in sitting with axial collapse and excess tension around the center (not apparent in this model) and neck – because the proximal limb girdles are not active. b) Allowing the weight to shift slightly onto the (R) sit bone frees the (L) sit bone and point of shoulder to draw back (4th patterns) and initiate the movement in concert with the head, which remains poised at the top of the spine. Axial FP4 controls the center.

Limb movements functionally connect through a well-controlled center.

For this reason, exercises such as Cat/Camel (Ex. 21) adopt an asymmetrical base of support; active limb movements are unilateral or asymmetrical, as in, for example, Wide wings (Ex. 19), Half Sphinx to Amphibian (Ex. 20), Windmills (Ex. 28c); and Spreadeagle (Ex. 44).

Widening

Anxiety and defensive postures constrict the center and bring the body and limbs forward in its protection. The axis becomes contracted and shortened; breathing and core control mechanisms suffer.

In movement therapy we aim to encourage elongation of the spine and a three-dimensional open center. Fundamental pattern control is facilitated by "widening" the lower rib cage, the sit bones, and the points of the shoulders. Thinking of widening the ears facilitates the first head pattern.

Widening the elbows or knees also helps release tight limb myofascia, as seen in Fig. 8.8.

"Going back"

Our daily lives involve us living a lot in our front body and "going forward" – walking, using our hands down in front, reaching. Occupations are increasingly sedentary, and technology based. Postural collapse in sitting and relative overactivity of the anterior shoulder girdle and arm myofascia lead to the spine becoming bowed down by the forward hang of the head and upper limbs. We begin to lose the sense of the back body and the space behind us. We lose the sense of readily "going back" in movement.

All the first fundamental patterns involve going back – the breath, the lower rib cage in controlling the axial FP, the sit bones, the points of the shoulders, and the head.

When people rely upon inferior tether strategies, their postures and movements will be second pattern

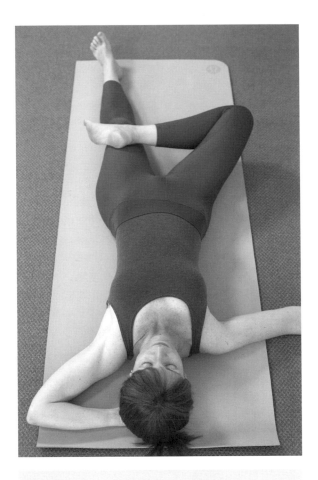

Figure 8.8

Matchsticks. Both proximal limb girdles are active in 1st pattern to aid opening and widening, and also tissue release. The focus is on working the center while encouraging the elbow and knee to "widen" and fall back. The limbs are supported by a block if the client is quite restricted and having difficulty letting go.

dominant and they will have difficulty with the first patterns. Hence, to aid flexibility in going back, we use passive poses to encourage "falling back" and release of anterior myofascial chain and joint stiffness. Even here there should be some active engagement of the 1st FPs (e.g., in Exs 1–4). "Matchsticks" is another variation on a theme (see Fig. 8.8). The elbow or knee may be supported by a block, if needs be, to aid tissue release.

Active control exercises always involve some regions going back; it happens even in abdominal exercises – to the breath and lower ribs. In forward bending the sit bones go back, up, and wide to bring the upper body down and forward.

Understanding the tendency for second pattern dominance helps us be alert for the cues we need to give the client to facilitate better first pattern control. For example, expect that on all fours they will show poor backward weight shift and little ability to lead movement back from the sit bones/tailbone; the ribs will hang forward, the anterior shoulder girdle will invariably be somewhat "locked," and they will either hang the head or poke the chin forward. Control of first patterns corrects this.

All the exercises provided in Ch. 7 involve going back in one way or another. Can you pick the important elements to cue in each? (The only exception is some foot exercises in Ex. 58.)

Stretching

Whether you are in a rehabilitation setting or teaching a yoga class, tight limb myofascia and insufficient, imbalanced proximal control are going to be common problems to deal with. In stretching, we need to ensure that the tail (the limbs) does not wag the dog (the spine).

The spine is often the victim in many common limb stretches. A variable combination of "end gaining," impoverished sensory perception, and inadequate deep system support and control through the proximal limb girdles and spine leads to stretches that are poorly localized to the limbs. Instead, they often create more stretch and strain in the spine – particularly lumbar, as well as reinforcing dominant anterior shoulder girdle activity and stiffness in the thoracic spine – and neck tension (see Figs 5.33–5.38).

By varying both the torso and the limb postures in various and ingenious ways, and engaging the FPs here, we can improve both primary/pelvic core control and release tight limb myofascia at the same time. Gravity does the work: we are simply surrendering to it and aiding the release by discreetly activating "key points of control" (the FPs) to fine-tune access to the tightest tissue vectors. Working in this way actively involves the nervous system in active elongation of tight myofascia, aiding neuroplasticity through focused attention. We both improve proximal patterns of control and achieve effective release throughout the myofascial envelope at the same time. This is exemplified in Matchsticks (Fig. 8.8) – and Exs 2, 4, 39, 41, 53, 56, and 57.

Forward bends

Whether from sitting, kneeling or standing, forward bends should always be initiated from the pelvis rotating forward on the femoral heads. The sacrum carries the spine and head forward. The lumbar lordosis should be controlled through the movement until the end (Fig. 8.9a) – when the top spine folds forward.

It is a basic functional pattern that all your clients will have difficulty doing well. Stiff hips and tightness of the hamstrings and posteroinferior myofascial chain are endemic to low back and pelvic pain – and most of the community.

The fundamental control comes from pelvic FP1 integrated with the Axial FP. Shoulder FP1 is also lightly engaged to open the top chest and "maintain the line."

We initially break up the forward bend pattern in different ways to improve its variable control and achieve myofascial release. Spinal alignment is always worked for (see Exs 7a, 10, 16, 22, 23, 30, 32, 35, 37, 38, 50, 52, 53, 56, 57, and 60).

Forward bends are a staple of yoga practice. Most Westerners are stiff in the hips and tight over the whole posteroinferior myofascial chain. They are also invariably "end-gainers," with their sights on how far they can move rather than how well. Holding excess tension is common, with little attention paid to the process of the movement.

Chapter 8

A problem in large, poorly supervised classes is that the client is not set up to make change in the pose. Poor pelvic initiation and spinal collapse, with excess tension and flexion in the upper spine, are common. The movement is initiated from the head and upper limbs rather than the pelvis. The lower back and pelvis are strained and leg release is ineffective (Fig. 8.9b).

Using sufficient props and the correct cues is important. Whatever the configuration of the legs, elevate the sitting base of support (such as folded blankets, blocks, a bolster or firm cushion) so that the hips are higher than the knees. The weight must be borne through the tops of the sit bones so that the pelvis can move into first pattern. If this is still difficult, place a support under the knees. This releases tension off the hamstrings so that the sit bones are freer to move. Being mindful of yielding the weight to the support, initiating from the first pelvic pattern, and the head–tailbone connection in lengthening the spine is important in the pose (Fig. 8.9c). Some of your clients may also require some sort of anterior support for the top body, such as an upturned bolster or a chair. This is not to collapse into, but provides the support some need to help them focus on the inner unit and leading from the ischial tuberosities to enable the hip/pelvic fulcrum to lead the movement.

Asymmetrical leg positions help bring the client out of sagittal dominance and open up the posterolateral myofascial chains. Support under the knee, if needed, helps yielding to the base of support.

Back bending

Spinal extension is always limited in people with spinal pain disorders – in some regions more than others. Regaining it has to be done in a stepwise, judicious fashion.

Not all parts of the spine naturally extend equally. Because of the anatomical geometry, it is freest in the neck and low back. However, this freedom relies upon functional support from the related proximal limb girdles integrated with control of the center.

Back bending requires control of the shoulder FP1 with the axial FP, which is fundamental to opening the thorax. Control of pelvic FP2 opens the front hip and thigh. The neck and low back become the weak link without these fundamental elements of control.

A common myth is the "too extended spine." Most seemingly extended spines are held up by the thoracolumbar extensors because intrinsic mechanisms are lacking (see Figs 3.10 and 3.19a,b)

Patient populations commonly have a stiff thorax and poor control of the center and proximal limb girdles. Unless checked by correct cueing, asking for extension will invariably result in simply more CCP activity over the thoracolumbar junction and little or no movement through the thorax and shoulder girdle, plus increased neck tension.

In kneeling, poor control of the center and opening of the anterior hip and associated myofascia is compensated for by increased CPC activity and shunting the lower thorax forward; this is particularly so in the posterior PXS subgroup (see Fig. 3.18).

We initially work to improve extension and prepare for back bending by more passive poses to open the front body, shoulders, and hips (see Exs 2, 3, 14, 39, and 41). Bear in mind that even in these poses, we still attend to control of the center and activating the relevant FPs – particularly the first shoulder pattern.

Early active patterns of preparatory control get movement into the thorax and shoulder girdle and open the front hip (see Exs 12, 13, 17–22, 25, 27, and 28). More advanced opening and control is in Exs 42–47, 51, 55, 56 and 60.

Sitting on a large gym ball and carefully lying back over it is a pleasing way to open the front body in a relaxed and supported manner (Fig. 8.10a).

More dynamic control can be achieved in kneeling or half kneeling with a bench or chair behind. Bear in mind that the fundamental control comes from

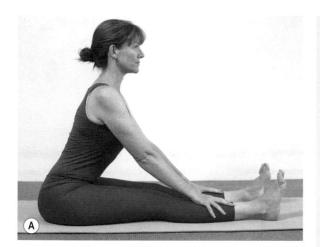

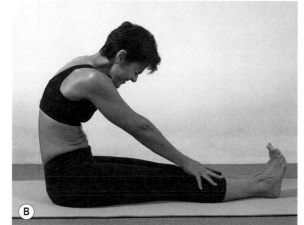

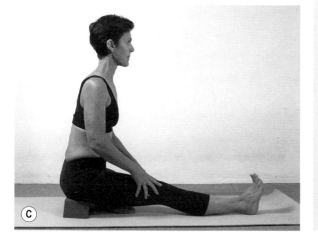

Figure 8.9

Forward bends. a) Effective pelvic control creates a fulcrum at the hips which brings the body forward while alignment is maintained. This should be the focus rather than trying to get to the feet, which should only occur at the very end of the pose – if one is proficient. b) Without effective pelvic control the client tries to pull themselves forward: the spine collapses, the neck and shoulders are tense, and the "dome" increases. c) Bringing the pelvis higher on a support assists the client to achieve better pelvic control (see Fig. 5.40). Placing a block under the knee can also help offload the hamstrings more, and placing a chair in front of the client can help slightly support them while they action all the 1st patterns – including the shoulder (not shown). It is more a case of how well the pose is controlled than how far someone can reach forward.

shoulder FP1 and pelvic FP2 integrated with the axial FP (Fig. 8.10b). A further supported variation can be from kneel sitting on a small stool with the hands resting on blocks if needed (Fig. 8.10c).

Bear in mind that those yogis who can beautifully come into the advanced poses such as Urdhva Dhanurasana have been usually been practicing for many hours each day, and over many years. Be patient, rather than becoming a patient! Master the parts, and the whole will come together.

Bridging

This is a popular exercise which works the glutei in inner range and mobilizes the whole spine. The prompts usually ask for initiating the movement with tail tuck, bringing the pelvis into posterior tilt and lumbar flexion – and controlling this through the movement.

Yet people with spinopelvic pain disorders are usually good at working the pelvis this way. What they cannot do is bring the pelvis into a neutral position and maintain the lumbopelvic lordosis while unloading the pelvis. This requires control of the first pelvic pattern. Hence Ex. 35 (Pelvic hovercraft) specifically works for control of this important pattern.

When they are proficient at this, we then incorporate it into a bridging sequence – initiating and finishing in a first pelvic pattern hover. The second pattern may need encouraging to bring the pelvis high and not overwork over the back ribs, particularly in a posterior PXS client. Clients need to learn smooth transitions from first to second pelvic pattern and back into first pattern.

To help mobilize the thorax and shoulders, I like to do bridging with the arms up above the head: they slide away on the roll up, the chin drops, and the neck lengthens. The arms remain here on the roll down, as you really ask for segmental movement sequencing and bringing as many of the vertebrae and lower ribs back, wide, and in contact with the support as possible – then, at the end, reaching the tailbone long and back to hover in first pattern – then landing. And repeat.

Pelvic control can be further challenged by three other moves. Spread the arms out to the side:

- Maintaining the hover position: brush both buttocks to the right side of the mat without rotating the pelvis. This requires first and third pattern control and movement through the hip sockets. The (R) waist lengthens and the (L) shortens. Repeat side to side. There should be weight shift

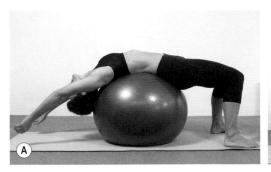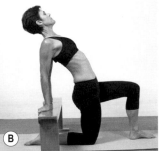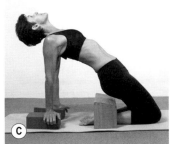

Figure 8.10
Back bends. a) Over a ball. b) Half kneeling with a bench or chair behind. c) From a kneeling/meditation stool.

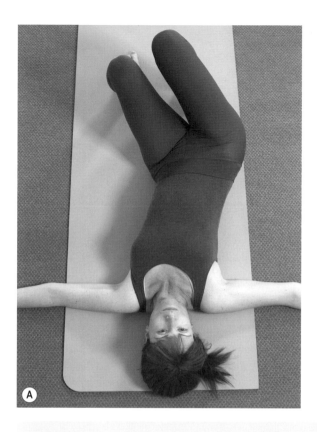

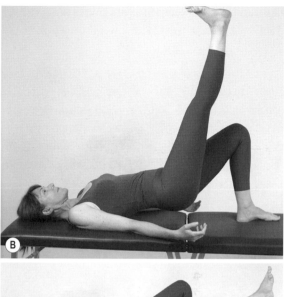

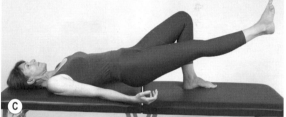

Figure 8.11

Bridging sequences. a) Pelvic lateral shift and rotation to land on one buttock. b) Challenging ability to maintain pelvic FP1 in half bridge with hip flexion and knee extension. c) Further challenge while lowering and raising an extended leg.

through the shoulder blades and movement through the thorax (see Fig. 7.35b).

- Shift the pelvis to the right, as above, and now rotate it so as to land only the (L) buttock. This requires the fourth pelvic pattern control. The weight will also shift onto the (L) scapula and rotation sequences through the spine. The movement is repeated from side to side (Fig. 8.11a).

- Pelvic hovercraft challenge: the pelvic hovercraft control is maintained while allowing the pelvis to lift more (about half way up) while flexing one hip, progressing to extending that

knee (Fig. 8.11b) – and further challenged by lowering that leg to the ground (Fig. 8.11c).

The glutes

Specific training of these are the flavor of the month within both the therapeutic and fitness industries. It is important to be alert to potential problems here. See Ch. 3, Pelvic inferior tethers, and Ch. 4, Third pelvic fundamental pattern.

The glutes commonly work reasonably well in inner range. Many clients feel the need to constantly stretch and release theirs. Clinicians know that tense, tight, and tender glutes are a common finding in their clients with lumbopelvic and lower limb pains.

The gluteal tendinopathy aficionados advise against inner range exercises such as "Clams" as they appear to aggravate the condition (and have probably contributed to it). When the glutei dominate movement patterns (especially the gluteus maximus), the pelvis is pulled into posterior tilt, which in turn brings the SIJ and lumbar spine into their vulnerable end-range positions.

For functional strength, the glutes need to work collaboratively with the LPU in efficient pelvic force couple control – particularly eccentrically – and into outer range. Control of the first and third pelvic FPs and exercises such as "Cat" in Cat/Cow (Ex. 21), Pelvic hovercraft (Ex. 35), and Lateral weight shift pattern (Ex. 49) begin this journey.

While positions A and C of Ex. 45 (Slow heel kicks) activate the glutes in inner range, the point of this exercise is to challenge AFP core control and the ability to control anterior pelvic rotation to support hip extension – and balanced activity between the lateral and posterior glutes in controlling hip rotation. The glutei learn to be team players in functional patterns.

Other exercises aim to tune up the pelvic core and rebalance the regional myofascial system: asking for elongation of the gluteal and associated myofascia through active control of the pelvic patterns, such as Ex. 22 (Supplicant pose), Ex. 53 (V to Z stretch), and Ex. 57 (Prone piriformis stretch).

Learning to control the forward bend pattern (Ex. 32) is an excellent functional workout for both the core and the glutei in controlling the pelvic rotation through range. In addition, in Exs 45b (Slow heel kicks in standing) and 54 (Butt booster) the glutei work really hard in outer range on the weight-bearing side to control the level symmetrical pelvic position.

Squats

Squats are a popular fitness and therapy exercise. It is important how they are done. When my patients with back pain (or any lower limb pain syndrome) report doing squats, I always look at their form: it is usually contributing to the problem (see Figs 3.15 and 5.32).

Ideally, the pelvis rather than the knees should initiate the squat – as in Ex. 32. Flexible hips and ankles allow the pelvis to move back and anteriorly rotate on the legs – the spine maintains its alignment. The toes face forward or slightly out.

When pelvic or core control is underactive, the inferoposterior myofascial chain dominates. It commonly lacks slide and flexibility, and the hips and ankles are usually stiff. Lack of hip flexion and ankle dorsiflexion means that in a squat the pelvis rolls into posterior tilt and the spine is pulled into flexion (see Fig. 5.32). "Just back stiffness" is likely to be the first symptom. However, the stress on the back will feed into the posterior myofascial tightness, and eventually result in pain symptoms.

Improving first pelvic pattern control under load will improve squat kinematics and pain. This includes during simple functional activities such as Sit to stand (Ex. 30).

Standing sequences

Standing desks are becoming popular, but if you cannot sit properly you will not stand well! There are more functional links in the kinetic movement chain to control; we need to help clients regain their sense of the vertical axis. By regaining control of important key phrases of movement, we rebuild spinal control.

The FPs are initially relearned in "low gravity" postures and then reintegrated into patterns of increasing upright control and complexity. This helps the client enlist more natural patterns of postural control which are enduring and adaptable, and allow freer movement – in sitting, kneeling, and standing. We work from the ground up.

The pelvis plays a key role in control, as do the feet in standing. An effective foot–pelvis functional connection supports the spine from below and frees the upper body for spatial reach and expression – and upper limb righting reactions that are also needed for standing balance.

We always work in bare feet. It is important to ensure that the feet are correctly placed so that the body weight is evenly distributed through them. This optimizes function higher up.

The basic standing position is feet narrow hip width apart, with toes facing forward so that the outer border forms a straight line ahead (see Fig. 3.35b). The client is made aware of distributing the weight through the "foot tripod" (see Ch. 2, Feet, Ch. 3, Other common features of altered movement, and Ch. 7, Ex. 58). Clients usually need prompting to unlock the knees and bring the weight down into the outside heel and the ball of the little toe, to spread the toes, and to reach the big toe medially. This redistributes the weight and helps activate the foot intrinsics. Aim to keep this basic foot template throughout the movement.

Standing sequences particularly drill integrated activity between the pelvic and axial FPs – and their integrated activity with the shoulder patterns – in the three planes of movement. The pelvic patterns are worked in more dynamic control of weight shift and support for limb movements.

Whatever the chosen leg configuration in standing (feet together, basic position, stride, abducted, step, single leg), it is important to first attend to a neutral and active base of support in the foot, and attempt to maintain this while initiating movement from the pelvic patterns. For example, in Ex. 32 (Forward bend pattern): look for control of foot centration, hip rotation, and driving the movement from the pelvis rather than pushing the knees back (which can be a very

entrenched habit). The knees should track forward in line with the second toe, not roll in (see Fig. 3.35a).

The spinal alignment should be maintained during sagittal weight shifts via the first and second pelvic patterns (see Fig. 7.32). If it is not, it is a sign of poor pelvic control and stiffening the legs. When drilling the third patterns in lateral weight shift, look for the spine and thorax adaptively following the pelvis (see Fig. 7.49b) while still maintaining sagittal alignment, and adaptable control through the feet and knees. When working the fourth patterns, look for underlying support from the first and third patterns.

We work a lot with the knees in flexion to "break up" the common habit of locking them. Locked knees lock the pelvis. Even when the knees are extended – they should be "soft".

The standing sequences "tune up" pelvic control so we can simultaneously stand on one leg, support the axis, and move the other limbs for locomotion or more complex sporting activities, such as tennis or kicking a ball.

The movement options in standing are only limited by your creative insights as to what are achievable functional challenges. The principles of the fundamental pattern blueprint underlie all imaginable moves.

Walking well

Many Westerners have lost the natural art of walking. The exercises in this book address various elements of function which help contribute to better walking one way or another.

Walking is a great form of whole-body natural exercise, provided that there is adequate underlying function: a flexible spine, plus good core and pelvic control on a flexible hip/pelvis and legs. Contralateral rotation of the pelvic and shoulder girdles creates opposite arm and leg swing. The spine transmits movement between the girdles and acts like an energy transfer and storage system – a decoupler between the proximal limb girdles which coils and uncoils, spring-loading the fascial system. Foot propulsion links into pelvic rotation and an energy efficient system for moving us forward. Ideal walking patterns are rhythmical and "easy" ; they conserve energy and enable endurance without fatigue.

I am always fascinated when I see a person of African heritage walking – relaxed, erect, having good leg stride and significant proximal arm swing. Any loads are carried on the head. They have grace and poise, and their movement has a lightness, freedom, and elasticity about it (Fig. 8.12).

In contrast, many Westerners are tense, bowed, have a short leg stride and insignificant (or no) proximal arm swing. Any loads carried are held in front or to the side of the body and the shoulders pull forward.

The foot–pelvis connection does not provide good propulsion. There is little rotation through the axis. In fact, it is as though they walk up to themselves rather than past themselves. Some appear to almost pull themselves along with their arms; their movement looks labored and heavy.

Dissecting out someone's faults in walking can be tricky because there is a lot going on: all links in the movement chain are operative. Disturbed function in one part will affect the freedom and efficiency of the whole system.

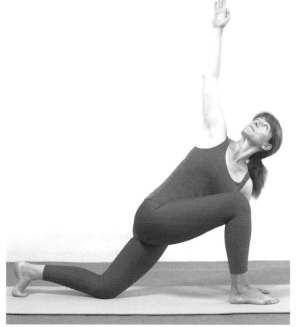

Figure 8.13

Poses such as "Bear Trikonasana" integrate many of the Key Moves principles: improving integrated control between axial FP1 and FP4 in maintaining spinal alignment with axial rotation; opening the hips/pelvis/inferior myofascial chain and the thorax/shoulder girdle; working with asymmetric poses and breaking up the holding patterns; controlling effective grounding through the base of support and so on.

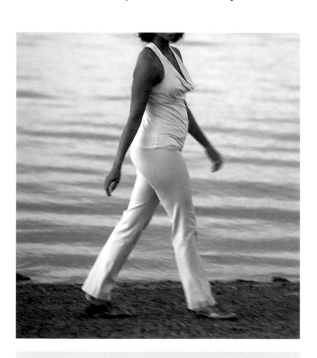

Figure 8.12

The art of natural walking – note the free arm swing and easy leg stride.

The common problem is a stiff spine and pelvic/hip joints. Reduced pelvic/hip rotation diminishes leg stride and rotation up through the spine. Lack of extension and rotation through the thorax and shoulder girdle further compromises erectness and the ability for backward shoulder rotation and relaxed arm swing. Compensatory spinal control and mid-lumbar "wind" result, which can fan a variety of hip, knee or leg pain syndromes.

Clients often ask: "how can I walk better?" This is a difficult question. As a simple guide I say: "Breathe down, float your head tall, and point your thumbs out to the side as you let your arms swing freely from the shoulders – particularly backward. Think of having a spring in your step – and most importantly, enjoy it." But this is, of course, easier said than done.

The objective of the exercises we prescribe is to prioritize the restoration of function in various key parts, such that the whole system is better optimized. Improving spinal, proximal girdle and limb joint, and myofascial mobility all contribute to efficient and easy walking (Fig. 8.13).

The most important aspects of control in walking are effective single-leg stance, propulsion, and limb swing. This requires control of triplanar pelvic rotation and good functional links between it and the spine, shoulder girdle, and foot. Propulsion requires adequate calf strength, hip and knee extension, and a freely rotating pelvis. The hip extension phase is said to stretch iliopsoas, readying its contraction to swing the leg forward. The freer the proximal limb girdles and spine, the better the limb swing and movement through the whole spine.

Chapter 8

Recommended reading

Avison JS (2015) Yoga: Fascia, anatomy and movement. Edinburgh: Handspring Publishing.

Black M (2015) Centered: Organizing the body through kinesiology, movement theory and Pilates technique. Edinburgh: Handspring Publishing.

Earls J (2014) Born to walk: Myofascial efficiency and the body in movement. Berkeley, CA: North Atlantic Books.

Farhi D (2000) Yoga Mind Body and Spirit: A return to wholeness. New York: Henry Holt.

Frank C, Kobesova A, Kolar P (2013) Dynamic neuromuscular stabilisation and sports rehabilitation. Int J Sports Phys Ther 8(1):1–11.

Grilley P (2012) Yin Yoga: principles and practice, 10th edn. Ashland, OR: White Cloud Press.

Hackney P (2002) Making connections: Total body integration through Bartenieff Fundamentals. Abingdon, Oxon: Routledge.

Myers T (2014) Anatomy Trains: Myofascial meridians for manual and movement therapists, 3rd edn. Edinburgh: Churchill Livingstone/Elsevier.

Scaravelli V (2012) Awakening the spine. Yoga for health vitality and energy. London: Pinter & Martin.

Schleip R (ed.) (2015) Fascia in sport and movement. Edinburgh: Handspring Publishing.

Constructing a class

Classes are a great medium for enabling us to appreciate the interconnectedness of functional movement: how improving control in one part can influence the whole system.

The specific focus of the Key Moves approach is initiating and moving more from the "deep" myofascial system, and "letting go" of excess superficial myofascial tension to improve spinal flexibility and movement ease. Reconditioning the deep postural system provides better foundations for a healthy, fit, strong, and robust musculoskeletal system.

We continue to work with the FP blueprint (Ch. 4). Improving your clients' skilled performance helps redress the common movement "faults" and features of posturo-movement dysfunction (Ch. 3), enabling them to move more naturally – and move out of pain. It is important that classes do not constitute a "Simon says…" circus where anything goes. Your clients will try to do what you ask, but it is *how* they do it that matters: so that dysfunctional patterns of control are not reinforced.

The effective therapist appreciates the need to explicitly cue the patient in such a way as to "set up" the correct response in the FPs both prior to and during the movement task. For example, the ability to differentiate and isolate hip flexion from lumbar flexion is an important functional pattern for spinal health. Simply asking the client to bend the hip in supine will invariably result in their adopting their usual strategy, which likely also involves posterior pelvic tilt, lumbar flexion, and dominance of superficial rectus femoris over iliopsoas/LPU activity. What we need to do is sequentially cue the patient to achieve a neutral pelvis via pelvic FP1, maintain a stable pelvis while folding in the groin so as to

maintain the lordosis, and to breathe(!) (see Ch. 7: Ex. 10, Isolating hip flexion).

The skilled therapist is familiar with the dysfunctional patterns of control (see Ch. 3) and is able not only to anticipate these but to counter them by correct cues to improve the movement pattern.

When the movement task is appropriate, the cues are correct, and the clients can adequately respond, they usually will not experience any pain. Any complaint of pain should be immediately investigated as it is generally due to incorrect performance. You also need to ask yourself questions, though. Is the task beyond the patient's abilities? Does it need modifying? Does the patient require different cues or props to improve the action?

Bear in mind that releasing tight myofascia and working to improve joint mobility invariably creates some discomfort. This is different to pain. The client is directed to focus on the diaphragmatic breath to ease discomfort and facilitate release in the tissues.

As the FPs become reestablished and more animated, they are integrated into a diverse array of functional movement patterns and more challenging exercises. This includes connecting them into sequences of movement, transitioning between postures, and sustaining postures for longer while maintaining correct alignment. No matter what the movement, the FPs always play a role.

Fig. 9.1 attempts a simple diagrammatic summary of the Key Moves approach to rehabilitating spinal pain. Note that reestablishing the fundamental patterns is at the heart of the approach. The FPs are then progressively reincorporated in a stepwise fashion

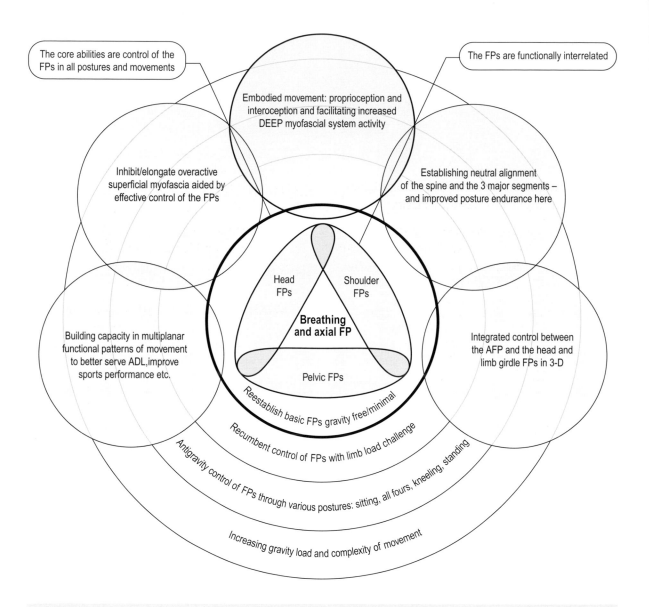

The core abilities are control of the FPs in all postures and movements

The FPs are functionally interrelated

Embodied movement: proprioception and interoception and facilitating increased DEEP myofascial system activity

Inhibit/elongate overactive superficial myofascia aided by effective control of the FPs

Establishing neutral alignment of the spine and the 3 major segments – and improved posture endurance here

Head FPs

Shoulder FPs

Breathing and axial FP

Pelvic FPs

Building capacity in multiplanar functional patterns of movement to better serve ADL,improve sports performance etc.

Integrated control between the AFP and the head and limb girdle FPs in 3-D

Reestablish basic FPs gravity free/minimal

Recumbent control of FPs with limb load challenge

Antigravity control of FPs through various postures: sitting, all fours, kneeling, standing

Increasing gravity load and complexity of movement

Figure 9.1

This schematic diagram attempts to simplify a complex subject. It offers a blueprint of the Key Moves approach to guide the rehabilitation of spinal pain disorders. The four groups of Fundamental Patterns (1. axial FP, 2. pelvic FPs, 3. shoulder FPs, 4. head FPs) are the core abilities which are initially reestablished without/with minimal gravitational loading. The large circles attempt to show the stages of the rehabilitation process where control of the FPs is *appropriately challenged* over time by increasing the gravity load and complexity of movement. At the same time the five most basic and interrelated principles (overlocking small circles) are operant through all stages of rehabilitation. 1. The focus is upon interoception and proprioception to facilitate improved activity and endurance in the deep myofascial system and sensorimotor learning; 2. working for improved axial alignment and increased

Figure 9.1 *continued*
postural endurance here; 3. integrating patterns of control between the four groups of FPs to improve motor skill and movement freedom; 4. down-training superficial myofascial overactivity and addressing restrictions in the joint and myofascial systems through control of the FPs; 5. building capacity in 3-D functional patterns of movement to serve the requirements of activities of daily living (ADL), sports performance, etc. Hopefully the circles can help you to see the interconnectedness of everything!

into postures and movements which involve increasing gravity load and movement complexity.

The following text constitutes is a detailed proforma for conducting a Key Moves preliminary program. The practitioner is hopefully now familiar with the concepts and due to space constraints, this section utilizes short forms and abbreviations (see the glossary on pp. 358–360).

The "KEY MOVES"®

Therapeutic exercise and movement program for spinal pain and injuries

Preliminary module

The suggested exercises and sequences are presented as a guide for the practitioner.

The 10 week program consists of 10 hour-long classes which introduce the client to the Fundamental Patterns (FPs) of control, natural movement sequences, and begin to work into joint and myofascial restrictions.

In general try to follow the program content – attempting to cover both the important basics which require competency before moving to level 2 – as well as some variety in "free and easy movements" to aid perceptual experience, enjoyment, etc. However, you may find that there are more exercises listed than the class can reasonably cover. You should progress the class at the rate that the participants can manage – hence the amount that you cover and rate of

progression will vary. Changing motor behavior can take some time.

Be prepared to manually guide key points of desired control – and at times to passively "give" the required movement to your client so they can experience its correct "feel" in order to replicate it.

Classes usually begin with a "coming down" passive posture to improve spinal flexibility and aid improved breathing patterns and internal awareness as a prelude to various deep system drills.

Many of the exercises are described in Ch. 7, but further information may be provided below. The action of the exercises not covered in Ch. 7 is briefly described here.

For each class, one exercise is prescribed as homework – given as a printed handout.

Watch points: These are an aid to help sharpen your observation skills: to anticipate and guard against further entrenching the adverse habitual responses that we do not want – and to facilitate those we do.

Chapter 9

Lesson 1

Introduction to the Key Moves® approach and experiencing spinal movement patterns which are deep system dominant

Equipment: Chair; pillow/s.

General introduction

We begin this session sitting on a chair. This is also useful time to observe habitual postural behavior. The following reference points provide background information. On day 1 only spend about 15 minutes on this: introduce the group and only cover the most basic points. What you do not cover in L1 you will talk about in later classes.

- Healthy control of the spine ensures one is not only healthy with no pain but also that one looks and feels good! Have you ever wondered why there is a pandemic of back pain, and also hip, knee, shoulder problems? Poor spinal control including that of the "core" is usually associated with these so called "old age" symptoms.

- Why is this so? Our modern lifestyle is *increasingly sedentary* – including work and leisure – and involves lots of time in flexion, particularly in sitting. (We all develop really bad habits here – POINT OUT GROUP TENDENCIES.) We are underactive and gradually lose variety in movement, which starts to diminish our available movement repertoire. The brain becomes understimulated and lazy and alters the program to the muscles producing *less ideal posture and movement patterns*. Some muscles overwork and others are "weak" – shy or lazy. This results in uneven contribution from the muscle team – and the spine is particularly vulnerable.

- Then we start to get various "injuries" for no apparent reason – or commonly when we try to exercise, "get fit", pursue sports activities, etc.

- Conceptually, the muscles of the body fall into two basic groups

  ○ *Deep* – Have important basic actions: hold us up against gravity; breathing; balance; skilled movement; light flexible dexterous effortless graceful movement. Good posture. **These tend to be *underactive* – "shy" muscles.**

  ○ *Superficial* – Provide actions with effort; increased tension; "fight and flight;" trying too hard; strength. **Tend to be *overactive* and constrict movement**. These are the ones that everyone is already overusing which then leads to the need for stretching because they are so overactive – "the bully" muscles.

  ○ The Goldilocks analogy is useful here: to function well we *need balance between the two systems* so that overall the superficial group are not too strong (tight) and the deep group are not too weak (flabby) – but *"just right."*

- **Why is imbalanced muscle activity of the spine a problem?** Because the spine is the central supporting "column" of the body involved in everything we do. As it has lots of bones, and hence joints, it is particularly vulnerable to changes in its muscle control. The joints which join each vertebra can become inflamed and sore. There is a big nerve right beside each joint. When the joint is inflamed this also inflames the nerve, which can lead to local and referred pain (like a sore tooth). Many painful joints in the body are often related to the spinal joints being chronically worried by the simple everyday postures, repetitive movements and activities, e.g., sitting at a computer, carrying the shopping, gardening.

- As both our research and science have shown, ALLEVIATING MUSCULOSKELETAL PAIN IS NOT ABOUT "GETTING STRONGER" BUT ABOUT "GETTING SMARTER" – i.e., being able to alter usual movement behavior and gain better CONTROL.

These classes rebalance the muscle system and restore the basics needed for healthy movement.

- **Bothered and inflamed spinal joints** will indirectly or directly affect the adjacent nerves and result in various symptoms:

  - feeling stiff; old and creaky; poor energy and "get up and go"

  - local discomfort or pains in the back

  - pains being referred into the limbs by that nerve, e.g., hip pain, knee pain, shin splints, etc. These are often construed as "sports injuries" or "old age."

- **Muscle control problems that you will predictably all have in common:**

  - can't "posture" yourself well without a sense of effort and fatigue

  - don't breathe properly!

  - generally hold and move with excess tension

  - can't get movement sequencing through the spine

  - stiff spine, hips, and shoulders

  - → we address all these issues in the classes.

- It is important to recognize that the spine functions as a whole – poor control in one region always influences other regions, e.g., some of you may have neck pain and not appreciate that this is partly related to poor control of the pelvis and lower spine. Everyone does not have both neck and back pain or stiffness, but many people do.

- **Common myths/misconceptions** about therapeutic exercise for the back abound:

  - "core control" is currently popular – this concept is often very misunderstood and incorrectly taught, creating lots of problems

  - there is a misconception that "beneficial exercise" needs to be strong, effortful, and hard work

  - however, exercising in this way can make the "tension" muscles work harder – makes you **tense, tight and stiff** – and is why you **want/need to stretch all the time**

  - stretching has become synonymous with exercise and is usually given prime importance. However most stretching is poorly performed as *deep control is poor and the spine is not protected* – further weakening it.

  - generally the important role of the fascial system is not considered in exercise.

- **The "Key Moves"® Program of therapeutic Exercise and Movement:** is about helping you to ***move out of pain*** – by relearning *fundamental movements which naturally move and protect* the spine during everyday activities, and particularly during challenging and strenuous activities.

Regaining control of these basic patterns of movement not only allows for a pain free healthy back and being able to enjoy an active life, but you will also feel more energetic and supple. It involves inner control/awareness.

- **Strength training:** *It is good underlying deep muscle control* which underpins the attainment of flexibility and real strength. Without this the large superficial "tension "muscles are forced to compensate – and this creates stiffness and poor patterns of control and renders you vulnerable to injuries.

Importantly: Just by looking at "how" someone moves we can gauge the relative activity level and performance quality in each muscle system.

We begin "at the beginning", relearning where these inner deep muscles are, and how to activate them in many and varied ways. This involves tasking your brain more than your brawn! We call them "brain exercises": *you will learn to work "smarter" – not harder.*

Demonstration

Demonstrate bony landmarks on skeleton – spinal curves; the bowl of pelvis, tailbone and ischial tuberosities. Relationship of thorax and pelvis. Explain pelvic and abdominal diaphragms and the "canister" which supports breathing and postural mechanisms (aided by illustration charts).

Practical: movement experience

Position: Supine, legs extended and arms by side; pillow(s) behind head – ensure a "neutral" head position, especially if kyphotic/stiff:

1. **Body wave** rock from rhythmical *plantar flexion* and APR (many will try to overuse dorsiflexion which is linked with PPR). Look for movement up though the spine. This provides a good indication as to how much muscle tension holding patterns are operant if they "can't get the rhythm." Note how the head moves automatically – C/C/J flexion on APR (may need to support some heads on a pillow if very stiff kyphotic, though this will lessen the movement).

Watch point: Dominance of dorsiflexion with PPR and L/P flexion and chin protrusion. Gross "overkill movement." We want movement gently sequencing through the spine *from APR*.

Position: Crook lying, arms abducted to 90°, palms up.

2. **"Rag doll"** – **(Ex. 12)**: Lateral arm reach with "look" and head rotation. Focus upon "feeling" movement get into spine *between shoulder blades*. Draw attention to the following:

   • if they relax the outer muscles they get further – "play with it"

   • move slowly and fully in a sensual way

   • allow the breath to come freely.

Watch points: Disturbed breathing; increased tension ULG and probably CPC over T/L/J.

3. **"Clock on the wok"** (briefly!): Have the center point between lower symphysis pubis and umbilicus; 12 o'clock is then the umbilicus, 6 o'clock the S/P. Focus the movement coming from *low down*. Circle through clock face clockwise and anticlockwise with various challenges (up/down; side /side; diagonals). Make sure of *small* (and gentle!) movements, localized, *low and slow*. Be aware how the rest of the spine follows and adapts to the movement.

Watch points: Ensure *that they do not punch into this movement too much* by pushing through the feet with butt clench, thus "overdoing" L/P flexion and PPR – a predictable tendency! Beware of a tendency for CCP behavior in 3-6-9 arc and try to cue to inhibit this. Spend more *time on localizing the 3-6-9 arc* – to segue into the feeling of PFP1.

4. **Pelvic FP1** – **(Ex. 7a)** (this is actually moving to 6 o'clock in the above exercise). Demonstrate on the pelvis. Draw the front pelvis/hip sockets closer together so that you feel the LOWER belly firm. At the same time spread I/Ts; *reach T/B long* and allow it to point down toward heels on the floor. This is achieved by co-activation of the LPU – in particular LM and Tr. A and eccentric PFM. What does the breath do? Low back should arch at the *base* (not cinch or throw from T/L CPC strategy which will be the tendency). No pushing from heels but feel the movement coming from *inside* the pelvic bowl and very low back and front. They may feel slight discomfort. Reassure them that this is to be expected as the joints are stiff going into this pattern of movement and muscles unused to moving this way. Gently and slowly explore the movement = *beginnings of "core control."*

*You may have to "give" some the feel of the movement by passively moving thighs caudad so the pelvis rolls into APR. Note how the chin drops when you do this – this is desirable.

Watch point: Beware of attempting the action from CPC rather than PFP1 –and/or butt clench and pushing with the feet.

5. **Diaphragmatic breathing – (Ex. 1):** One hand on sternum; other over LPU. Simply become *aware of their pattern of breathing* and initially do not change anything. Helps instructor to know what they are dealing with.

Breathing with a relaxed abdominal wall in and out through the nose.

Then begin to focus them on gradually letting the air *down* to the belly from inside without UCB. "Allow the center and lower body to open and expand in 3-D" (an exercise in "being" rather than "doing"); through habit we often tend to constrict it. Make sure that they are not pushing the belly forward. *Let exhalation be passive* – and longer – and let any tension go.

Draw attention to breathing rate pattern (in for 2; out for 3; pause for 1, etc.).

Focus upon relaxation around body particularly the three "stress/tension regions" during exhalation.

Focus also on lateral and posterior basal expansion *without any lift of the chest and accessory muscle activity:* "breathe down/back into the floor;" "allow your mid back to relax/fall back into the floor." **(Homework)**

Helpful Br. Mantra: "Nose, low, slow, let go". "Breathe *down and back* – not up and forward."

Watch point: Tendency to "over-breathe" – both rate and volume – and to lift the chest.

Position: Prone arms loosely up above head; head in N position or most comfortable.

6. **Backward pelvic rotation – (Ex. 16)** *initiated from I/Ts* reaching the T/B long and back.

Watch point: try to lessen the general tension in the body, arms and legs - and "find" the pelvis here. This is covered in more detail in lesson 2.

Chapter 9

Lesson 2

Looking at the "core": the axial FP and beginnings of specific motor control relearning

Comprehensive background material can be found in Chs 2, 3 and 4.

Equipment: Chair; pillow(s); wheat-bag (or filled with sand – approx. 25 × 70 cm); anatomical charts for demonstration; drinking straw; hand mirrors and/or balloon.

Position: Crook lying head supported (if kyphotic they will need more height).

- Ask about how they felt after last week. Any questions?

1. **Learning to understand, activate and sense the three elements comprising the deep "abdominal canister"** (utilize skeleton and charts).

* DO NOT GET TOO STUCK WITH THIS SECTION – it is really an **"awareness exercise" to help focus their perception "internally" and of the LPU** – in healthy function the elements never work alone (except probably the diaphragm).

Diaphragm

Holding excess muscle tension in the body disturbs how it works. *D inhalation should be natural.*

2. **Diaphragmatic breathing – (Ex. 1):** Head well supported, one hand monitoring "no lift" in the upper chest. Good breathing patterns are *basic to "core control."*

Place a sandbag over belly and notice it lift here – *or* can place it over upper chest and notice NO lift here.

Be aware of Br. pattern during the day, aided by the mnemonic: **Stop** – check chest and shoulder position and any neck tension; **Drop** – shoulders and breath down via the D; **Flop** – relax all over.

Mention desired pattern and rate:

"Slow": – through the nose not mouth – longer exhalation.

"Low": in the body/pelvis.

"Let go": all the tense outer muscles on exhalation.

**If someone just "cannot get it" you can try "Sensing the diaphragm"* by: bringing the legs into high hip flexion feet on the wall – or feet resting on a chair such that there is *full support/contact of thoracolumbar spine on the surface.*

- Make sure shoulders fall back and that neck is supported in neutral and comfortable.

- Focus on what the diaphragm automatically does and go with it – descending down through the body to create bilateral basal and slight abdominal expansion – and see if they have a better sense of it and it feels easier.

- Expiration is passive and "relaxing" – "letting go."

3. **Focus upon exhalation:** In general we want this to be *longer* than it usually is:

- *"Passive"* with extended expiration and *relaxed post expiratory pause.* APXS may find this hard to do as upper abdominal wall (UAW) can be very hyperactive. If so, encourage relaxation of LPT by "holding more open" with hands. PPXS are loath to exhale and bring the chest back/down into contact because of poor abdominals – may need to facilitate this.

Watch point: Ensure that on the subsequent inhale after the post expiratory pause they do NOT lift the chest – but that D comes down inside.

- *"Active exhalation"* engages the LPU – in particular Tr. A and PFM. Ask for a large "sshhh" while *palpating iliac fossae* and noting the natural activity of *lower a*bdominals and IAP here – which should be enough to also *bring the lower* *thorax caudad/down* – and then stay down! This is particularly difficult for PPXS – it may take weeks to "get." If so, you can also try "blowing out" through pursed lips. Similarly a "hiss", cough, laugh, etc., or blowing out through a drinking straw. Watch that APXS do not overactivate UAW. Rather, you want to feel this action come **from below** from *pelvic floor with lower Tr. A* – **not at the waist with CAC**. *Draw attention to the natural "automatic" LPU activation of "the core" when breathing out like this.* Perhaps even try some "OMMS" or other sounds.

Using active exhalation like this helps them initially "feel" IAP. Eventually they need to "keep it on" irrespective of the breath cycle.

Watch point: That the chest does not lift on the next inhalation – it stays caudal.

Pelvic floor

Diaphragmatic breathing and particularly active exhalation activates the PFM!! *Stress that PFM do not work alone but as part of a synergy in various patterns of movement control.* A lot of specific overactivation of these muscles alone can cause problems. Pelvic girdle pain research is increasingly showing overactive PFMs. *It is more functional to work the PFM like this – with Tr. A and/or D in Br. cycle and IAP.* Getting good D activity naturally reflexly activates the PFM.

Transversus

Works beautifully in active exhalation. Explain specifically that you *want lower rather than upper ALAW* engagement. As an important part of the LPU, Tr. A is involved in many functions and movements including *breathing, pelvic and postural control.* Cueing single muscle activity such as "drawing navel to the spine"; "drawing up and in" will tend to increase CAC behavior in APXS group – and "suck in" and thorax lift in PPXS. Therefore also demonstrate/facilitate other Tr.

A actions here via the LPU in a variety of its functional patterns of movement control – while palpating the LPU activity in the inguinal fossae:

1. *Active exhalation* – want *lower* more than upper ALAW activity (APXS will predictably go into CAC). *To monitor*, place one hand over the LPU and the other over the upper ALAW to check against this. Note the longer the exhale the more the LPU works.

2. "'Set' the muscles under your middle fingers (palpating in the iliac fossa)."

3. "Widen the sit bones."

4. "Draw the ASISs closer."

5. "Narrow between the hip sockets."

6. "Reach the tailbone long."

Note that in 1 and 2 the LPU is activated as part of the breathing/"core" cycle. And in actions 2–6 the LPU is also activated in pelvic patterns of movement such as PFP1. Note how imagery helps this.

Position: Supine, calves on a chair, with drinking straw, hand mirror and/or balloon handy.

Sustained activation of all LPU elements together to *develop IAP* with regular D Br.

This is the critical part of healthy "core control" – and necessary to control "the center."

Need a "neutral" thorax position where the thorax and pelvis become aligned over each other so as to optimize their ability to generate IAP.

We work for the correct action in stages:

1. *Bring thorax into an "expiratory position."* Place both hands over the LPT. Breathe out bringing the thorax into the caudal/expiratory position – *without posteriorly tilting pelvis more.* Ideally the posterior LPT is in contact with (or aiming for) the support surface. May need to increase head

support for cervical "neutral" and comfort. The task is to keep the thorax "down" here – and breathe diaphragmatically – with neck and shoulders relaxed.

2. *Sustained generation of IAP: with thorax maintained in "expiratory position"* as above.

- Place index or middle "cocked" finger in each iliac fossa and "allow/direct the breath to your hands" – you should feel a sustained *firming or "engagement" of the LALAW* under your hand = the natural reflex response of the Tr. A and PFM when the diaphragm is active in antigravity situations = IAP! If not getting it, try for positive expiratory patterns such as exhaling through a drinking straw. To help provide "the sense of" the right IAP action, stronger activity is required to fog a mirror or blow up a balloon.

- The task now is to maintain this firming in the inguinal fossa (IAP) while breathing "normally" (rate, rhythm, etc.). Watch for shortening the out breath which will tend to occur if they are a hyperventilator and/or the abdominals are either over- or underactive, and rest of the LPU synergy is "weak" and not used to sustaining postural support *while also* allowing the breath to oscillate to and from the "center."

- And further, if they are reasonably mastering the above, while still maintaining the above, they can now also widen the lower ribs and direct the breath both down, laterally (and back in a PPXS client). This will not be possible for many to begin with. *Only try this progression here if you have an advanced group.

Watch points: Loss of thorax position; loss/inability for sustained IAP; disturbed breathing pattern; clenching buttocks and thighs; tense neck and shoulders.

*This exercise is known as **"Pinning the beetle 1"** (Ex. 5)** – also done in supported high hip flexion – legs up wall or on chair. (**Homework**)

PRONE: Arms up, elbows wide to form a U around head: which needs to be comfortable – either neutral with support through forehead and bridge of the nose – or rotated.

3. *Place a sandbag across posterior LPT.* Focus upon D Br. – *Br. down* into the pelvis and "widening the center" and PBB. You should see some expansion of the LPT and slight PPR as the PFM automatically contract as the D descends. Focus on rate: slowing the outbreath and increasing expiratory pause in association with "letting go;" and not hurrying/gasping for the next inhalation.

Watch points: You do not want to see "Pectoral Cinch" and accessory breathing muscle activity.

4. *Engage IAP.* See if they can achieve and maintain an "open center" while continuing to breathe regularly as above. Monitor with a finger placed in the iliac fossa.

Watch points: Inadequate movement/expansion over the lower pole of the thorax – or if able to expand, they are not able to sustain this while breathing regularly.

Lesson 3

Activation of the axial FP with D Br. and basic pelvic control via pelvic FPs

Equipment: Chair; pillows/blankets; low flat firm cushion; spiky pod; yellow ball.

SUPINE:

1. **Constructive rest position – (Ex. 2a):** Folded blankets or two pillows lengthwise (or bolster if look more accomplished*). Make sure you ensure their pelvis drops back toward APR – from L/S/J.* May need to place small/flat cushion under pelvis if very stiff/irritable. Also ensure *head and neck are neutral.* May need to support outer thigh with blocks etc. if hips stiff/painful. Draw attention to gently engaging PFP1 to help hips open. Encourage yielding their body weight to the support and sensing the breath coming down and back.

Watch point: Adequate support if needed; pelvis; thighs if stiff hips – and head if stiff thorax; shoulders? – want C/S neutral so that they can completely relax and sense the breath here.

2. **Temperature check rotation in side lying – (Ex. 13):** Most will need a small pillow under head to ensure a "N C/S"; if stiff, have bolster/pillows behind to rest top arm when moving back; if hips/pelvis stiff may have cow cushion or pillow(s) between knees. Repeat other side.

Watch points: Ensure the uppermost *point of the shoulder leads the arm movement back*; care that they are not wringing the waist CCP activity.

This is a good daily exercise to do upon waking; after bolster; to relax, etc. **(Homework)**

SUPINE: Heel support on chair, hips and knees supported in 90° flexion. Head supported on a spiky pod (more head support needed?).

3. **Pinning the beetle – (Ex. 5):** Coordinating abdominals and breathing. If centering the thorax is difficult (PPXS) attempt the action through exhalation *without the pelvis posteriorly tilting.*

Watch point: Want relaxed legs and buttocks; ribs to come back without pelvis going into more PPR; shoulders and neck relaxed; no lift of thorax on inhale; sustained IAP while allowing the breath to "come naturally."

CROOK LYING: (Flat cushion(s) under head).

4. **Pelvic FP1 – (Ex. 7a):** Beware movement is not coming from "two storeys too high" via CPC – it is important to initiate from I/Ts and T/B and feel LPU active. Place one hand behind the back over *the low L/S and lumbosacral junction to feel LM and the lordosis* shape and help monitor this, while other hand is over the lateral valley of the iliac fossa to monitor a "setting" through the LPU. Maintain this "N" lordosis; engage and sustain IAP while D Br. This is tricky to begin with.

Watch points: The ALAW should "firm" and not "balloon"; *movement is led from the pelvis* moving into APR, *not by thrusting lower ribs forward.* The spine follows the movement.

*If you have a group that find AFP control very difficult this may be as far as you get in this class.

SIDE LYING: N spine and hips flexed about 80° or so with top shoulder in slight BSR; yellow ball between knees.

This series of movements initiate spinal movements from the base of the spine through the pelvic FPs. Watch for initiation in the sit bones and tailbone and sequencing through the spine – we do not want CCPs to dominate and be further entrenched here.

5. **Engage AFP and sustain while performing PFP1 and PFP2.** Place top palm over the ipsilateral LP1 to monitor both relaxing superficial

mms and sensing P/L expansion under hand. Try to sustain this while performing PFP1 to *ensure that they stay soft and open here* and spine gently moves while regular D breathing. PFP2 usually dominates and needs little encouragement.

Watch points: Do not want movement attempted through CPC for PFP1 and butt clench for PFP2.

6. **Forward/backward knee slides with top leg - initiating from the top I/T (PFP4).** Note how the movement wave travels up through the whole spine. Feel the movement coming low via the LPU <u>from</u> the I/Ts and hip socket and note how the pelvis rotates also. On the leg shortening in particular, the top shoulder should also fall back and the head rotate slightly - (and vice versa on the leg lengthening).

Watch points: Inability to relax the buttocks and legs and so gain good LPU activity – particularly leg "shortening/backslide" via the *top I/T rotating and reaching back and wide;* undesirable CPC increase.

Repeat Exs 5 and 6 lying on the other side.

Lesson 4

Beginning to stretch while activating the fundamental patterns of control

Equipment: Bolster or pillows; low flat firm cushion; spiky pod; KMCRB introduced.

Note: *Correct placement of the KMCRB* (see Ch. 8 and p. 309). This is placed over the LPT. *It does NOT wrap around the waist.* Fit all clients correctly before the class.

1. **Constructive rest position – (Ex. 2a):** With bolster/blankets/pillows depending upon client flexibility. Legs in simple cross leg; arms spread.

Watch points: support arms/leg and head if needed; ensure N head and neck and D Br.

2. **Rotation in side lying – (Ex. 4):** Most will need a pillow under head to ensure a "neutral C/S"; if stiff, have bolster/pillows behind to rest top arm. If hips/pelvis stiff and/or L/S discomfort place a small/flat cushion or pillow(s) between their knees: focus on PBB and improving AFP control.

• Repeat other side. This exercise is actually also retraining AFP4.

Watch points: "Central disconnect" between thorax and pelvis because of inadequate centering of thorax over pelvis through the initial active exhalation – and/or inability to keep it there while breathing. This is prerequisite to achieving and sustaining IAP and D Br.

CROOK LYING: With head on spiky pod; KMCRB on.

3. **Axial FP with arm challenge – (Ex. 33):** If the thorax is well controlled, the range of arm elevation may be quite restricted due to thoracic stiffness and tight anterior chest wall myofascia.

Watch points: Ensure *maintenance of thorax position and D breathing throughout the arm movements.* The LPU has to constantly work here.

4. **Isolating hip flexion – (Ex. 10):** This really drills pelvic FP1 control in both creating a neutral stable pelvis and flexing the hip principally from LPU/I/P activity. Repeat with other leg.

Watch points: Inadequate PFP1 and loss of lumbo-pelvic neutral; using superficial hip flexors – (this is evidenced by the knee being held in 90 degrees flexion instead of the foot dangling); loss of active extension in the straight leg. Some will find it difficult to achieve good hip flexion.

5. **Smart hamstrings stretch – (Ex. 37):** Further challenges LPU control in both maintaining a stable neutral pelvis and the thigh in the vertical position. Monitor lordosis with 1 HBB.

Watch points: Avoid "getting into battle" – poor N pelvic control – and where thigh loses vertical as the heel rises – and over-relying on ULG "lock-in" strategies, breath hold and tension.

PRONE:

6. **Prayer stretch – (Ex. 14):** May not feel much in the stretch – but will coming out of it.

Watch points: Ensure adequate position and "letting go" in ULG – that elbows go as high and as close together as they can. If too sore place a small/flat cushion or blue square cushion under their chest; inability to O/C, direct the breath low, slow and let go.

7. **Backward pelvic rotation – (Ex. 16):** Head rotated to the right if possible – otherwise face down. If stiff: place cow cushion under chest – or a blue square cushion.

Look for the movement initiated from I/Ts and the movement wave traveling up through the thorax, opening of the ipsilateral shoulder and slight head movement. The more they can relax the limbs and upper body the better. Repeat other side with the head to the left.

Watch points. Poor pelvic rotation and hip hiking. You may need to guide the correct feel of the pelvic rotation – and check that the LPU is on. Check do not use CCPs or push with the ULG as both will block the movement through the spine. **(Homework)**

8. **Sphinx – (Ex. 3):** Check buttocks and legs are relaxed. Warn them that some L/S discomfort is to be expected, but to keep bringing the breath to it and softening and lengthening the spine on each exhalation. Place a pillow under pelvis if anxious.

Watch points: Check they are not "locking in" with the ULG; hanging the head; tensing and holding the breath against the discomfort of the stretch.

9. Rotation in side lying if time allows.

Lesson 5

Deep system activation: focus on thorax, shoulders, head and neck

Equipment: Bolster or pillows; low flat firm cushion; spiky pod; yellow ball; KMCRB; 1 large block.

- **Questions after last lesson?**

1. **Constructive rest position – (Ex. 2a):** On bolster or pillows. Ensure that they work the pelvis into the correct APR position off the edge through PFP1. Support legs (? pelvis) as necessary. Also ensure scapulae are repositioned down and back and spread the arms in sufficient abduction to feel a stretch across the front chest and shoulder. Yield their weight to the support surface. **(Homework)**

SIDE LYING: ?Yellow ball between knees – find a "neutral spine" with no rotation, with hips flexed toward 80–90° as able without robbing an attempt for lumbopelvic "neutral." Support the head on a flat cushion if preferred/needed.

2. **"Southern Cross" and circles with the elbow.** "Place top hand on its shoulder and imagine you have a light shining out of your elbow! – *moving from the scapula and* reaching the elbow long, "draw" a cross on the ceiling with your elbow." Begin with protraction/retraction *emphasizing full exploration of retraction*; then elevation/depression *emphasizing full exploration of elevation* such that the side ribs begin to open. Then go to joining each point on the cross making a circle. Allow the head and rest of the spine to follow the movement. *Focus mostly upon the up/back arc of the circle.*

Watch points: This should be free and easy – motor control is less important here – but be alert for habitually neurological diminished range into elevation/extension more than actual limitation.

3. **PFPs 1–4 in side lying:** Best to start with pelvic FP4 (forward/back knee slides) while keeping

the "center open" with posterior basal breathing A/A and monitoring over the top LPT for no CCP activity while performing PFPs – with focus on *T/B and I/T initiating the movement* and movement sequencing through the spine.

Watch points: Look for ability to relax/disassociate the legs/buttocks and initiate movement from the I/Ts in the pelvis; ability to inhibit CCPs.

4. **Scapular control:** Lying as above, top hand by side resting on pelvis – *keep a "soft relaxed arm"*:

- Retract scapula only and return to neutral (no CPC) – repeat few times, etc. (SFP1).

- Retract scapula and rotate the head in the same direction to "look"– repeat (SFP1/4).

- Move scapula up and down to come closer/farther from ear. Let head adjust to the movement. Ideally feel "stretch" at scalene web on caudal movement (SFP3).

- Circle scapula fully backwards then forwards allowing spine to adjust to the movement.

The scapula movement should bring in some thoracic and cervical movement.

Watch points: Neck tension and/or arm "lock-in" – either adduction and/or flexion which limits scapula travel.

*Repeat exercises 2–4 in opposite side lying.

SUPINE CROOK LYING:

5. **"Shoulder hopscotch":** Crook lying, arms spread, palms up. "Imagine your spine is lying on a line. See if you can lift that area of your spine between your shoulder blades to either side of this line, rather like what you would do to adjust a puckered piece of clothing under you" (or cue "lift and shift your nipples") so get *lateral flexion of UPT.* The BOS for the action becomes the head and the elbows/forearm.

This is a combination of SFP1 and 3. The movement is *initiated from the LSS and through the "dome"* – and not via CPC at the T/L/J. The KMCRB helps engage the AFP and' inhibit this. "Looking down" can aid desired pattern of C/S N with sternal lift and LSS engaged, while at the same time inhibiting tendency for dominance of long cervical extensors, U/T and L/S when asking for LSS. Some may need you to passively "do the movement" to get the feel of it.

Watch points: Beware of CPC compensation strategies – i.e., here, we are looking for closed chain movements of scapula and upper T/S.

6. **Head FP1** (see Ch. 4 – p. 120; also see Ex. 11 p. 205) = occipital flexion on C/S "neutral" rather than mid C/S flexion.

Head on front part of a spiky pod: Start in PFP1 with chin drop and cervicocranial flexion.

- Begin to slowly and fully nod occiput up and down with the eyes accompanying the movement direction, focusing on the movement coming *principally from C/C/J levels*. "Try a discrete nodding as though you were saying "yes." Getting them to "look" with the eyes will make a difference to the movement, i.e., "look up"/"chin up"; "look down"/"chin down." Repeat a few times. Emphasize the discrete C/C/J DNF/nodding action.

- Sustain the DNF occipital flexion/nod with PFP1 while D Br. – and then add tri-planar eye movements *while holding the occiput stable in this position.*

7. **Latissimus dorsi stretches in supine crook lying:** Engage LPU and move pelvis slightly into PFP1 and hold it here while drawing lower pole of thorax down and back on a full exhalation and hold to engage the axial FP (Ex. 5) – and widen into the KMCRB. Then bring palms over

each elbow and without losing pelvic or thorax position *engage the LSS to position scapulae down and back*; (SFP1) and then explore bringing the arms overhead trying to let them relax back toward the floor on each exhalation. Best to give support to arms with a block if shoulders are tight. Aim to feel shoulder stretch.

Watch points: Avoid losing thorax position, tensing the neck, disturbed breathing.

8. **Half supplicant pose – (Ex. 22):** If the client has stiff shoulders rest the head on a block/spiky pod so that C/S is N. Yield to the base of support in the knees which are abducted *with big toes together. Focus on elongating the spine from and Br. to the T/B; reaching the I/Ts back, wide and up; while at the same time bringing the lower ribs back and widening the LPT – and D Br slowly.* Soften and lengthen and expect/chase feeling of stretch in the dome and shoulders while also being aware of LPU engagement below the belt – "Find the peace in the position." *It is a good idea to go around the class and place a belt in their groins – and distract the pelvis up and back to facilitate the idea of APR and the feel of folding in the groin, etc.

Watch points: Inability to let go butt and shoulder clench; poor activation PFP1 and pelvic APR; breath holding; neck tension; loss of thorax alignment; poor AFP and PBB and O/C.

Note: Initially engaging the AFP to O/C tends to induce T/B tuck; I/T lift might result in CPC. Both tendencies should gradually lessen with adequate IAP generation and improved ability in thoracopelvic spatial control.

Lesson 6

Working the AFP or "core" in functional patterns

AFP in gravity eliminated postural pattern → maintaining it in sitting with PFPs and SFPs; transitioning to standing

Equipment: Chair; hand mirror; spiky pod; KMCRB; drinking straw.

SUPINE: Heels supported on chair in the 90/90/90 degrees flexion hips, knees, and ankles; active feet; thighs vertical; neutral hip position; spiky pod under head for neutral C/S. Allow 20–25 minutes to cover Exs 1–4.

1. **Establish correct D Br. "gravity free"** with relaxation and inhibition of any UCB. Hold hand mirror and "fog it" through active exhalation = automatic LPU activation. Want a sustained long exhalation. The poorer the IAP generation, the less fogging there will be.

2. **Move into "Pinning the beetle" – (Ex. 5):** *Sustain the posture, IAP and a regular breathing pattern.* Note that the body is in the same configuration as when sitting.

3. **Try to gradually widen the LPT (2nd stage AFP)** and sustain while breathing out through a drinking straw. If this is going well you might try fogging a mirror and/or blowing up a balloon to get the sense of IAP needed for these. Do not be surprised if many cannot do it.

Watch points: No lifting of the thorax on inhalation; ability to sustain an "open" LPT on the active exhalation driven by the LPU – palpate for this action in the inguinal fossa.

4. **Challenge to "Pinning the beetle" – (Ex. 33):** *
   If the group is slow omit this:

Continue a/a and *maintain thorax position sustaining IAP and regular D Br. and* slowly unweight the legs

one at a time. If someone is very dysfunctional and stiff and control unlikely, support them more with heels on the backrest of the chair in high hip flexion – or legs up the wall.

Watch points: We are aiming for the thoracolumbar junction making contact with the surface to enhance the stability of the diaphragm's attachments in order to help facilitate its optimum function and contribution toward generating IAP. This is achieved either passively (legs supported) or actively through adequate and balanced activity between the diaphragm and abdominal wall for optimal IAP to provide stability for psoas activity.

UNSUPPORTED SITTING ON A CHAIR: Ensure KMCRB are on.

5. **Healthy sitting – (Ex. 23):**

   - From habitual/collapsed sitting → move into "sit up straight." Note how this is invariably accomplished with little pelvic movement and by *a CPC strategy* which inhibits contribution from the inner support mechanisms and is costly both energetically and functionally.

   - Learning "how" to sit up properly whereby the "core" naturally switches on:

This actually involves the *ability to activate and combine all the first fundamental patterns of the torso!* (See Fig. 4.2.)

We do this in stages as it is important to sense and control each step:

   - **Finding the correct pelvic "neutral" BOS through PFP1:** Gently roll onto the back of the sit bones so the T/B tucks under – and note how the spine collapses; then "sink" the sit-bones and slowly roll right onto the front of them as you also think of widening them apart (PFP1) – note how your spine gets an "inner lift" and arches from the base. This may feel difficult and/or weird but it should be natural Ideally the T/B points slightly back when PFP1 is naturally active and there is a *neutral L/S lordosis*. Maintain this N pelvic position.

- **Then focus on the center body and ability to engage the AFP:** Place the hands around the LPT and the KMCRB (thumbs pointing behind) and attempt to gradually widen the LPT and O/C as was practiced in supine. The generation of optimal IAP helps to balance the thorax over the pelvis – monitor LPU activity in the iliac fossa. If the lower ribs are still thrown forward via CPC activity ask for more expansion *back and wide* into the thumbs (over KMCRB buttons) to facilitate the CPC letting go and allowing the thorax to move back slightly – without losing the lumbopelvic position, i.e., driving for a *N thorax stacked over a N pelvis.*

- **Focus on centering the shoulder girdle on the thorax:** Rest the hands on the thighs. Gently move into SFP1 – imagining widening the points of the shoulders and bringing the top breastbone forward and broadening the nipples to activate the LSS and target the "dome" area – without losing IAP and the O/C posture and compensating with a CPC strategy. Encourage awareness of the pelvic BOS and widening of the LPT to facilitate optimum "lower cylinder switch on" which helps inhibit ES splinting and CPC.

- **Attend to balancing the alignment of the head and neck over the torso:** Gently drop the chin, "float"/lift the superior/posterior occiput and glide the head back (especially those with APXS). Note the relationship between the T/B and occiput – when the T/B is back the head can move back and the chin drop which is associated with a centered occiput.

- Let your awareness travel to each area making the necessary small adjustments – *continuing to focus on D Br. in concert with O/C, gentle elongation of the spine, while widening collar bones, waist and sit bones and remaining supple trying to attain/ maintain that oh so tricky N alignment!*

Watch points: The correct pelvic position and the ability to open the center are the key to everything else. Keep the focus on what is happening under the KMCRB – want CCP activity to let go and to be able to generate adequate IAP to O/C instead. As simple as this seems, it is difficult to readily sit like this because of axial stiffness also limiting corrections. Paired with this is the chronic deep system dysfunction, hence postural adjustments even to the perturbation of breathing are difficult. In general, habitual usual unsupported sitting has been in collapse with "core" switch off – or by employing global dominant CCPs in order to "hold themselves up." An adequate pelvic BOS and optimal IAP are critical in supple lift and support of the spinal column. The KMCRB has been developed to help this. **(Homework)**

1. **Fundamental shoulder patterns:** Hands on pelvic rim. Reestablish a neutral pelvic BOS, "open the center" and achieve neutral axial alignment A/A:

- From axial "collapse" and sternal drop (= SFP2) come into SFP1 by widening the front points of the shoulders and the elbows, allowing the manubrium to come forward and lift slightly (not with CPC!). The scapulae come back and move caudad while the nipples widen. *Arms must stay soft and elbows do not pull back* via teres/ infraspinatus cinch.

- "See saws" (SFP3). Try to retain SFP1 as an underlying posture for this.

- BSR and "look back" (SFP4). Again retain SFP1 as a basic posture for this.

Watch points: Correct sitting postural alignment underlies the ability to do these well. SFP1 is the most difficult to achieve and sets the stage for SFP3 and SFP4. In particular one is working the shoulder girdle while also being able to control the center and avoid CCP activity.

2. **Lateral weight shift in N sagittal alignment – (see Ex. 49):** *"Sink" one I/T and lighten the other and allow the weight to laterally shift through the pelvis and creating lengthening of the ipsilateral side body* with PBB. The movement is *initiated in the pelvis through PFP1 and PFP3* and is followed by movement sequencing through the whole spine while receiving internal support from IAP (axial FP3). Cue for increased expansion over the ipsilateral LPT/"center." The whole torso slightly side bends – but ensure sagittal alignment of whole spine and breathing are maintained.

Watch points: The movement *must be initiated in the pelvis* and the spine free to follow. We do not want a "leaning tower of Pisa" or initiation from QL/CCPs which happens when the pelvis does not initiate the movement. When the action is correct, the entire "core" is really "on"!

3. **Sitting forward weight shift via PFP1.** Ensure action comes *from the hips/pelvis – while N torso alignment and an O/C are maintained.* We want the spine to be free to make the small necessary compensatory segmental adjustments to the changes in the center of gravity. Gently oscillate back/forward.

Watch points: Ensure m*ovement is initiated through PFP1* – not by the head/shoulders – or the ribs via CPC.

4. **Sitting to stand – (Ex. 30):** The main action is in the pelvis. Try to avoid "plonking" onto the seat when sitting down. Go up and down repeatedly – *feeling the connection between the I/Ts and the heels* – noting that as the heels *"yield"/press down, the I/Ts find it easier to widen and lift.* Also

make clear the need for the I/Ts to spatially *come back* in order to lower to sit.

Can try various arm positions – wide, forward, back, etc.

***Emphasize strongly the importance of this pattern in everyday ADL** – sit to stand, toilet, bending over, etc.*

Watch points: Head and shoulders leading the movement rather than the pelvis. Watch axial alignment, particularly of thorax on L/S as they will tend to "jack-knife" with ES (CPC) – countered by adequate IAP/abdominals and with elongation of the whole spine.

Chapter 9

Lesson 7 | **Working into extension prone – spine and proximal limb girdles**

Equipment: Bolster; pillows; blue square pillow (approx. 6 cm high); wheat-bag; spiky pod; KMCRB.

1. **Constructive rest position – (Ex. 2):** Ensure correct position and comfort.

2. **Rotation in side lying – (Ex. 4):** Head support if needed. Try for 80° hip flexion but ensure L/S is neutral (support between knees?). Topside hand monitors over the pectorals for no inspiratory lift. Underside hand monitors sustained IAP.

PRONE LYING: Over a square pillow to support just below breasts to S/P: KMCRB on; wheat-bag over LPT; spiky pod support for forehead head in neutral; arms 1/2 up to form a U around head.

3. **Coordinating breathing, IAP and pelvic movements:** Relax the body, especially the shoulders, and notice what happens in the pelvis with the breath cycle – (inspiration creates I/T *inflare*; exhalation creates *I/T outflare* with T/B *lift*). After a few cycles gradually widen/expand the LPT into the KMCRB and wheat-bag (tailbone will drop slightly). *Try to stay wide over the LPT* while actively exhaling, feeling how *PFM and lower Tr. A initiate* this. Keeping the center open during the respiratory cycle requires sustained IAP which can also modulate to the breath cycle. Make conscious of LPU/ALAW engagement. Repeat a few cycles and then see if they can now slightly widen and lift the I/Ts on the exhale (PFP1), i.e., **are focusing on O/C and Br. and PFPI and Br.**

Watch points: Ensure they do not tense arms and legs while practicing this.

4. **Activating LSS singly in A/U:** Focus on staying wide under the KMCRB and wheat-bag so that the center remains open while drawing the front point of one shoulder back to roll the scapula around the chest wall toward the spine while also slightly depressing it so that LSS engage and C/S is longer on that side. The hand remains relaxed and the elbow lifts. Repeat a few times. Try moving the elbow cephalad/caudad. Repeat alternately.

Watch points: Take care they do not flip into using pecs when asked for retraction/depression. Most will tend to employ abnormal synergy of tensing the arm +/- engaging the pecs/ACMs with I/S and teres whenever they get a chance or when the going gets tough.

5. **Happy neck exercise – (Ex. 17):** Still ensure expansion back and wide over the LPT.

Watch points: Do not allow the arms to tense, the elbows to pull in or the neck to tense and shorten – or CPC. Ensure a regular breathing cycle can be maintained.

6. **Mini-press – (Ex. 47a):** Allow caudal weight bearing point to be the S/P. Relax the legs and let go any "butt clench". Ensure the center remains open and maintain normal Br. pattern.

Watch points: Tendency to "lock-in" with ACMs and lose SFP1, LSS and scapular stability; inability/loss of C/S neutral; initiating with CCPs rather than LSS.

SUPINE CROOK LYING:

7. **Rag doll – (Ex. 12):** Do this at any stage during class if someone is finding the time in prone tiring. Engage the AFP and try to isolate the movement to the UPT – and then return to prone sequences.

PRONE over blue square pillow:

8. **Slow heel kick – (Ex. 45a):** Hip extension prone.

Watch points: Inability to sustain an O/C and correct postural stability pattern in PLGs – and particularly sustaining so and inhibiting CPC occurring as the leg lifts; inability to initiate the leg lift from PFP1 – going into PPR; disturbed breathing, neck and shoulder tension.

TAKE OUT: Blue square pillow (leave in if someone is particularly anxious about extension).

9. **Sphinx – (Ex. 3):** Work for elongation and "dropping the spine" with anterior torso opening on the expiration, particularly above the umbilicus, while also trying to widen under the KMCRB. Engagement of LSS will help sternal opening. Try and work for softness, lengthening and opening of the central torso in the position over a couple of minutes. Explore micro-movements in the pelvis and shoulders. Reassure them discomfort is to be expected – and that six-month-old babies can do this easily!

Watch points: Guard against holding patterns in the breath, shoulders and center.

10. **"Praying mantis" – (Ex. 18):** It is important that IAP is somewhat engaged to limit CPC behavior. Allow the head to passively roll ipsilateral with the movement. This is a nice movement to initiate with LSS and help inhibit I/S and teres overactivity and pectoral dominance. In keeping the elbow up, pectorals, teres and I/S have to lengthen while LSS shorten. Do unilaterally a few times each to feel the pattern – then alternate.

Watch points: The elbows are a dead giveaway here. If they drop, the person is trying to push with the hands and use "pecs punch" and a dominant ACM/I/S synergy. Instead of engaging LSS they have learnt to overuse I/S and teres as "adductors" in an attempt to stabilize the scapula – thereby pulling the scapulae more laterally. Often, suggesting "imagine your hands are on some scales and that you don't want to see the reading increase while doing the movement" can help them alter the response. (**Homework**)

Chapter 9

Lesson 8

Deep system movements and control recumbent and on all fours

Alignment in W/B and relationship of head and T/B; weight shift and maintaining control of a "neutral" spine, "core"/ breathing and pelvis with limb load

Equipment: Wheat-bag; small/flat cushion; bolster; KMCRB; spiky pod. *Some may like knee pads.

Remind them that adequate switch on of the deep muscle movements, ensures they can safely stretch and exercise. Ideally, movements are effortless precise, slow and smooth.

1. **Constructive rest position – (Ex. 2):** Crossed legs and 1 HBH – elbow growing wide and the point of the shoulder falling back (support elbows if anyone has "a shoulder problem").

SIDE LYING:

2. **Rotation in side lying – (Ex. 4):** Focus on D Br, control of the center and "letting go" on exhalation. This is a good "daily" spinal flexibility exercise – especially to wake up a stiff spine in the morning.

It should always be done after using the bolster (Ex. 2) – or Sphinx (Ex. 3).

PRONE:

3. **Shoulder backward rotation (Ex. 46a,b):** Can they feel the back arm being lifted as they O/C?

The challenge is to stay soft in the arm (and legs) while engaging SFP4 ipsilaterally to come into BSR and subsequent spinal rotation – including head rotation – which brings them into side lying. If shoulder range of movement is limited try with the HBS.

Repeat back and forward slowly. Repeat with the other arm.

Watch points: SFP4 must initiate the rolling – difficult with overactive tight pecs. *Keep the focus on*

continuing to come back with the point of the shoulder. If FSP4 is initially engaged the tendency is for it to drop out early – and they will try to use CCPs and/or hooking the big toe and stiffening the leg.

ALL FOURS: You really need to be alert for central and limb girdle "lock-in" strategies here.

4. **Finding a "N" spine (limbs in *slight* contralateral pattern = important):** Place a wheat-bag over LPT to encourage better opening up under it. Hands are slightly forward of shoulders.

Build a good open BOS in the hands to help engage the LSS with soft arms and collar bones and elbows *wide* toward achieving a neutral shoulder girdle via SFP1.

Knees hip width apart, thighs vertical; lengthen entire spine from head to tailbone; focus on head in line with T/B; open "the center" back and wide under the KMCRB and sandbag with AFP to help lessen CPC. Draw attention to trying to maintain pelvis neutral while doing this. Encourage widening I/Ts and T/B elongation and feel LPU engaged. Focus on "sinking" through hands and knees and O/C with the breath.

Watch points: "Proper" all fours is a very challenging position for most dysfunctional people. Most will go into habitual inferior tether "lock-in" patterns – hence we aim for proper "core"/Br. patterns and PLG control is critical! Even so, they will find it difficult to inhibit overactivity of pecs, U/T and L/Scap. However, unless we start to work for it they will find achievement difficult. Depending on class ability you may need to limit the time you spend on all fours.

5. **Key Moves® version of "Cat/Camel" – (Ex. 21):**

• CAT: As above: and add in PFP1 to initiate the *weight shifting backwards and the spine sequentially lengthening from the T/B to create a nice lumbopelvic curve where the groins deepen – and the weight through the arms lessens.*

• CAMEL: Move into FPP2 to initiate the weight shifting forwards – movement sequences through the spine into flexion including the head. The weight increases through the arms without overly activating the ACMs. *Focus upon widening and lifting under the KMCRB.*

Watch points: The spinal movement and weight shift is *initiated from the pelvis* without the ribs coming forward during PFP1/BWS; and without pecs cinch and arm lock on PFP2/FWS.

6. **Forward and back weight shift in all fours while maintaining a neutral spine and open ©:**

The aim here is that while moving, the head and T/B remain aligned and level in a N spine position, while at the same time the center is "open" through adequate AFP and D Br.

Prepare by establishing a "neutral" all fours alignment *and specifically "open the center"* through the AFP by expanding into the KMCRB and sustain this while doing the following:

Reach back with T/B through PFP1 bringing the hips into full c/c flexion. Draw attention to the *I/Ts widening and lifting* to help the tailbone lead the movement.

Then rock forward leading with head *without losing control from LSS in SFP1 – the* scapulae should remain © and the abdominals need to work more to keep the LPT stable. Draw their attention to widening the elbows and consciously engaging LSS as they move their weight forward over the arms.

Watch points: This seemingly simple movement can be quite difficult to organize. Watch out for lock-in strategies in the PLGs and ©. The client needs to be able to disengage the "inferior tethers" which he has relied upon for control – in favor of the first fundamental patterns in the trunk and PLGs. A useful analogy is as to "imagine that the trunk was a table set for dinner and do not upset the glasses!" This challenges control of alternate weight shift through the proximal girdles with a well organized "center."

7. **Further challenging control in all fours:**

"Hula hoop" – imagine a hoop is suspended so that it encircles the LPT with about 2 inches distance between it and the body. *Attempt to make the LPT make contact around the hoop while keeping the center open.* The IAP + F/LF/E/LF circular movement (axial FP 1–4) at T/L/J helps break up habitual "central holding patterns."

Watch points: The limbs and the "inferior tethers" over the PLGs and center need to able to disengage to allow movement freedom.

8. **Hip extension in all fours – (see Butt booster: Ex. 54):** *Ensure PFP1 is achieved and maintained through the movements* – plus maintain alignment and an O/C.

Through a well-controlled PFP1, *shift the weight well back* – focusing on widening and lift of the I/Ts – and slide one leg back as far as possible *without the T/B dropping.*

Ensure the weight stays back; now lift that leg and *keep reaching the heel and T/B long with the hip in N rotation.* The leg lift should be initiated through the I/T with pelvis staying level and the center remaining open. *The weight bearing I/T really needs to work up, back and wide.* Butt burn is usually a sign that the action is right!

Watch points: Poor PFP control (particularly APR) in the movement sequence and a tendency to rely upon CPC and limb-lock strategies for control. This exercise really challenges the ability of the "inner" LPU to control and stabilize the pelvis in 3-D against the actions of the larger "outer" myofascial slings. When pelvic control is deficient, we see that on the leg lift, the body weight will shift *forward to engage the arms more in control; and/or the pelvis will tilt and rotate and hip extension will be in ER.* Hence, to regain control, you will really need to *cue backward weight shift through PFP1, engaging LSS and controlling the front ribs through IAP, etc.* (see Fig. 3.21b).

9. **Baby supplicant pose – (Ex. 22):** *"Ground"* the knees and relax the buttocks and PFM and draw pelvis back over the legs via PFP1 and *keep it active here.* Work for *spinal elongation and alignment with an O/C while D Br* so as to achieve a sustained stretch in the T/S and "dome" and the shoulders and arms. Think of the *T/B reaching up and back* as much as possible to draw the body back away from the shoulders. Use the breath to try and soften and let go in the stretch. Try to work for some LSS/SFP1 here to help the ULG girdle disassociate from the T/S (widen and drop nipples). *It is important that this is in combination with an O/C with D Br.*

This is quite different to the "Pose of the child."

Watch points: Bringing the pelvis too far back does not allow APR and the I/Ts to widen and lift. Attempts to lift the T/B result in CPC and loss of alignment and internal spinal support. This pose really challenges the ability to combine the AFP with PFP1, SFP1 and HFP1. Take care they do not cinch with pectorals – which will round the thorax and shorten the C/S. **(Homework)**

If you use a belt in their groins, it helps facilitate the feeling of the correct pelvic movement initiating spinal elongation, hip flexion, and thoracic and shoulder opening.

Lesson 9

Working upright in sitting and kneeling

Establishing a vertical axis through effective deep system support and control

Equipment: Chair; spiky pod; KMCRB.

SUPINE: Head on a spiky pod; hips and knees at a right angle supported by heels on chair; toes, knees and I/Ts in line.

1. **Pinning the beetle – (Ex. 5):** Ensure that in bringing the thorax back the pelvis is not tipped back. This exercise is drilled one way or another in most classes lot to improve control of "the center."

2. **Latissimus dorsi stretch:** *Maintain the above task* and cupping palms over elbows, engage SFP1 and bring the arms above the head bringing awareness of "letting go" the tightness in the fascia around the UPT/ULG as "the center" remains controlled against the arms dropping back.

Watch points: Loss of "center" control; fighting the stretch with disturbed breathing.

3. **Basic abdominal exercise for a healthy spine – (Ex. 33):** Still *maintaining thoraco-pelvic alignment and an organized "center"* slowly lift alternate arms; then alternate legs in hip, knee, and ankle flexion 90°. The limb load challenge must be appropriate to ability. If someone cannot control "the center" unweighting a leg – *just stay with them better mastering basic "center" control.*

Watch points: Clients tend to focus more on "bigger and better" with the arms and legs and lose quality control of "the center." Here we are not only challenging the ability to organize "the center" but building its capacity and endurance – yes strength! If control of the center is lost the point of the exercise has been lost – we need in Kolar's terms "to go back" and more soundly establish the basic pattern before trying to put it under load challenge. *The challenge must be commensurate with the client's ability to maintain proper control.*

4. **PFP1 and PFP2 with legs in the 90/90/90 hip/knee/ankle flexed position:** The task is to be able to relax the legs and buttocks and then isolate pelvic movement independent of the legs and "the center." You would like to be able to see the pelvis rotate back and particularly forwards.

Watch points: Clients in general find difficulty in dissociating pelvic movement from the trunk and legs. The tendency is to tense the legs and buttocks rather than move the pelvis – except into PPR – little happens movement wise! – and/or they attempt FPP2 from a gluteal/hamstrings synergy rather than the LPU. And when attempting PFP1, a CPC strategy dominates.

5. **Prayer stretch in kneeling – (see Ex. 14):** Facing a chair, elbows supported on front of seat, shoulder width apart, palms together. Open "the center" and maintain while engaging PFP1 to reach the T/B back so that the spine lengthens from head to tail. The body weight shifts back and the stretch is felt in the shoulders and UPT.

Watch points: Loss of alignment and "center" control; blocking the BWS through holding the pelvis in PPR through "butt clench" and excess leg tension.

6. **Half kneeling iliopsoas stretch – (see Ex. 55):** Using chair for (minimal) support on the side of the kneeling leg. Keeping 90% of the weight back over the kneeling leg, bring the pelvis, spine, thorax and head in alignment over that leg. Here we want PPR through PFP2 to open the front of the kneeling hip while *maintaining thoraco-pelvic alignment and between thorax and ULG.* This requires the ability to combine

the AFP with PFP2 and SFP1. This is different to a lunge.

Watch points: Over-reliance on arm support; tendency to bring the weight forward over the front leg with poor control of PFP2 so that the I/T does not move forward under the trunk – poor control of the AFP means that the front ribs spill forward and the alignment is lost.

SITTING ON A CHAIR:

7. **Healthy sitting – (Ex. 23)** (also see "sitting" in lesson 6): The ability to "sit up" without tension by engaging the FPs. Find a neutral pelvis through PFP1; a neutral spine; neutral shoulder girdle and head with hands over the LPT. Engage the AFP by *pushing lower ribs out sideways into hands and sustaining this* while continuing to PBB. LPU has to remain active to do this – check they have an active BOS through PFP1 and legs are relaxed.

8. **Head fundamental patterns (Ex. 26):** Ensure a N spine is sustained as above. These very discreet movements of the head on the neck are best done in front of a mirror for added feedback.

9. **Fundamental shoulder with head patterns with spinal movement (Ex. 25):** The movement locus should be the "dome" and above with minimal *CCP behavior – helped by activating the AFP and controlling an O/C. The head should also be involved in all these FSPs.*

SFP1: with upper thoracic extension, manubrial protraction and head FP1.

SFP2: with upper thoracic and head flexion – the head moves into HFP2.

SFP3: try to maintain ULG in sagittal N (via SFP1) with *upper thoracic lateral shift and side bending* (not at the waist!). The head moves into HFP3.

SFP4: try to maintain ULG in sagittal N (via SFP1). Want UPT rotation and S/C joint lifted and clavicles wide – not waist wind through CCPs! The head moves into HFP4.

Watch points: Poor localization of the movement; related to inadequate inferior BOS and control of "the center" means the action occurs three storeys too low around the T/L/J via CCPs.

10. **Lateral weight shift pattern with one hand on head – (Ex. 49):** With an active N pelvis through PFP1 and also well supported by the AFP, place one hand on *the top* of the head trying to maintain alignment. Draw the scapula slightly back/ inferiorly through SFP1. Ensure that the neck remains "soft and long" and the head "floats free – and D Br. is free. The LWS pattern *is initiated in the pelvis.* The spine follows the pelvis and the LPT laterally shifts and expands, the ipsilateral ribs opening more *while sagittal spinal alignment and an O/C is also maintained.*

Slowly grow the ipsilateral elbow to the ceiling (i.e., to lengthen the weight bearing side). Sustain the action with relaxed D Br. Repeat other side noting movement sequencing from the pelvis up through the spine.

Watch points: A poor pelvic BOS and initiation from here means the spine remains locked "centrally" via CCP activity with excess tension around the neck and shoulders. Lateral shift/side bending in the spine helps unlock CCPs; however, this also needs to occur with an O/C and the spine aligned in the sagittal plane. *Adequate control and stability of "the center" here also allows the armpit chest to lengthen in order to grow the elbow to the ceiling* – otherwise they will shrug and tense the ipsilateral shoulder and neck. (**Homework**)

<table>
<tr><td>

Lesson 10

</td><td>

Sitting to standing: working in standing – weight shift through pelvis, balance, etc.

</td></tr>
</table>

Equipment: Chair; spiky pod; KMCRB.

SUPINE: Feet on the chair and the KMCRB on.

1. **Pinning the beetle – (Ex. 5):** With wide "open center" sustained while D Br. – and *no* chest lift – CHECK PERFORMANCE OF EACH CLASS MEMBER. This exercise sets the stage for healthy sitting.

SITTING ON A CHAIR:

2. **Healthy sitting – (Ex. 23):** Establish a N axis and an O/C.

3. **Core challenge in sitting – (Ex. 48):** The task is sustaining a N spine and AFP control with no loss of stability with the leg action – and the upper body remains relaxed.

Watch points: Adequate AFP activity is critical in providing stability for the spine against the torque created by psoas flexing the hip. If inadequate, CCPs will dominate – stability and alignment will be lost – the lower ribs will move forward and/or the subject will lean back or to the side. Shoulders will tense/lift and breath holding is likely.

4. **Hamstring release in sitting – (Ex. 50a,b):** The task is to gain and monitor a stable APR through PFP1 against the tug of the tight (and often hypertonic) hamstrings and posterior myofascial slings in the leg during some knee extension.

Watch points: The pelvis will tend to roll into PPR because of poor LPU activity and PFP deficiency – and posterior/inferior myofascial restrictions. The ability to perceive pelvic movement is generally poor – hence we usually need to primarily focus awareness of this.

5. **Sit to stand – (Ex. 30):** Achieved through FWS via PFP1 (previously drilled in lesson 6).

6. **Awareness of personal habitual standing pattern:** *How* do they "naturally" do it? What is ideal? Generally the difficulty is controlling pelvis in space. *DEMONSTRATE:* Spatial position of pelvis will determine the posture of whole body. Because the deep muscles are not active enough in many people they compensate by taking the lazy route. Essentially, there are two main problem tendencies. Either a tendency to shift it forward and hang (APXS), or clench the buttocks and lock in the pelvic "inferior tethers." Either way the spine loses its "lift" and the head hangs forward. This is probably the most common. Otherwise the tendency is to bring it behind more behind (PPXS) which may give the impression of "good posture" as the chest appears more open (despite thoracic kyphosis often). However this achieved by a strong "cinch" at the T/L/J (CPC). In both extremes there is usually the presence of a "dome" with T/S stiffness, etc. How someone stands is a dead giveaway as to state of their deep core muscles. When they are deficient it is common to see people standing with the toes turned out, legs wide apart, knees locked, clenching the buttocks with the tail tucked under and the torso collapsed – or "hanging" on one leg. Check this out next time you are in a public domain.

7. **Healthy standing – (Ex. 31):** Standing should be dynamic – building deep system support from the ground up. As in ideal sitting, standing well automatically fires up the deep system. It involves being able to co-activate all the first patterns in the torso. For many, of course, this will take time to do well – but we need to start somewhere.

Cue them into feeling each step:

- *Foot position* – parallel, narrow hip width apart; fan the toes and create a *short foot tripod* (see Ex. 58). The feet and ankles and legs should be adaptable and *dynamic.*

- *Knees unlocked*, top front thighs back/centered; allow legs to do small adjustments.

- *Achieve a "neutral" pelvis – which is in slight APR.* Cue them to relax the buttocks and PFM: try to sense ischia being able to freely minutely swing back and forward. In the correct pelvic neutral the T/B is slightly back and the LPU automatically engages as the pelvis tips into slight APR. Monitor LPU and IAP at iliac fossae

- *Elongate the spine* – press *down* through the heels and "float" the head away from the T/B – to aid firing of the LPU and postural reflexes for inner axial *lift. Check head does not go into HFP2.*

- *Open "the center" and D Br.* – be aware how "good" AFP control tends to bring the pelvis slightly forward and into PPR. Try to stabilize the pelvis against this.

- *Center the ULG on the thorax* – and the head over this: through SFP1 and HFP1.

- Try and feel a sense of *inner lift/buoyancy* and softness here whist appreciating *how different it feels "inside."* Keep focusing on the D breath coming and going.

- Suggest to clients they be aware of "how" they habitually stand and try and replicate this correct position through the day, e.g., standing in the bank queue, traffic lights etc. **(Homework)**

- A correct N standing posture is the basis of more challenging exercise in standing.

Watch points: There is a lot to take in here! And clearly it is not all going to happen at once. Correct foot position, unlocking the knees and unclenching the buttocks are probably the easiest to do at home alone.

8. **PFPs in standing:** Placing the middle fingers on the I/Ts helps focus on these leading the movement. Try to maintain a sense of the above standing alignment with these movements. And also try to ensure the © remains open – and that PFP1 is maintained while doing PFP3 and 4.

Watch points: The feet will tend toward abduction, external rotation and pronation. Overcoming habitual butt clench and stiffening the legs can be difficult to inhibit initially. As the PFPs become better established, more varied movement options become possible.

9. **Forward bend pattern – (Ex. 32):** Pelvic sagittal plane weight shift through PFP1 and PFP2. Feet are wide and ll. Place hands on I/Ts so subject can feel them lead the movement *back, wide and up through PFP1. Find the connection between the heel/sit bone.* When correct, both LPU engagement and a stretch in the hamstrings is also felt. Looking at themselves in a mirror helps to open the top chest and ULG during the action. Both limb girdles are working back while an "open center" and alignment is maintained. Watch that knees and ankles do not roll in. Can they sustain the forward bend with an O/C and D Br.? Is the neck soft and long – chin back? Is the ULG "open"? FPP2 brings the pelvis forward to stand up. Repeat a number of times. **(Homework)**

Watch points: Tendency to lock the knees which locks the pelvis. The APXS group in particular have a poor idea of pelvic posterior shift/APR and tend to go into a "total flexion pattern" in the torso. Or, the pelvis may shift back but in general it rolls into PPR as they have usually been over-reliant upon butt clench for inner range control. The LPU needs to develop *adequate capacity in PFP1 for the I/Ts to drive the movement* – which then necessitates eccentric lengthening in the glutei and hamstrings through range to overcome the resistance in the posterior inferior myofascial slings.

10. **Forward bend pattern with a broomstick:** (if time allows) – to check out whether alignment was as they thought. Place broomstick over sacrum holding it with 1HBH and the other HBB – ensure *contact with both T/B and occiput and maintain this* while repeating forward bend patterns.

11. Lateral weight shift pattern – (Ex. 49): Maintaining sagittal alignment, practice lateral pelvic control here – *sustaining the (R) pelvic elevation* while lightly tapping the (R) toes – appreciating how the *LPU and glutei work together* to control the pelvic position.

Wrap up:

Recap on preliminary program: introduces the basic deep system movement vocabulary which is necessary in correctly performing more challenging, movements and stretching.

The physiotherapist will suggest most appropriate ongoing classes to match the level of the individual's competency.

Suitable ongoing class levels:

Level 1: For those clients that struggled a lot in preliminary – particularly sorting out correct D Br. patterns and AFP – and coordination between them – content closely resembles preliminary.

Level 2 and on: Incorporates the FPs into a variety of exercises and movements aimed at building better strength, control and flexibility. As control of the basic FPs is mastered we progressively challenge them in further movement control.

Options to do more than one class a week (some do three).

Class satisfaction surveys handed out.

Glossary of abbreviations used in preliminary program and exercise class descriptions

A/A:	as above
ACMs:	anterior chest muscles
ADL:	activities of daily living
AFP:	axial fundamental pattern
AIR:	anterior innominate rotation
ALAW:	antero-lateral abdominal wall
Ant:	anterior
APR:	anterior pelvic rotation
APXS:	anterior pelvic crossed syndrome
ASIS:	anterior superior iliac spine
A/U:	arms up
BBB:	bilateral basal breathing
B/F:	back and forward
BOS:	base of support
BPR:	backward pelvic rotation
Br:	breathing
BSR:	backward shoulder rotation
BWS:	backward weight shift
© -	"the center" or centrated/centering
C/c:	closed chain
C of G:	center of gravity
CAC:	central anterior cinch
CCC:	central conical cinch
CCF:	cranio-cervical flexor mms
CCPs:	central cinch patterns
CPC:	central posterior cinch
C/C/J:	cervico-cranial junction
CN:	counter nutation

C/S:	cervical spine
C/T/J:	cervico-thoracic junction
D:	diaphragm
D Br:	diaphragmatic breathing
DMS:	deep muscle system
DNF:	deep neck flexors
E:	elongation or extension
EO:	external oblique
ER:	external rotation
ES:	erector spinae
Ext:	extension
E/Ab/ER:	extension abduction/external rotation
F/Ab/ER:	flexion/abduction/external rotation
F/Ad/IR:	flexion adduction/internal rotation
F:	flexion
FBP:	forward bend pattern
F/E:	flexion/extension
FPR:	forward pelvic rotation
FSR:	forward shoulder rotation
FWS:	forward weight shift
Gluts.:	glutei
GMS:	global muscle system
HAH:	hands above head
Hams.:	hamstrings
HBB:	hand/s behind back
HBH:	hand/s behind head
HBN:	hands behind neck
HBS:	hands by side
HOH:	hands on head
H/R:	home routine
HVS:	hyperventilation syndrome

I/Cs:	intercostals	**PFPs:**	fundamental pelvic patterns
IO:	internal oblique	**PFP1:**	fundamental pelvic pattern 1
Ipsi:	ipsilateral	**PFP2:**	fundamental pelvic pattern 2
IR:	internal rotation	**PFP3:**	fundamental pelvic pattern 3
I/S:	infraspinatus	**PFP4:**	fundamental pelvic pattern 4
I/P:	iliopsoas	**PIIS:**	posterior inferior iliac crest
I/T (or I/Ts):	ischial tuberosity	**PKB:**	prone knee bend
KMCRB:	Key Moves® Core Retrainer Belt	**P/L:**	postero-lateral
LAW:	lower abdominal wall	**PLG:**	proximal limb girdle
LD:	latissimus dorsi	**PPR:**	posterior pelvic rotation
LF:	lateral flexion	**PPXS:**	posterior pelvic crossed syndrome
LM:	lumbar multifidus	**QL:**	quadratus lumborum
L/P:	lumbopelvic	**Quads:**	quadriceps
LPT:	lower pole thorax	**RA:**	rectus abdominis
LPU:	lower pelvic unit	**R Cuff:**	rotator cuff
LWS:	lateral weight shift	**RF:**	rectus femoris
L Scap:	levator scapulae	**ROT:**	rotation
L.S.:	layer syndrome	**SA:**	serratus anterior
L/S:	lumbar spine	**S/C:**	sterno-clavicular
L/S/J:	lumbosacral junction	**SCM:**	sternocleidomastoid
LSS:	lower scapula stabilizers	**SFPs:**	fundamental shoulder patterns
LWS:	lateral weight shift	**SFP1:**	fundamental shoulder pattern 1
MBD:	minimal brain dysfunction	**SFP2:**	fundamental shoulder pattern 2
N:	neutral	**SFP3:**	fundamental shoulder pattern 3
Nu:	nutation	**SFP4:**	fundamental shoulder pattern 4
NPRM:	normal postural reflex mechanism	**SGMS:**	systemic global muscle system
O/C:	open center	**SLMS:**	systemic local muscle system
OTC:	open the center	**S/P:**	symphysis pubis
PBB:	posterior basal breathing	**SUI:**	stress urinary incontinence
Pecs.:	pectorals	**Tr. A:**	transversus abdominis
PFM:	pelvic floor muscles	**T/B:**	tailbone (coccyx)

Chapter 9

T/L:	thoracolumbar
T/L/J:	thoracolumbar junction
T/S:	thoracic spine
UAW:	upper abdominal wall
UCB:	upper chest breathing
ULG:	upper limb girdle
UPT:	upper pole thorax
U/T:	upper trapezius
W/B:	weight bearing
↓:	decrease/down
↑:	increase/up

Basic requirements for ongoing class participation

Many clients will have difficulty reestablishing a healthy diaphragmatic breathing pattern and/or the axial FP. It is perhaps the most difficult competency to master; hence, retraining this is an ongoing feature in all classes where it is always drilled in one way or another. However, some clients may really struggle with it in the early stages of rehab and require additional/considerable one-on-one tuition to manage these basic patterns before safely joining the ongoing class streams.

Unless reasonably established, it can be difficult for clients to "find" the correct action and integrate this with the movement task at hand. To assist this, the Key Moves Core Retrainer Belt has been designed to help further facilitate improved patterns of adaptable "core control."

Fitting the Key Moves Core Retrainer Belt (see also Ch. 8)

These are introduced in the 4th preliminary class and are worn during all ongoing classes to aid in more effective control of the center through all postures and movements.

It is important that this is correctly placed and with the correct tension.

It is NOT worn around the waist! It is worn over the lower pole of the thorax: the xiphisternum is at the top and the bottom sits above the umbilicus. The two "buttons" are placed at the bottom of the Velcro strips and sit each side of the spine over ribs 10–12.

"Goldilocks" tension should prevail: let it be sufficient to provide proprioceptive feedback, but not so much as to constrict the lower rib cage. A guide is being able to easily place a hand underneath it. Its purpose is to act as an "aide-memoire" – to remind the wearer to "let go" superficial myofascial tension under the belt while at the same time expanding it laterally.

Directing attention to one button is also used to encourage lateral weight shift and additional associated expansion of the lower ribs on that side during certain movements. It is probably most useful in the APXS client who finds lateral expansion of the lower thorax more difficult.

To optimally benefit the PPXS clients, they need some ability in repositioning the thorax posteriorly in relation to pelvis via good expiratory/abdominal activation in order to generate adequate IAP – and inhibit lifting the chest in inspiration. The posterior buttons particularly encourage *posterolateral* expansion of the lower pole of the thorax in PPXS clients.

For those PPXS clients in whom repositioning the thorax inferiorly and posteriorly is initially really difficult we have been recently experimenting with placing 2 soft balls (approx. 6.5 cm diameter) one each side over the lower 3–4 ribs (in lieu of the buttons). They are encouraged to "sink into them" and sense expansion against them. These appear to be helpful in the early recumbent retraining of the AFP. Obviously they are too bulky to be worn in movement.

Class theming

While each class drills the FPs in a variety of ways, it does so within an overarching class theme. These themes aim to redress the common deficits which were described in Ch. 3: targeting various aspects of lost control, such as improving alignment, extension, breaking up the holding patterns, lengthening the sides, weight shift and rotation and so on.

Improving these various aspects of control and reintegrating them in movement will contribute to improved performance overall.

We work for control in the three planes. Good sagittal control underlies effective control in the other two planes (lateral and rotary movements).

Three early/mid stage classes have been recorded/videoed so that you can get an idea of the class theme, structure and flow. These can be accessed via their related embed code.

1. **Sensory enrichment: waking up the deep system and integrating articulated spinal movement:** Listen to the recording

Password: keyapproach

This class includes Ex.#: Supine: #s 1; 2; 7–9 = PFPs in unusual leg position; 12; 34; wriggly worm; 5; 6; side lying: #s 4; 39; Prone:#s16; 44; 46; Kneel sitting on a stool with sustained AFP control, 1st pelvic shoulder and head patterns and "neutral" alignment.

2. **Working the center with the pelvic FPs:** See video 1

Password: keyapproach

This includes Ex. #: Supine: #2: plus alternate leg slides; side lying #4 + PFP4; Supine: #s7; 8; 9; 5; 6; 33; 10; 37; 35: and additional bridging sequences; Prone: #s16; 45a; 46b; All fours: #s 22a; 54; Finding neutral alignment in kneeling; 55; Standing: #31: and progress to PFP 1 + PFP3 sustained with foot tap; 32.

3. **Working the center with the shoulder and head FPs:** See video 2:

Password: keyapproach

This includes Ex #: Supine: #2; Side lying: #13; Supine: #s5; 33; 12; 11 (Head FP1); side lying on under arm with forward/back arm slides; side lying top arm up and lengthening and shortening the arm; Prone: #s14; 17; 18; 42; 3; 20; 47; 22b; Sitting: #s 23; 25; 28; 43; 23.

Further class themes

I hope that by this stage you can appreciate how the fundamental patterns provide the foundations of control in healthy spinal movement: and that reincorporating these FPS into postures and a variety of movements produces tangible client benefits: movement freedom, less pain, improved balance and a general improvement in "self" and wellbeing.

When the Key Moves principles are born in mind with an understanding of the deficits we aim to rectify (Ch. 3), you can appropriately prescribe and monitor performance in the exercises drawn from the inventory in Ch. 7.

And further, being guided by the preceding chapters in this book, and the examples I have provided in the preceding classes, you will begin to think about class "themes": and which exercises would suitably contribute to reestablishing these various lost aspects of control.

Over time, you may well discover other exercises which encompass the Key Moves principles and which might also be responsibly incorporated into your classes.

I have listed below further themes which you might like to start thinking about when planning a class. They are not ranked in any particular order or importance. All aspects matter. When I see certain "weaknesses" in a class, this will often bring about the theme for the next week's classes.

In the future I plan to video further classes which in time will be available on my website: www.keyapproach.com.au

In the first listed class theme, I have suggested possible exercises you might incorporate. Most are listed in Ch. 7: but there are many more feasible exercises and "moves" beyond those listed in Ch. 7. Some of these other exercises are included but only briefly described here. Of necessity, I have used shorthand prose and abbreviations so you may well need to refer to the glossary above.

1. **Focus on the pelvis: improving mobility and control, and releasing inferior tethers.**

The following exercises may be appropriate for those with reasonable control: #2: still over bolster with stand feet, spread arms → I leg F/Ad/IR with ipsi A/U → 2 feet together + PFP1 with arms spread → #38; Supine crook lying: body wave rock into *APR*; 1 leg F/Ab/ER + stand other foot on underneath foot + PFPs = #7, 8, 9; Crook lying: #10; 37; 38 repeated without bolster support. Side lying: under leg ext and top leg flexed 90° + top leg F/Ad/IR → E/Ab/ER to stand foot behind (repeated FPR/BPR); Bottom leg Flexed 90°+ top leg ext: + monitor stable N pelvis with alt top leg hip flex and ext behind line of body → sustain N pelvis with RF stretch engaging SFP1; side sitting: PFPs 1-4 → # 53; Prone: #16 with head rotated R and L; 15a,b,c; 45a; all fours: #22; 56a → bear trikonasana (see Fig. 8.13); Standing: #32; 31 →45d; 60a.

2. Lengthening the sides: supine, side lying, kneeling, and standing.

3. Targeting mobility in the "dome" and shoulder girdle with control.

4. Rotation: breaking up the holding patterns, spinal sequencing, weight shift and opening the myofascial envelope.

5. Extension through transitions to standing.

6. Feet focus: mobilizing and "grounding" through various weight-bearing poses.

7. Chair class: controlling the center against the proximal limb girdles.

8. Kneeling and all fours sequences.

9. Various sitting posture sequences particularly focusing upon forward weight shift.

10. Standing sequences.

11. Connecting the FPs in postures and transitions between postures.

12. Ball class: integrating the Key Moves principles.

13. "Staying in it": FPs in sustained postural control with release in the myofascial envelope.

More advanced poses

Being able to pick up key deficits in less ideal movement is an important skillset of the artful movement therapist.

The FPs are basic components of natural movement, and their lack is noticeable in people with less optimal function and spinal pain. This is also common to see in many yoga classes. Hence it makes sense that they be reintroduced into yoga practice at all levels to optimize opening the tissues and forming the ideal "shape and line of the pose." An accomplished yogi automatically engages them, e.g., crossed leg sitting with a flexible neutral spine is naturally easy. On the other hand, a deskbound Westerner will usually find this really difficult to do correctly: hence their practice can usually be greatly assisted by incorporating the FPs into this and other poses.

In Yin yoga, the poses are sustained to allow myofascial opening. Adding "key points of active control" via the FPs greatly enhances the tissue release.

Many of our clients have disconnected bodies and reduced self-awareness. The combination of kinesthetic awareness (proprioception, interoception, and exteroception), improving deep myofascial system activity and reintegrating the FPs in movement provides a vehicle for helping the client reconnect with his body and rebuild more effective patterns of spinal support and control.

When the spine can assume an easy and adaptable verticality it can serve us well as an effective sensory corridor between the CNS and the periphery. This promotes an ability for enhanced self-regulation and better balance in the nervous and myofascial systems: which in turn offers ideal joint protection and contributes to enhanced spinal health and well-being.

The Key Moves is a biopsychosocial approach to rehabilitative exercise for spinal pain.

The method aims to improve spinal function and pain by changing movement behavior. This requires the patient's focus and paying attention to how and where they move. More a neurophysiological approach to exercise, it looks at the *quality of control* rather than concentrating on strength and conditioning.

Making change involves working with the senses and more highly integrated movement.

People with spinal pain exhibit altered sensory processing – of interoception and proprioception and a diminished ability to sense their own body and movement accurately. They display disorganized posturo-movement control which becomes habituated and "feels normal." Marked pain can lead to fear of movement, and stress anxiety and depression also frequently coexist. Movement commonly involves excess tension and effort, and becomes coarser and more stereotyped. Over-challenging the client increases this and dulls the senses. Function suffers. Our task is to understand how this impinges upon spinal health, see it and help facilitate change.

"Working-out" vs "working-in"

The media and advertising industries have fostered the belief that being fit is about "looking good." The fitness industry has mushroomed, yet musculoskeletal health often suffers. Injuries and feeling physically bad in order to look good is commonplace.

Working out

This is a lot about discipline and pushing oneself hard to burn calories for weight loss, often for cosmetic, superficial results. Toning, body sculpting, and strengthening is prime and there is a preoccupation with going for the "burn" and building muscles mass. The process frequently involves isolating single muscle groups and working predominantly in the sagittal plane – yet usually with little attention to alignment. The approach does not address movement function. It is quantitative and "end gaining:" how many reps, how much weight is lifted, and so on. Little attention seems to be paid to *the process or quality in the activity.* The assumption is that the person organizes their movement well, so getting stronger is what is needed.

Yet what is often strengthened is an unhealthy pattern (or multiple patterns) of control. The spine is the victim. Stiffness and pain ensue. Adopting this approach in rehabilitation is unlikely to yield results for someone with spinal pain.

Working-in

This is prerequisite to changing movement behavior and improving spinal health.

It is a more qualitative, process oriented approach to exercise. Focusing inward – "finding oneself" – experiencing the body from within – sensing the feel of a movement, one's weight, and moving lightly and naturally with more ease. It involves mindfulness and the practice of "meeting oneself" at the point of resistance or difficulty. Many of our clients need to be assisted and reminded to connect with themselves – to find the inner self and appreciate and experience the body in economical, easy movement.

Embodied movement and interoception

The sensory nervous system is a vital contributor to our movement and general well-being.

The fascial continuum is the richest sensory organ as it possesses a diverse and extensive innervation field which contributes to the senses of interoception,

Chapter 10

proprioception and nociception – and our emotions (Craig 2003; Bordoni and Marelli 2017). The integration and processing of these sensory signals enables our sense perception and body awareness.

Interoception is the ability to sense our inner landscape – to perceive our "inner being" and know how we feel inside. This can be our "gut feelings" – e.g., of discomfort, fullness, pain, constriction, "feeling uptight" – or a sense of internal spaciousness, connectedness, and general well-being.

Interoception is involved in many physiological systems, e.g., the cardiorespiratory, gastrointestinal, and nociceptive systems.

Interoceptive sensibility is fed by information from small sensory nerve fibers which are particularly plentiful within the fascial matrix including that of our body cavities, around our organs and in the skin. These inputs with afferents from the autonomic nervous system are processed in the insula and share other connections within the CNS. Through interoceptive refinement we can develop a fuller sense of our self – both psychologically and physically.

The science around interoception is now substantial and could justify a chapter on its own. Most of it has addressed embodied cognition, which infers that a person's thoughts, knowledge, beliefs and understanding are strongly influenced by aspects of that person's body and its related sensations – beyond the brain itself.

Interoception and stress are closely associated by the bidirectional transmission of information on the brain–body axis. We all know the feeling of "butterflies in the stomach" when we are nervous, and how easily our breath can flip into "stress mode" or become constricted (I was mortified to see my breathing pattern in the videos I recorded in Ch. 9!). Chronic or excessive activation, e.g., an acute psychological trauma or chronic stress, leads to sympathetic nervous system upregulation and this can induce malfunction and dysregulation of these information

processes – with altered perception of body sensations and the generation of physical symptoms and pain which may in turn facilitate further stress (Schultz and Vögele 2015).

Improving interoceptive awareness can be helpful in improving our ability to "self-regulate" and experience self-empowerment – in lessening anxiety and depression – particularly in the area of managing chronic pain (see Moseley 2003).

Studies looking at embodied movement are comparatively few and have tended to examine its effects on depression and anxiety. Forms of mindful movement include dance therapy, Tai chi and Qigong, Feldenkrais, Body Mind Centering, Continuum Movement and streams within yoga and Pilates

A low back pain study comparing the effects of Feldenkrais against a Back School found comparable results (Paolucci et al 2017). A disappointing outcome given the Feldenkrais focus upon "awareness in movement." A RCT of breath therapy in patients with chronic low back pain showed more encouraging results (Mehling et al 2005). (See Ch. 1: How effective are exercise interventions for spinal pain?, p. 4)

Breathing is uniquely situated at the intersection of body and mind and has been described as the "bridge to embodiment". It is probably the most important resource for enabling our ability to self-regulate and adapt to the changing environment – particularly in regard to managing stress.

The diaphragm is perhaps the most important myofascial entity in the body as it serves so many significant functions – namely breathing, internal spinal postural support through IAP – but also phonation, expulsion, organ massage and as a venous/lymphatic pump. Respiration exerts significant effects on body chemistry and metabolic balance. The diaphragm also influences CNS function and cognitive processing (Varga and Heck 2017) and can raise the somatic pain threshold, decreasing pain perception (Bordoni et al 2018).

The function of the spine and diaphragm are mutually interdependent in both health and dysfunction. A well-organized vertical spine is the sensorimotor conduit between the CNS and the periphery and also supports optimal diaphragmatic function. The diaphragm is emotionally sensitive in its response to stress and mechanically sensitive in that when spinal postural support and control is deficient, its function is compromised.

Dysfunction of the internal body canister or "core" is a major finding in people with spinal pain – where activity in the diaphragm, pelvic floor, and transversus is delayed, inadequate, poorly sustained and coordinated (Hodges 1999; Janssens et al 2013; see Ch. 2, p.25; Ch. , p.60, and also my review paper on the "core" (Key 2013). There is also an excellent review of the diaphragm and its changed function in failed surgery for back pain (Bordoni and Marelli 2016).

What is underused becomes underrepresented in the CNS – cortical reorganization occurs where loss of discreet representation or "smudging" in the sensorimotor cortex is apparent (Schabrun et al 2017).

The ability to redirect breathing and the internal pressure change mechanisms and *enhance patterns of axial deep myofascial system activity* is at the core of the Key Moves approach.

Changing the brain's habitual motor responses requires "new" and added sensory inputs. Developing interoceptive literacy is a valuable tool to assist clients to connect with the inner topography of their bodies, to be able to sense and manipulate the internal cavity pressures and volumes and create shape change of the torso.

The spine is also "internal." Relying a lot on interoceptive and proprioceptive awareness, the fundamental patterns (FPs) are a vehicle for priming the sensorimotor cortex of the brain to aid sensorimotor learning and spinal motor skill development. The client's attention is directed inward to sense and feel specific yet varied and discreet motor actions – "micro-movements" of the spine, head and proximal limb girdles.

The Key Moves is a mindful movement exercise program which rebuilds the foundational patterns of control for enhanced movement.

In some respects, particularly in the initial stages, we underload the gravity system so that sensory processing has a freer rein and clients can better reorganize their habitual responses. We help them to reexperience and relearn what was once natural and automatic, but which has gradually been lost from the movement repertoire.

Moshe Feldenkrais was a pioneer in movement therapy who understood about neuroplasticity long before it became common parlance. He was interested in how we learn, and developed "Awareness through movement," which explored natural patterns of movement while drawing attention to the sensations of the movement both during and afterwards. Long before the advent of functional MRI scans, he understood that even thinking about a movement primes the brain to organize a more refined response. Reintegrating "natural" movement patterns breaks up habitual crude "holding patterns."

As therapists, we assist clients to be involved in their self-care. We point the way and provide the tools to aid the client's self-empowerment to manage their own problems. Clients are prompted to notice aspects of movement, encouraged to practice awareness about changing habitual provocative postural behavior: to be mindfully alert and observant about their body, relaxed, sensitive, and responsive. And as "practice makes perfect," they are urged to practice FP activation and simple "key" movement phrases through the day.

We attempt to help our client experience and get the movement pattern right before asking for increased load and strength. If we over-challenge they will do the best they can – and invariably revert to habitual "more primitive" control and excess effort.

When clients understand the role of poor postural and movement patterns in the genesis and perpetuation of their spinal pain – and have the opportunity to experience and develop "sensitive movement" – they can move out of pain and enjoy better freedom of movement. They are assisted to self-regulate, to rebalance nervous and myofascial system activity to improve spinal function. Well-being is promoted and pain becomes a thing of the past.

As disturbed postural control and breathing patterns underlie all spinal pain problems, probably one of the best way to improve this and practice mindfulness is to sit (properly) and meditate, focusing on a relaxed upright neutral spine, an "open center" and the slow internal breath. The mind/body becomes reconnected.

Paying interoceptive attention to the breath has been shown to improve functional plasticity in the insular cortex, the region of the CNS which appears to support present moment awareness (Farb et al 2013).

Incidentally, an 8-week program of resisted inspiratory muscle training in a cohort of back pain patients showed improved inspiratory muscle strength, an increased reliance on proprioception in postural control and improvement in their back pain (Janssens et al 2015).

Changing posturo-movement behavior is a journey. Small shifts in understanding can make enormous changes to outcomes. The ability to deconstruct movement into component parts and progressively sequence "proper embodied technique" reaps large rewards for both therapist and client.

Motivation, a conscious mind, and thoughtful practice can create significant change.

Recommended reading

Franklin E (2012) Dynamic alignment through imagery, 2nd edn. Leeds: Human Kinetics Publishers.

Myers T (2014) Anatomy Trains: Myofascial meridians for manual and movement therapists, 3rd edn. Edinburgh: Churchill Livingstone/Elsevier.

Porges SW (2011) The polyvagal theory. Neurophysiological foundations of emotions, attachment, communication, self-regulation. New York: W Norton and Co Publishing.

Schleip R, Jäger H (2012) Interoception: A new correlate for intricate connections between fascial receptors, emotion and self-recognition. In: Schleip et al (eds), Fascia: The Tensional Network of the Human Body. Edinburgh: Churchill Livingstone, Elsevier.

References

Bordoni B, Marelli F (2016) Failed back surgery syndrome: Review and a new hypothesis. J Pain Res 9:17–22.

Bordoni B, Marelli F (2017) Emotions in motion: Myofascial interoception. Review article. Complementary Medicine Research 24:110–113.

Bordoni B, Purgol S, Bizzarri et al (2018) The influence of breathing on the central nervous system. Cureus, June 01: https:// www.cureus.com/articles/12790-the-influence-of-breathing-on-the-central-nervous-system

Craig AD (2003) Interoception: The sense of the physiological condition of the body. Current Opinion in Neurobiology 13(4):500–505.

Farb NAS, Segal ZV, Anderson AK (2013) Mindfulness meditation training alters cortical representations of interoceptive attention. Social Cognitive and Affective Neuroscience 8(1):15–26.

Hodges PW (1999) Is there a role for transversus abdominis in lumbo-pelvic stability? Man Ther 4(2):74–86.

Janssens L, Brumagne S, McConnell A et al (2013) Greater diaphragm fatigability in individuals with recurrent low back pain. Respiratory Physiology and Neurobiology 188:119–123.

Janssens L, McConnell AK, Pijnenburg M et al (2015) Inspiratory muscle training affects proprioceptive use and low back pain. Med Sci Sports Exerc 47(1):12–9.

Key J (2013) The "core": Understanding it and retraining its dysfunction. J Bodyw Mov Ther 17(4):541–559.

Moseley GL (2003) A pain neuromatrix approach to patients with chronic pain. Manual Therapy 8(3):130–140.

Mehling WE, Hamel K, Acree M et al (2005) Randomized, controlled trial of breath therapy for patients with chronic low back pain. Alternative Therapies 11(4):44–52.

Paolucci T, Zangrando F, Iosa M et al (2017) Improved interoceptive awareness in chronic low back pain: A comparison of Back School versus Feldenkrais method. Disability and Rehabilitation 39(10):994–1001.

Schabrun S, Elgueta-Cancino EL, Hodges PW (2017) Smudging of the motor cortex is related to the severity of low back pain. Spine 42(15):1172–1178.

Schultz A, Vögele C (2015) Interoception and stress. Review. Frontiers in Psychology July (6):1–23.

Varga S, Heck DH (2017) Rhythms of the body, rhythms of the brain: Respiration, neural oscillations and embodied cognition. Consciousness and Cognition 56:77–90.

INDEX

Note: Page number followed by f and t indicate figure and table respectively.